PRAGMATIC BIOETHICS

Edited by Glenn McGee

VANDERBILT UNIVERSITY PRESS

Nashville and London

R
725.5
.P73
1999

Library of Congress Cataloging-in-Publication Data

Pragmatic bioethics / edited by Glenn McGee.
    p. cm. -- (The Vanderbilt library of American philosophy)
  Includes bibliographical references and index.
  ISBN 0-8265-1320-4 (cloth)
  ISBN 0-8265-1321-2 (pbk.)
  1. Medical ethics. 2. Bioethics. 3. Medicine--Philosophy. 4.
Pragmatism. I. McGee, Glenn, 1967- II. Series.
  R725.5 .P73 1999
  174'.2--ddc21
                                        98-25317
                                        CIP

Manufactured in the United States of America

39002230

CONTENTS

ACKNOWLEDGMENTS

Although not all the chapters in this volume were written in concert, it is obvious at once that work on pragmatism in bioethics is part of a conversation that began long ago in many places. The Society for the Advancement of American Philosophy has in so many ways given birth to pragmatic social philosophy. Many of the scholars represented and cited here, as well as their teachers, participate in this unique and growing society. Its founders, too, shaped and nurtured the possibility for bringing philosophy into the clinical setting.

In particular, John J. McDermott of Texas A&M University was among the first philosophers of our era to venture into the clinical world as a scholar of philosophy and medicine, pragmatism and phenomenology, and his example in many ways, as engaged participant and scholar, made possible the pursuit of this and other projects. A capable mentor and friend to many, he aroused the curiosity and concern of philosophers about working in the world, yet he also continues to this day to be one of the most capable interpreters of the voices of pragmatic philosophy. All who worked on this project are in one way or another in his debt, including myself.

This project would not have come to be without the support of Vanderbilt University, the University of Pennsylvania, and the Greenwall Foundation. Vanderbilt's bold initiative in publishing works on American philosophy—and the lengths to which the press has gone to extend the reach of philosophical literature—made possible conversations that led to many of these chapters, to the volume itself, and to the continuing presence of bioethics at philosophical meetings about pragmatism. In particular, I am ever in the debt of my friend and teacher John Lachs, whose stewardship I cannot hope to repay. Charles Backus has made the Classics in American Philosophy series a remarkable opportunity for reconstructing the study and discussion of American philosophy, and his vision and cooperation are already bearing fruit.

Finally, this book is a direct product of support from the Greenwall Foundation's core support grant to Penn Center for Bioethics, a grant dedicated to facilitating the study of the relationship between social science and bioethics. The participants in the Greenwall Seminar on Social Science and Bioethics were unwitting participants in the construction of this volume, and I am particularly grateful in this regard to Arthur Caplan, Peter Ubel, Charles Bosk, Mildred Cho, and Jonathan Moreno. Jon Moreno has worked particularly hard to shape and advance ideas about the role of consensus in bioethics and in naturalized philosophy, and he was as much a collaborator in this enterprise as a contributor. Vanderbilt University Press and I are also grateful for permission granted by The Johns Hopkins University Press to reprint the article by Joseph Fins, Matthew Bacchetta, and Franklin Miller, "Clinical Pragmatism: A Method of Moral Problem Solving" (chapter 3 of this book), which first appeared in the Kennedy Institute of Ethics Journal 7, no. 2 (1997): 129–145.

Many whose voices are not reflected here were nonetheless helpful to me. Specifically, James Fowler, James Gustafson, George Agich, Eric Juengst, David Magnus, Paul Root Wolpe, Renée Fox, Margaret Pabst Battin, James Wilson, Richard Lewontin, John Robertson, Dan Brock, Daniel McGee, Anthony Graybosch, Stuart Rosenbaum, and participants in two sessions of the Society for Advancement of American Philosophy helped with review of manuscript sections or shaping of the agenda.

This volume owes its form to Garth Green, a staff assistant at the Center for Bioethics and doctoral candidate in anthropology at the New School. Mr. Green's careful coordination of the conversations reflected herein made this volume come to life. His careful editorial eye and many suggestions contributed much. My graduate and undergraduate students at Penn read versions of several of the chapters as well and contributed to the bibliographical assembly required for a book that stakes ground for taking a new approach.

Philadelphia
May 1998

INTRODUCTION

GLENN MCGEE

The twentieth century has seen overwhelming advances in biomedical science. There is truth in the Whiggish history that brags of this century's discovery of long-sought scientific grails. Science and medicine have developed tremendous momentum toward solving research problems that scientists first posed in the 1890s. The fruits of this labor are apparent every year.

In 1997 more than 148,000 patents were issued for new devices, drugs, procedures, plant genes, and tests for human genes. Several hundred thousand peer-reviewed articles were published that year in *Cell, Science, Nature,* and two thousand other journals of science and medicine (including sixty-four science, medicine, and nursing journals that made their debuts in 1997), covering several dozen varieties of science and medical research. Scans of the human brain promised new bounty in solving problems of mental illness once thought intractable. As efforts to map and sequence the human genome raced ahead, corporations began to patent the parts for future home genetic testing kits that would allow families to test at home for unseen ticking genetic timebombs such as genes associated with Alzheimer's disease or Huntington's chorea.

Progress is the order of the day at the end of the millennium, too, and 1997 showed some hints of the extraordinary change that will be coming in the next century. The headlines of 1997 read like tabloid visions or science fiction. The U.S. Supreme Court ruled that there are no constitutional protections for one who wishes to kill oneself with the assistance of a physician, while the people of Oregon voted—twice—that physician assistance in dying is appropriate and even merciful. It was announced that more than 10 percent of American schoolchildren now receive drugs for attention deficit disorder and that the use of antidepressants by children had increased 250 percent in a year.

Also in 1997, a lamb was cloned from the nucleus of an adult sheep's somatic cell, causing worldwide hysteria about the possibility of human cloning and prompting funding of a U.S. presidential commission on bioethics. Through transgenics another sheep was produced from an engineered nuclear implant to produce in her milk the human clotting factor necessary for treatment of hemophilia. Headless tadpoles were made to grow through a technique that could conceivably be applied to mammals. Nuclei taken from rats, sheep, and pigs were for the first time implanted in enucleated cow eggs and successfully developed to the blastular stage, prompting concern about the environmental and ethical issues posed by radical interspecies cloning soon to come.

In the realm of human science, a sixty-three-year-old woman underwent in vitro fertilization with a donor's egg (after she lied about her age to a fertility clinic) and gave birth, and a family in Iowa began the month of December with seven new babies produced by the side effects of a routine fertility medication. Three children of perfectly fertile couples were born through in vitro fertilization because the couples elected to use a new technology, preimplantation genetic diagnosis, to discover and eliminate embryos that carry hereditary diseases. Studies purported to show links between sex and longevity, between pregnancy and breast cancer, and between 377 newly sequenced gene mutations and dozens of diseases. Scientists also began to take seriously the idea that the human genome is much more malleable than previously suspected, susceptible not only to "random" mutations at the level of individual cells, but also to more predictable influences of our environment. One case in point is the mutation most commonly associated with prostate cancer in men.

Ironically, just as the interpenetrative relationship between genes and the environment was becoming more clear, in 1997 the United States led all peer industrialized nations in risks to human health caused by malnutrition, the toxicity of our air and water, and loss of life due to iatrogenic illness. A single pregnant woman employed part time in Houston was most likely to receive her pregnancy care in one of Houston's two remaining emergency rooms and would have little or no access to genetic testing, whereas a wealthy couple in Philadelphia would be expected to use medical services to enhance the genes, teeth, character, and educational opportunities of their child.

In 1997 the proportion of Americans using managed health care plans increased more than 500 percent as health insurers swarmed around the new market created by cutting the salaries formerly drawn by American physicians. Meanwhile, surveys and studies showed that, although patients were not suffering from managed care, they did not really bene- fit, either. The creation of a new market in primary health care, more- over, did not cure the inability of America to care for fifty million of its citizens who are uninsured and ineligible for federal or state-funded medical aid. And, although Jack Kevorkian made possible the suicides of another nine residents of Michigan, the average dying or demented elder in the United States was condemned in 1997 to expensive, inadequate, boring, and sometimes dangerous nursing home care—a kind of aging that might make Kevorkian's plans seem palatable.

It is obvious, then, why bioethics has seen such recent growth. In 1997 bioethics played a critical role in shaping many of the discussions of new and difficult-to-regulate technologies. A small discipline—if it really is a discipline—bioethics struggled in 1997 to meet the demand for discussion of bioethics in churches, schools, the media, and scholarly fora. Everyone wants to talk about emerging social problems in medi- cine, and with good reason. There is little sense among those working in bioethics or medicine more generally that we are on the verge of solving the problems associated with genetic and reproductive technologies, human subjects research, care for the aging, or distribution of health care services. The problems are likely to get more thorny rather than more solvable. Clinicians receive some training in bioethics today, but most clergy, physicians, nurses, social workers, insurance executives, genetic counselors, and lawyers charged with educating the public and facilitat- ing public discussion about ethical issues in health care say that they are undertrained and overworked today and anticipate that the situation will get worse rather than better.

At the bedside, too, emerging and timeworn questions about clinical medicine continue to provoke conversations about ethics. How can we help our mother make a decision about Dad's cancer treatment? Should I sell my sperm? How should we think about our gestating fetus while we await the results of the amniocentesis, and what if it shows Down's syndrome? My mom can't live in my house, but I don't want her in a home; what can I do? How do we do research on kids to find better ther- apies if kids can't give consent and might be hurt? Ethicists facilitate conversations about these questions, but studies show that there is no consensus among ethicists about even the most routine ethics cases, and there are perhaps five hundred clinical ethicists on the planet at any rate. By classical American philosophical measures, health care is perhaps the area of public life most overdue for creative and methodical analysis.

Whether to resolve a problem that must be handled on an emergency basis or to develop a hospital policy, people are asking for advice about moral matters, and it is unclear how that advice should be provided, by whom, and in what form.

Who will provide the new century with leadership in solving problems in the areas of ethics and medicine? The bulk of the work in examining, regulating, providing education in, and finally reconstructing American science and medicine will likely not be performed in departments of philosophy. American philosophy departments are shrinking to a few faculty working in core areas, and what was once called applied philosophy has largely moved out of the philosophy departments into professional schools. American philosophers John Dewey and William James found a way to handle the dilemma of the public philosopher by inventing new institutions and different career tracks. Today, though, such opportunities are rare; for every successful center for the study of bioethics there are a dozen that exist only on paper due to budget cutbacks. Successful work in professional school settings comes at a price: Members of the medical school or science "team" can feel uncomfortable criticizing their fellow team members' work, are frequently on "soft" funding, and are compelled to meet the formidable requirements of scholarly production in medical settings.[1] Philosophers who finally attempt to meet unrealistic or inappropriate production or diplomacy demands, "going native," are ill suited to provide comprehensive analysis of health systems or social relationships.

In the high-technology tertiary care medical setting, funding, glory, and research production frequently orbit the areas of research that are trendy rather than those such as public health, nursing, basic science, and other critical fields that touch almost all lives. A bioethics scholar is little help to policy makers or society if her work illuminates a tiny corner of a tiny but provocative practice in an ultra-advanced medical setting that most patients will never see. Similarly, in the medical setting little reward is pinned to teachers—even at a time that interdisciplinary teaching and the training teachers are coming to be perceived as the most felt demands of our advancing society.

How should the field of bioethics think and act in a time of social crisis? What is its academic responsibility, if any, as a discipline? These are questions about the emphases of the field, its identity, and its method. In this volume one kind of answer to these questions is advanced. The authors of the chapters in this volume argue for a reconstruction of our institutions and professions that deal with health, disease, medicine, and science.

The Abuses of Pragmatism

At the end of the millennium interest has again turned to pragmatism. The classical American philosophy of pragmatism evokes false worship and derision today from many quarters. Scientists, drug companies, and politicians invoke pragmatism in defense of expedient but costly actions. In biomedicine in particular, pragmatism has been hailed as an approach to "utilizing the media to mollify public concerns."[2] At the same time, in Canada, the Caribbean, and in much of Latin America, American philosophy has sometimes been perceived as the philosophical arm of U.S. colonialism and melting-pot ideology, a big-stick "reconstruction" of American philosophy written by professors within elite U.S. universities.[3] In the field of biomedicine, Leon Kass and others decry pragmatism as a thoughtless advance toward whatever ends serve expediency.[4]

Is there a pragmatic method for resolving problems of the public and the professions, or is pragmatism merely an ad hoc historical depiction of the writings of William James, John Dewey, and a few other philosophers? Are there any non-negotiable, bedrock social values that might usefully be elucidated as a theory called pragmatism? Those who are most critical of pragmatism in medicine and ethics have complained that the philosophy of John Dewey, William James, Charles Saunders Peirce, and their contemporaries lacks both a universal moral foundation and a simple method for action. Pragmatism, after all, makes no simple universal claims about how things should be. For pragmatism ethics is a matter of satisfying the complex demands of multiple individuals and groups in a contingent and changing world. There is no metaphysical dividing line between facts and values in pragmatic philosophy.

In contrast, the "principles" of autonomy, beneficence, and justice so commonly applied in bioethics today are simplicity itself, easily understood and steadfast in character. If there is a problem, facts matter, but principles are absolute. Keepers of the principalism flame will admit when pressed that even the most cherished bioethics principle, the autonomy of patients, is tough to use in complex situations.[5] However, Leon Kass and others argue that pragmatism is worse, because the philosophy of James and Dewey lacks both universal moral principles and the conservatism that those principles engender. As Kass wrote: "Simple pragmatism asks, will the technique work effectively and reliably, how much will it cost, will it do detectable bodily harm, and who will complain if we proceed with development? . . . Perhaps the pragmatists can persuade me that we should abandon the search for principled justification, that if we just trust people's situational decisions or their gut reactions, every-thing will turn out fine. Maybe they are right. But we should not forget the sage observation of Bertrand Russell: 'Pragmatism is like a warm bath that heats up so imperceptibly that you don't know when to scream.'"[6]

It may seem ironic, but even those who have devoted the most atten-tion to classical American philosophy—contemporary scholars of prag-matism—do not commonly defend a single pragmatic method. In part this is attributable to the plural nature of the concepts of pragmatism. Theories of ethics are typically associated quite closely with a particular person or book. However, there are many scholars whose compatible but distinct philosophical work might reasonably be classified as prag-matic, and determining which elements, works, and philosophers are authoritative or canonical for pragmatism could pose an insurmountable obstacle. But splitting hairs over who is responsible for which element of a scholarly canon while such enormous social problems continue unabated would be proverbial fiddling that would be ill suited to a phi-losophy of action and education.

A Quiet Renaissance

The obvious dilemma, then, is that pragmatism, whose claims about society and ethics speak directly to current debates about bioethics, has until recently gone undefended because its foes see it as a simple argu-ment for progress and its friends would rather concentrate on solving particular problems than elucidating master theories.

Those working on particular problems through a pragmatic lens have also had difficulty pointing to a particular element of their work that is pragmatic because pragmatism, unlike many theories of ethics, blurs the distinction between facts and values. Therefore, for pragmatic philosophers there are no pregiven universal principles that totally defy context and demand assent from all parties; ethics demands solution of a particular problem in all its dimensions. Pragmatism is not a simple ethics machine or a bucket of solutions that can be dumped on any emergent fire. Figuring out the solution to a complex social problem through pragmatic philosophy will turn out to be more a matter of immersing oneself in the details of the particular problem than studying Dewey's position on that problem. Therefore, pragmatic scholarship about particular social problems is seldom credited as such.[7] When one strays far enough away from the philosophical dimensions of a problem (traditionally defined), the method one uses to solve the problem becomes somewhat opaque. Calling one's solution pragmatic can seem a mere afterthought or gesture.

It is for this reason, too, that scholars of pragmatic social thought do not commonly fix on a particular chapter or book in James's or Peirce's or Dewey's work as "the method." Different parts of the enormous corpus of "pragmatic" philosophy are helpful for different kinds of problems. James Campbell writes that John Dewey "did not provide an explicit elaboration of his method in his writings; nowhere did he expressly put forth . . . a method of social re-construction."[8] Campbell concludes that Dewey's method, if we must identify it, is present only in a "series of hints and suggestions" in several key chapters on method in the corpus of his work.

The task of the authors of the chapters in this volume is to make manifest the outlines and dimensions of pragmatic philosophy so that elements of a pragmatic method for inquiry in bioethics can be ascertained and discussed. At the same time, the authors of the chapters in this volume represent a plurality of perspectives, identifying both different approaches to pragmatism per se and different ways in which pragmatic philosophy is expressed in the worlds of science and medicine. This volume represents a salient test of the viability of philosophical work for solving social problems. If philosophy can be put to this task, work in the American tradition of pragmatism should have among the highest of yields: Rooted in American culture, tied to American ideas about social and scientific progress and about health and disease, in many ways pragmatism is America's philosophy. If pragmatism has one obvious strength, it is its relevance to real life. Our purpose here is to catalyze a growing trend in American philosophy and in bioethics and to form a community of inquiry to debate, reform, and finally reconstruct aspects of personal, institutional, and social health care and science.

The Plan for This Book

This volume is divided into three parts, with chapters by twenty authors representing different disciplines and complementary approaches to the questions addressed in the volume. At one level the chapters in the volume quite clearly speak to the coherence of a single pragmatic core of methodical emphases and theoretical claims. Jonathan Moreno, Joseph Fins, Matthew Bachetta, Franklin Miller, Kelly Parker, and I concentrate on elaborating different aspects of a pragmatic method for research, policy, and clinical activity in bioethics. Mary Mahowald, Griff

Trotter, William Gavin, Micah Hester, and Bruce Wilshire make claims about how the work of particular philosophers in the classical American tradition can help reframe debates in bioethics and clinical medicine. Chapters by Beth Singer, Herman Saatkamp, Martin Benjamin, John Lachs, Jacqueline Kegley, John Lysaker and Michael Sullivan, and Marian Secundy focus on particular clinical and scientific areas of concern with a more general theoretical orientation.

PRAGMATIC BIOETHICS

ONE

The Pragmatic Method in
Bioethics

1 Bioethics Is a Naturalism

JONATHAN D. MORENO

IN THIS CHAPTER I argue that bioethics is a naturalistic philosophy in the sense associated with the tradition of American philosophic naturalism, and that the genealogy of bioethics as a predominantly American intellectual field helps account for bioethics as a naturalism. To offer these views is not to deny that there have been multiple intellectual influences on the origins of bioethics. It is patent that several faith traditions, especially Roman Catholicism, and several secular moral philosophic orientations, especially utilitarianism and deontology, have heavily influenced both the methods and the substance of modern biomedical ethics. It is also clear that bioethics has arisen in other national contexts, particularly in the United Kingdom and the Commonwealth countries, in western Europe, in some Latin American countries, and increasingly in central Europe.

Nevertheless, one of my premises in this chapter is that the social institution of bioethics has an undeniable American flavor and that bioethics is mainly an American field in its origins and, perhaps more controversially, in its style. By the latter claim I mean that bioethics emphasizes themes such as moral autonomy and pluralism and that in its practice, from calling for clinical ethics consultations to convening national ethics commissions, it is consensus oriented. In fact, a former director of the French equivalent to the U.S. National Institutes of Health has complained that bioethics commissions are so preoccupied with consensus that consensus is often forced on society.[1] Although consensus is not exclusively American, American society is exceptional in being autonomy driven in its ideology and pluralistic in its makeup. Perhaps for this reason, our public discourse is particularly preoccupied with the problem of achieving consensus.[2]

Few bioethicists—and not all philosophers—have a firm grasp of the views associated with American philosophic naturalism. Therefore, I first

5

need to explicate that philosophy, partly by distinguishing it from the somewhat more familiar epistemological naturalism associated with thinkers such as Willard van Orman Quine. I then move to an account of some ideas in ethical naturalism, after which I am in a position to explain more fully why I see bioethics as a naturalism.

American Philosophic Naturalism

Although pragmatism may be regarded as a philosophic method, American philosophic naturalism is a worldview most closely identified with the writings of Charles S. Peirce, William James, John Dewey, George Herbert Mead, and Clarence Irving Lewis.[3] Both pragmatism and naturalism have come to be identified as well with the writings of a more recent distinguished philosopher, Willard van Orman Quine. However, the similarities and differences between what may be called epistemo-logical naturalism and philosophic naturalism are instructive.

Both naturalisms reject foundationalism, the notion that knowledge must be grounded in a priori methods of inquiry. Versions of founda-tionalism are represented in many of the most influential philosophies, Platonism being the classic example. The naturalisms find the same essential flaw in all philosophies that appeal to transcendent essences or structures: These philosophies fail to see that knowledge can—and in the final analysis must—be understood as embedded in the world of our experience rather than in some separate realm of being. Foundationalism is not only a failure to apprehend knowledge as "a natural phenomenon that must be examined in its natural setting";[4] it is also a failure of nerve, a fruitless and even pathetic attempt to reach into some great and myste-rious beyond for answers that can be attained only within experience.

Part of the appeal of foundationalism lies in its promise that the key to knowledge can be found without doing the hard work of inquiring into the world as it is. Rather, according to naturalist philosophers there is no escaping the nitty-gritty of such work if any real knowledge is to be found. All else is a philosophical form of that emotional refuge known to psychologists as magical thinking. The classic critique of this poignant, ancient, but finally tragic quest for certainty is found in Dewey's critical work of that title.[5]

Both naturalisms thus agree that a satisfactory account of the nature of knowledge can be achieved only by attending to the methods and tech-niques exemplified within experience, and that by so attending an account can be given of the possibility of knowledge itself. In other words, the two great epistemological questions must be approached in a naturalistic spirit. The pragmatic element of this attitude should be apparent; indeed, it is a pragmatic temperament that leads one to a naturalistic worldview. Further, when one engages in a naturalistic inquiry into knowledge by examining the ways in which it is actually attained, one notes certain means and patterns that are more productive in the pursuit of knowledge than others. These lessons are inherently normative, in the sense that they provide guidance concerning the ways that the expansion of knowledge ought to be pursued. Some of these normative lessons have moral as well as instrumental implications, insofar as they provide counsel about, for example, the most economic and therefore least wasteful ways to pursue what can be known.

Epistemologic naturalism and American philosophic naturalism also agree that attention to the ways knowledge is gained shows a continuity between these means and the method of science itself. At this point, however, the two naturalisms begin to part company. The pragmatic temperament can be traced to a rejection of a "spectator" theory of knowledge associated with Cartesianism, the view that the observer stands apart from and over against the object of knowledge. The pragmatic naturalist understands that the knower and that which is known are in the same matrix, just as the inquirer is within nature and is one of its entities along with the object of knowledge, not outside of nature or fundamentally disconnected from the object.

Yet epistemological naturalism, for all its powerful contributions to modern philosophy, is too closely associated with causal theories of observation, such that causal processes are said to produce true belief-states. The psychological behaviorism of Quine, for example, is in the tradition of J. B. Watson and B. F. Skinner, who stressed a stimulus-response model that places observer and observed apart from each other in static relations. But the "behaviorism" of Mead and Dewey stresses the dynamic interaction of the knower with that which is to be known, the fact that the attitude (physical as well as psychological) of the inquirer influences the way the object is apprehended, just as the object influences the inquirer's experience. To use Dewey's phrase, the stimulus-response relation is not an arc, but a circuit.[6]

In rejecting epistemological naturalism, American philosophic naturalism also rejects the notion that the ultimate authority on the nature of the world is natural science, and that the only questions that can legitimately be framed about the world must be expressed in the terms of natural science. The philosophic naturalist stresses the method of science rather than the content of science. Too great an emphasis on the content of science can lead to scientism, which is the substitution of dogma derived from current scientifically validated ideas for the open-minded inquiry and critical thinking characteristic of the method of science.

According to the philosophic naturalist, science can flourish only through an active engagement of the knower with the known, operating within the same matrix in a dynamic interaction through which emerge the meanings that make knowledge possible. Moreover, the method of science does not result in only scientific information, and it is not used only in "scientific" contexts, for the method of science is mainly an intensified version of the pattern of successful investigation into any subject matter. Therefore, the meanings realized from inquiry may be the data typical of a scientific setting, but they may also be aesthetic signifiers or moral guides or some other type of information suitable to a certain type of inquiry.

Consistent with its conception of the dynamic interplay between the knower and the known within the tissue of lived experience, philosophic naturalism also emphasizes the experimental character of experience. Of course, not all experience is experimental in the systematic fashion of the method of science, but all experience is said to be continuous with that more intensified version characteristic of scientific inquiry. In fact, philosophic naturalists contend that scientific investigation is rooted in the same tendencies that are brought to experience in general: Stimulated by a problematic situation, the organism applies its various resources (prior experience, creative imagination, and so on) to the problem, implements a hypothetical solution, assesses the success of the endeavor, and, if necessary, formulates an alternative approach.

Philosophic naturalism's rejection of the notion that only science can give a legitimate account of experience has been embraced by another recent prominent philosopher whose views should not be too closely identified with naturalism. Richard Rorty rightly credits American naturalists, especially Dewey, for a pioneering critique of foundationalism.[7] In elaborating his own version of that critique, Rorty has attracted more attention to some of Dewey's ideas than has been given to them for over fifty years. However, Rorty does not accept the philosophic naturalists' positive doctrine concerning the nature of experience and the intellectual tools inherent in experience. Hence Rorty contends, with the naturalists, that the content of science is only one way of representing the world, that it does not have sole license to confer legitimacy upon experience; but he does not appreciate that the method of science as intelligent inquiry has characteristics that inhere in all experience. Therefore, he is left to conclude that science is merely one sort of conversation among many, with none having any particular claim to priority.

Philosophic naturalists, while they agree that there is no privileged representation of experience, find within the method of science ways of knowing that are characteristic of all successful modes of representing experience, including the aesthetic and the moral. That is, not only scientific explorations, but also artistic projects and ethical inquiries, exhibit qualities of intelligent examination of the material provided by experience, including purposeful efforts at interpreting that material, revising it so that it bears the imprints of the examination, and engaging in further reconstructions in light of previous results. In other words, there are no hard and fast lines between different forms of inquiry into the nature of experience; each bears some characteristics of the others. In turn, these modes of inquiry into experience identify generic qualities of existence that extend well beyond the self-limited conditions established by the terms of even the most erudite conversation.

One element that the notion of conversation does capture is the social, and this is an important feature of philosophic naturalism, which views the interpersonal dimension as crucial for all modes of representing experience. Inquiry, whether scientific, aesthetic, or moral, is viewed as a social enterprise. The role of community is perhaps most apparent in science, wherein the opinion of a single investigator is subject to scrutiny by many colleagues who have the opportunity to confirm or disconfirm the hypothesis that has been proffered. Only when the community of inquirers reaches a consensus can the matter be said to have been settled, and even then it is settled only until no further doubt is raised.

In aesthetic affairs the success of a composition is dependent on the judgment of a community of appreciation, and in ethics the soundness of a principle or maxim of conduct depends on the judgment of a moral community. In a still more general sense, all forms of representation, all symbol systems and modes of signification, obviously require the cooperation of a linguistic community. In this respect the early American naturalists such as Peirce and James anticipated Ludwig Wittgenstein's famous private language argument, while Dewey, Mead, and Lewis elaborated its sociological and logical implications.

Ethical Naturalism

The American philosophic naturalists wrote extensively about the implications of their views (which were by no means as uniform in their details as my very general summary might suggest) for many fields, including metaphysics, epistemology, logic, social and political philosophy, education, semiotics, and aesthetics. But it might well be that they had less to say about moral philosophy than any other field. The most comprehensive anthology of writings central to American naturalism in the past fifty years, for example, includes only two selections on ethics, one of which was included in a volume published in 1944,[8] the other originally published in 1965.[9]

One explanation for this relative lack of treatment of moral matters may be that American naturalists have been more interested in the process of inquiry, including inquiry into moral questions and the way society works out ethical quandaries, than in the big questions associated with classical moral philosophy, including What is the nature of the good? and What is the good life? Much of Dewey's theoretical ethics, for example, emerged through his writings on the nature of inquiry and community. Dewey's substantive ethical views appeared in his less technical essays—and in his social activism—related to concrete moral problems, such as his support of equality for women, his championing of civil liberties, and his opposition to American involvement in World War I.

Another reason for the paucity of commentary among American naturalists on ethical theory per se is that they do not accept the traditional agenda of moral philosophy, which engages in efforts to justify moral claims. The preferred form of justification is deductive, with one or more general moral principles comprising the major premise of an argument. But naturalists reject not only the a priori metaphysics of moral principles already noted, but also the abstraction from actual moral experience represented in this conception of justification. Simply put, unless we are engaged in a mere academic exercise, we do not confront moral problems separate from our daily lives.

Actual moral problems are living problems and problems of living; they are "contexted" or embedded in states of affairs. Reminiscent of Aristotle's conception of practical wisdom, naturalists contend that actual moral problems call forth a wide range of skills, including a capacity to generalize from previous experience and an ability to project imaginatively what it would be like to select one alternative for action or the other. Context also helps determine our moral obligations, for what is an evident duty in one state of affairs is not at all apparent under another. Consider, for example, how the environment has been elevated to a moral concern in a short time by public awareness of such phenomena as the fragility of the ozone layer.

It is clear that American philosophic naturalists cannot accept the notion, so important in so much modern ethical theory, that there is a discrepancy between facts and values. The celebrated naturalistic fallacy is a fallacy only if expressed in a fashion that begs the question, according to naturalists, for it is patent that in the world of experience moral judgment requires that one be informed of the facts. What kind of ethics is it that can afford to ignore actual states of affairs? One way to characterize the error inherent in the idea of the naturalistic fallacy is that it suggests there can be only one sort of relationship between facts and values—namely, a deductive one. The philosopher Owen Flanagan has noted that inductive and abductive processes are alternatives that the naturalist does well to select. Induction refers, of course, to generalization from previous experience, and abduction (a logic elaborated by Peirce) refers to the formulation of novel hypotheses based also on prior experience.

Even the idea that facts and values can be readily distinguished is doubtful, considering that facts are often, if not always, value laden and that values are often encountered as facts. The value-ladenness of assertions that are held up as fact is now a familiar phenomenon. Less familiar is the insight, associated especially with Dewey but also found in James's writings, that values are encountered in experience as features of states of affairs. The work of the cultural anthropologist is perhaps most consistently associated with values encountered in the field as facts in the worldview of a people. To turn this account upon ourselves (the inheritors of the western European worldview), the proposition that human rights are embedded in human dignity is so familiar as nearly to have lost its character as a value and claim authority as a fact.

Another prominent feature of ethical naturalism to which I have already alluded, but which may be brought out more sharply, is an emphasis on the situation or, perhaps a better term, the context of moral decision making. As has been said, what counts as a moral problem is tied up with a matrix of conditions that both define the problem and render it perceptible. For naturalists the context-dependent nature of moral choice is very nearly self-evident, for how else could any choice make contact with the issue at hand if it were not formulated in the light the actual circumstances? Critics of naturalism may deride this approach as an invitation to "moral relativism," since it suggests that general principles or rules will have, at best, limited applicability in different situations. Naturalists embrace this conclusion. They especially see general rules or principles as providing orientation and guidance, but also as carrying the seeds of dogmatism if not subject to interpretation in light of the facts of the case at hand. This position is entirely consistent with their view that inquiry requires openness, which is a methodological principle rather than a substantive general rule.

Similarly, naturalists regard choice as prior to rules in terms of actual experience. When faced with a concrete dilemma, moral or otherwise, people do not in fact consult theory, but "apply ourselves" to the problem. To be sure, this application of oneself includes application of what one knows about general rules, but it also includes application of one's experience with previous similar problems, as well as judgment, intuition, temperament, and "gut feelings."

In other words, we bring to bear on an actual problem the greater or lesser part of the totality of our experience. An individual who literally consulted an ethics textbook when faced with a concrete dilemma would rightly be regarded as either naive, obsessive, or simply lacking in understanding of the nature of ethical principles. Rather than implying a conclusion that must be drawn in particular cases, moral generalizations represent the retrospective aggregate insights gleaned from eons of human experience—or so we hope. Whatever wisdom inheres in such generalizations cannot be deductively transferred to a problem at hand; rather, wisdom in the form of judgment or what Aristotle called practical wisdom is also required in the assessment of the problematic situation with the aid of theory, rules, and principles.

By now it should be apparent why philosophic naturalists are not concerned with justification in the way that mainstream ethics has come to understand that as part of its mandate. Principles do not justify a means of resolving a problem, moral or otherwise; only experience itself can do that. And in the real world any resolution always has a tentative quality, is always subject to revision. Only in a metaphysical fantasy are solutions permanent. "The Good," therefore, is not a mere static thing, but a project, one that is undertaken not by isolated individuals, but by social individuals, generally persons working together, even if often at odds. The Good, that which is desirable, is an ideal that helps organize human energies, which are in fact engaged in continuous social reconstruction. Conflict is frequently a feature of this process, but so is cooperation. Both conflict and cooperation are largely superficial qualities of social reconstruction, however. What is more important is the quality of the deliberation with which we have entered into the reconstructive process.

Like any dimension that calls on the method of inquiry, reconstruction requires intelligence, and in the world of actual human affairs it requires social intelligence. A socially intelligent response to a problematic situation that seems to require reconstruction resembles the method of science. It requires, among other things, reliable information, an understanding of the problem, a plan of action, a purpose or "end-in-view," and a willingness to engage in a further reconstruction if the hypothesized approach proves unsatisfactory.

These are among the crucial elements of ethical naturalism. It now remains to see not only how the field of bioethics exemplifies these elements, but how at least some of the practices associated with it might be viewed as a vindication of ethical naturalism.

Bioethics as a Naturalism

"By their fruits shall ye know them." This biblical admonition was cited by William James in one of his many attempts to define the pragmatic method. In this section I take a pragmatic view of the field of bioethics, for in ascertaining exactly what bioethics is I am less concerned with how it is represented by its participants or commentators than how it presents itself as an institution, a set of social practices.

The "practice" of bioethics occurs in numerous settings and groups: case conferences, ethics committees, classrooms, institutional review boards, print and broadcast media, professional organizations, bedside rounds, governmental panels, and civic organizations—and these do not exhaust the list. These settings and groups do have some elements in common, among the most important of which is that all of them involve communication, usually within a small group. This underscores the fact that bioethics is a social activity. Even when the ultimate goal is communication about an issue with a large group, such as members of a profession or the public in general, discussion tends to emanate from a relatively small number of initial participants.

It may be said that characterizing bioethics as a social activity is trivial, since by naturalism's own lights any intelligent activity is social. But the sociality I am referring to here is of the more quotidian variety. Compare the creative process in the traditional humanities disciplines with that of bioethics. It is a commonplace that humanistic creativity, while obviously profoundly influenced by teachers and contemporaries, has an ineluctably individual dimension. Put simply, it is the rare important document in the history of philosophy that has more than one author, and one that does is often labeled a manifesto. Yet important writings in bioethics appear regularly with multiple authors without prompting surprise.

One might argue that the difference can be explained by the relatively more fundamental concepts that are dealt with in philosophy, which require individual reflection, as compared to the concepts dealt with in an applied field such as bioethics. Apart from the fact that it is not always easy to tell which idea is more basic than another—and the problem of explaining why one sort of reflection calls upon individuality more than another—this account does not conflict with the observation that bioethical work, even in its written form, has a social character that the traditional humanities tend not to have.

As I have argued elsewhere, the social character of bioethics is closely associated with its institutional functions. To see this it is necessary to distinguish bioethics from the traditional humanistic disciplines in another way. Humanities professors may—and arguably should—leave their students in a state of doubt about some great human issues, such as the meaning of personhood or the significance of death. The Socratic tradition renders this view of humanistic pedagogy more than respectable.[10]

Bioethicists, too, may adopt the posture of the perpetual critic, but only insofar as they occupy the role of professor. Put bluntly, those who leave the seminar room for the hospital conference room either drastically change their professional role or soon find themselves unwelcome or ineffective in the latter setting. Raising hard questions is important work, as is challenging prejudices and preconceptions and "speaking truth to power," but when action is required, as it is in virtually all the contexts in which medicine functions, the critical posture is simply not enough. Perhaps the most striking personal effect of bioethics on those who, like me, have undergone the transformation from humanities professor to bioethicist, is the way it forces those who might otherwise remain perpetual critics to "cash out" their views and take a position.

In framing matters in terms of their "cash value" I have made reference to the inherently pragmatic strain in bioethical practice. The naturalistic strain emerges insofar as the views that cash out do so influenced as much by the problem at hand as by any prior theoretical views that participants bring to the table. In other words, it is rare (in my experience at least) to hear an ethics committee member explicitly appeal to the problem of balancing autonomy and beneficence, for example. Rather the facts of the case, the medical uncertainty, the suffering involved, its human importance, the legal and administrative complexities, and other more immediate factors tend to overwhelm theory.

To be sure, theory is often brought to bear on the problem at hand, but far more gingerly than is normally the case in the textbooks. And when theory is brought to bear, usually by oblique references or the shorthand use of terms such as *self-determination*, it bears none of the earmarks of deductive moral argument so dear to the hearts of many philosophical traditionalists. Instead there is a tentative and "hand-over-hand" quality to many of these conversations, with ethical theory one foothold among a precious few others, including prevailing practices, theological paradigms, institutional policies, useful analogies, and the law. Other resources are previous cases, and adumbrations suggested by casuistry in moral reasoning by Jonsen and Toulmin, which has generated so much enthusiasm in the bioethical literature. These resources blend well with naturalism's emphasis on the moral guidance available in experience.[11]

When ethical naturalists survey instances in which moral problems have been solved, they find that the most important resources are those that dwell within the situation rather than those that are introduced from outside of it. Principles are viewed, along with theories and other generalizations, as reducible to hypotheses about the realization of desirable outcomes. Among the resources inherent in the problematic situation are moral values themselves. When an ethical course is unclear it is not owing to lack of moral options, but due to an excess of them. The challenge lies partly in ascertaining what outcome is both most desirable and within reach, then in constructing a means for its realization. Consider the example of physician-assisted suicide. What is wanted by all who dispute the matter is the most dignified death consistent with respect for life. Setting aside abstract recriminations about right and wrong, what concrete steps would be most likely to ensure the generally desired outcome?

I alluded to the casuistic explorations of Jonsen and Toulmin as compatible with a naturalistic bioethics. I now want to go further and argue that many of the arguments and accounts of bioethics are implicitly naturalistic, that the naturalistic orientation in bioethics is prevalent but unrecognized. A reliance on experience gleaned from previous cases is only one example, and one that has even been embraced by Tom Beauchamp and Jim Childress in the most recent edition of their influential text.[12] Other examples can be drawn from references to "species-typical functioning," as in debates about the meaning of health,[13] from attempts to rationally establish that fetuses have moral status through studies of fetal development,[14] from appeals to neuroanatomy in arguments about brain death,[15] or even from generic attempts to highlight values as proper parts of medical education because they are inherent in medical practice.

The whole of efforts to incorporate bioethics into policy creation, to render values explicit in public life and evaluate political structures in their light, as in the federal and state ethics commissions now so popular, can be seen as a Deweyan adventure. Bioethics is not only capable of being understood as ethics naturalistically pursued; it is already a naturalism in light of the kind of field it has become since its beginnings in the 1960s.

The last comment requires some elaboration. It may well be argued that the roots of bioethics include some decidedly non-naturalistic strands, especially the theological ethics that were so important to the beginnings of the field. The important role of theologians and their deon-tological orientation in the early period is undeniable, but what is note-worthy is that as the field grew in the 1970s, its style and mode of argument became decidedly more empirical or "consequentialist," and theologians and moral theology steadily lost influence. A sociological explanation for this shift might point out that the institutional environ-ment of bioethics changed from small conferences dominated by church-men in the 1950s and 1960s to major universities and government panels in the 1970s and 1980s.[16] Without celebrating or bemoaning these histor-ical facts, they can be noted as important forces in the naturalization of bioethics.

Bioethics, American Society, and Dewey's Legacy

Dewey liked to use the term *social intelligence* in his discussions of the importance of cooperative inquiry conducted in an experimental spirit. At the heart of social intelligence is the use of the best available informa-tion to craft improved living conditions. Today we might regard Dewey's call for socially intelligent action as best represented in the policy sci-ences, wherein a program is implemented according to expressed goals and in light of historic evidence, is evaluated, and then is redesigned in light of actual experience and the extent to which the goals have been achieved. In this respect Dewey and other ethical naturalists resemble the French *philosophes* of the eighteenth century, who arguably founded the notion of public policy.

Bioethicists, too, operate largely through policy reform and adjust-ment, whether at the local department or institutional level or through state or national entities. Even individual interventions—for example, the clinical ethics consultation—are part of a larger effort to enhance the prospects for more general change in the way medical culture deals with ethical issues. The bioethicist is in many respects a policy scientist—or, as some might prefer, a policy humanist.

Dewey's interest in the way values operate in problem solving stemmed from his concern to show that they are not merely abstractions, but are crucial in what we might today call policy making. Dewey thought of values as organizing principles for otherwise undisciplined energies. Values for Dewey were like vectors that galvanize and give shape and direction to energies that must be harnessed for effective social action. The ideas that values have an organizing function and that they have a practical role are perhaps most obvious in a pluralistic society like

that of the United States. Anyone who believes that values are not concrete, vital forces has never traversed with open eyes and ears the varie-
gated neighborhoods of a place like Brooklyn.

It is in such a cultural climate that ethical naturalism and bioethics
both flourished. In many ways bioethics practices what ethical naturalism preaches. Like the early New World settlers who brought an ancient
but abstruse intellectual tradition into the wilderness, bioethicists have
by and large been more impressed with what they have found in the
clinic than with the philosophies they brought with them. In its attempts
to find moral lessons in actual experience—and in its efforts to secure and
expand moral values for human enjoyment—bioethics reveals itself as
not merely pragmatic, but naturalistic.

Among the many fields in which Dewey attempted to apply social
intelligence, including education, race and gender relations, disarma-
ment, and industrial policy, medicine would surely have been added to
the list if Dewey had lived long enough to witness the technological
breakthroughs of the 1960s and 1970s. One philosopher who was
strongly influenced by Dewey, Joseph Fletcher, published a pioneering
work in the 1950s in which the promises and perils of modern medicine
were analyzed from a framework of "situational" ethics,[17] but prior to the
full rush of the new biotechnology and without the richness of naturalism as its philosophical background.

Although history did not permit Dewey to become the first bioethicist, it did allow him to articulate a dynamic philosophy that was well
suited to American society. America provided fertile ground for the most
dramatically new intellectual and social reform movement since the hey-
day of Continental existentialism and Marxian politics: bioethics.

2 Pragmatic Method and Bioethics

GLENN MCGEE

JOHN DEWEY spent much of his life reconstructing instituions in society so that they might better serve the common good. In his public life as a philosopher he revolutionized sociology, education, American aesthetic theory, and public health. However, perhaps his greatest challenge was an attempt to reconstruct and promote the practice of ethics and social philosophy in public life. His goal was to make philosophical tools more useful both in policy and in communal life. He created a method of working on social issues that he called a new logic.

"New" logic was probably a bad choice as a name for Dewey's social theory. Just about nothing inspires less public interest than logic. Pulse rates slow measureably at the mention of the word. Logic is, after all, traditionally understood as the furthest point from practice, a "science of necessary laws of thought, and . . . the theory of ordered relations which are wholly independent of thought."[1] They do not teach logic in medical school, and few Americans could be persuaded that politicians are logical, either. Logic is typically independent of practical and professional life, a "pure field" in which the "order" of the way that existence "must be" is articulated, often in a highly abstract and symbolic way.

Mr. Spock, the pointy-eared Vulcan of *Star Trek,* loved logic. And for many contemporary logicians logic is exactly what Spock took it to be: an unemotional glue of the universe, a tie that binds together matter and consciousness in an tidy language of order and completeness to which everything adheres. Although logic might normally be justified in terms of its ability to help us think more clearly, this feature is only an externality for traditional logic, not its matrix, purpose, or limit. However, John Dewey thought logic arises "within the operation of inquiry and [is] concerned with control of inquiry so that it may yield warranted assertions."[2] For Dewey logic is the way we control an inquiry so that it can deliver helpful conclusions that become good personal and social habits. John Dewey produced perhaps the clearest account of how pragmatism can revolutionize bioethics in his book about method, *Logic: The Theory of Inquiry.*

Dewey located logic in an "existential matrix of inquiry." His purpose was to highlight aspects of the subject matter of logic, which merely means the subject matter of our lives. The first aspect of this existential matrix is biological (*bios*-logical). Dewey saw that our lives involve environments and resources, and they operate at levels to which we often pay little or no attention. Part of this biological logic in which we are all invested is, for example, related to the simple brute fact that we have to eat and breathe to live. We ignore such facts at our peril; they are the basis of our sustenance and of our regular interrelations with our world. As Dewey wrote, "[N]ot even a hibernating animal can live indefinitely upon itself. . . . If there is a deficit balance [of resources used to resources obtained], degeneration commences. . . . The processes of living are enacted by the environment as truly as by the organism, for they *are* an integration."[3]

In clinical encounters, a lot hangs on understanding biology. Concepts of health and of disease are defined in terms of our best guesses about the biological limits of the human body. We say that one patient is dead, another one comatose, and still a third "infected" on the basis of assumptions and theories about what it means to be alive or dead, healthy or sick. Much of the time it is unnecessary to question such assumptions. I do not worry about my cholesterol or even notice it until my nurse practitioner points it out to me and calls it a problem. But when patients are ill, and when scientists design our most sophisticated experiments about human and animal physiology, assumptions about health and disease—about biology and the stability of the "brute" facts—are the most critical elements.

Sometimes we question biology. Science counts this among its higher-order tasks. When we try to slow aging, cure Alzheimer's disease with fetal tissue transplantation, or design "artificial" intelligence, the goals are framed in terms of understanding the basic biological context of life. If we say that infertile individuals have a disease, assumptions about what it means to be fertile will have to be made: Are we healthy in this regard when our testes or ovaries "work," when the gametes they produce work, when conception is possible, when gestation is possible, when birth is possible, when a family is made, or even when adoption is chosen? Knowing what having a disease or being in a healthy state *means* is very important to us, requiring both our most fundamental articulations of value and our best methods for investigation. Much of our energy in all major social institutions is devoted to satisfying what we call biological demands by means ranging from religious programs aimed at feeding the hungry to industrial production of heat in winter.

What logic and political theory say about human "nature" rarely takes seriously the biology of human life. John Dewey argued that our rational and intellectual lives as well as our "brute" lives arise within the context of the *bios*. Sick people are rarely autonomous, and reasonably alert sick people will commonly say that they value health more than self-governance, no matter what bioethicists say about the importance of autonomy. By emphasizing a libertine notion of rational choice that few sick or impoverished persons enjoy rather than the feelings and goals of sick people, bioethics has created a wholly unworkable paradigm for decision making. The focus is on figuring out how to cope with individual rights in the hospital rather than on responsibilities of families and caregivers to educate each other about their goals.

In contrast, the difficult-to-articulate value of "dignity" motivates many who are ill, and the desire for a death with dignity is often mistaken for libertine love of self-governance. The point is that it pays to notice the existential dimensions of being sick, made manifest in our inarticulate but crucial social and personal demands. Individuals may not place as much emphasis on food as on individual rights, but, as Berthold Brecht noted, they eat before talking about ethics.

When ethical theories are developed under the pretense that human moral action is purely rational, the result is abstract moralizing. Dewey began his logic with a simple but radical recognition: Any method that takes life as a context for its existence will have to begin with rigorous attentiveness to the processes and protocols of that life, to the logic that is already integral to *bios* (bio-logy). Reason that does not allow us to continue to live satisfactory lives within that context will not be reason that lives a long time, and our habits are linked to animal habits in exactly this way: "*Habits* are the basis of organic learning" such that "logic is rooted in the conditions of life itself."[4] The study of nature and of its logic constitutes an unavoidable part of our lives, so the logic of philosophy, argued Dewey, ought to follow suit.

The study of biology is frequently abstracted as well to an aggregation of valueless facts. Dewey's claim was that by studying and focusing on the habits of humans and their partners in constituent life on Earth, it is possible to think about both the scientific and the existential dimensions of what we call biology. Dewey thought that habits, as "organic structures," become "embedded in traditions, institutions, customs, and the purposes and beliefs they both carry and inspire," because, "as

Aristotle remarked, . . . Man . . . is a social animal."[5] Therefore, biological matrices of inquiry are overlaid by a second aspect of the existential matrix: culture. Human behavior is shot through with cultural images and meanings. Culture does not occur only in instances of art and polity; it is present as well in the form of narratives that we find ourselves living: "[T]o indicate the full scope of cultural determination of the conduct of living, one would have to follow the behavior of an individual throughout at least a day. . . . The result would show how thoroughly saturated behavior is with conditions and factors that are of cultural origin and import."[6]

This saturation evidences itself, for example, in language, which interacts with our more brutish biological demands to produce a complex and interrelated cultural matrix. As Dewey wrote: "Even the neuromuscular structures of individuals are modified through the influence of the cultural environment upon the activities performed. The acquisition of language . . . represents an incorporation within the physical structure of the human beings of the effects of cultural conditions . . ., modifications wrought within the biological organism by the cultural environment."[7] This interrelation also evidences itself in symbolization and in devices or "technologies" with which and by means of which we live our lives. Like language, they texture our ways of seeing ourselves and others and provide a context—in fact, many overlapping contexts—of meanings within which we find ourselves navigating on a daily basis.[8]

Much of bioethics is narrative about the social realm of medical and scientific action. Jeremy Rifken has a narrative about how humanity is moving from one stage of science to another more overwhelmingly engineered stage. His narrative engages and animates many who protest the advance of science and technology. Hans Jonas, too, made claims about the movement of social action into a new realm of engineering. Joel Feinberg's claim that children have a right to an "open future" is situated in an analysis of the stages through which human development must pass. When we argue for ways of satisfying our demands, the role of social thought is frequently to give a history of human action that seems to lead to the present moment, as though the momentum of our argument was building all along. This is one way in which language, at a meta level, organizes and energizes more brutish demands in human life.

Together the biological and cultural spheres form the *ethos* within which Dewey's method for bioethics operates.[9] This *ethos* is what Dewey calls common sense. Common sense is the atmosphere of culture within which we find ourselves grappling to devise remedies of varying kinds and efficacies in order that we might bring a sense of settlement, fulfill-ment, or stability to our culturally bound lives.[10] "Common-sense solu-tions" to life's problems can be intelligent or not so intelligent. The less intelligent solutions produce a feeling of settlement without resolving matters in a way that satisfactorily links our actions (means) with the consequences (ends).

According to James Campbell, examples of such solutions include rationales for action based on "custom or tradition, obeying political authority, accepting some divine will, conforming to the wishes of the wealthy and powerful, resorting to partisan politics, and so on."[11] These "methods" of solving problems were, for Dewey, "vestiges of a time . . . when the practice of knowing was in its infancy."[12]

Although these less-than-intelligent methods may not be suitable to give us a unified understanding of the methods of social inquiry, they do intimate an important fact about social problems: Our culturally laden problems come to us laced with multiple "feelings" of problem-aticity to which we must be attentive. In other words, we must resist the tendency to explain away the "felt" aspects of a problem for clarity's sake lest we be led astray to the imagined indifference of unintelligent thinking. As Dewey wrote: "In ordinary language, a problem must be *felt* before it can be stated. If the unique quality of the situation is *had* immediately, then there is something that regulates the selection and the weighing of observed facts and their conceptual ordering."[13]

Pragmatic solutions to bioethical problems begin with what William James called a "genuine" problem that is felt to be urgent and momen-tous. This feeling is fixed on the problem's existential (biological + cultur-al) matrix. Intelligent solutions are made by integrating scientific method with social inquiry. Although these may seem to be divergent enterpris-es, it is scientific method that forms the axis of Dewey's method. Dewey married the teleological[14] sense of social thought with the rigorous atten-tiveness of "less qualitative" scientific endeavor. As he explained:

The subject matter of science is stated in symbol constellations that are radically unlike those familiar to common sense; in what, in effect, is a different language. Moreover, there is much highly technical material that has not been incorporat-ed into common sense even by way of technological application in "material" affairs. In the region of highest importance to common sense, namely that of moral, political, economic ideas and beliefs, and the methods of forming and confirming them, science has had even less effect. . . . Science is a potential organ for *organizing* common sense in its dealing with its own subject-matter and prob-lems and this potentiality is far from actualization.[15]

Here Dewey emphasizes the differences between the traditional roles of science and common sense, turning finally to suggest that it is science's ability to organize social and political thought to which we must turn in our method. Even more clearly, Dewey wrote that social concerns "cannot be solved apart from a unified logical method of attack and procedure. The attainment of unified method means that the fundamental unity of the structure of common sense and science must be recognized, their difference being one in the problems with which they are directly concerned, not in their respective logics."[16] It is the business of method to fashion solutions through intelligent integration of existential context with scientific method and common sense.

Warranted assertability, logic's ability to "work," will be defined within these limits. So, too, will acceptable goals and purposes. The purposes of traditional logic, attached to assumptions that "suppose it can find a final and comprehensive solution," will not work within these matrices. Such a logic, Dewey thought, simply "ceases to be inquiry and becomes either apologetics or propaganda."[17] Therefore, present logics as taught by philosophy departments will not do: "[I]n the main," Dewey wrote, "we are asked to take our choice between the traditional logic . . . and the new purely symbolistic logic that recognizes only mathematics . . . not only separated from common sense, but . . . independent."[18] A logic that does not claim itself as a part of method and inquiry into the conditions of life is useful only as a distracting game for professional thinkers; Dewey's logic is about making society better through intelligent action in an existential matrix.

The goal of a methodical or "patterned" reflection on method is to figure out how to think about the testing of experiments and actions in the context of deliberative or judicial inquiry. A pragmatic understanding of successful thinking is required in order to see the way that Dewey's analysis of method works. He provided this in the second section of the *Logic,* in which he attempted to relate the structure of inquiry to "the construction of judgments." He thought that the goals of successful inquiry attach to those of successful common sense: "We know that some methods of inquiry are better than others in just the same way in which we know that some methods of surgery, farming, road-making, navigating, or what-not are better than others."[19] Therefore, successful methods, methods whose epistemology works, are "the methods which experience up to the present time shows to be the best methods available for *achieving certain results,* while abstraction of these methods does supply a (relative) norm or standard for further undertakings."[20]

A bit later Dewey wrote: "Only those things . . . that have connection and bearing upon this life enter into the meaning system. There is no such thing as disinterested intellectual concern with either physical or social matters."[21] Method cannot be created without involvement, as well as awareness of context. Inquiry takes this involvement in a patterned way and uses it to direct or control the transformation of "an indeterminate situation into a determinately unified one."[22] In this sense we "undergo" inquiry when we work on a problematic situation by examining it for the purpose of some objectives[23] in relation to our own investment in the problem.

Inquiry is always aimed at judgment, tied to decision, and accompanied by action. The "undergoing" of inquiry is purposive and invested; it is the process by which we arrive at decisions that tie us to actions in the world. We sometimes choose the form of our transformation in the reflective atmosphere of method. Intelligent method, as I have already noted, converts an indeterminate situation into one that unifies our efforts with the desired results; at the same time, successful inquiry gives us a road map for future efforts. Therefore, intelligent inquiry that has worked in the past "fruitfully leads" or points to the future.

Whatever we do, we must not put off or distance decisions about important issues. Inordinate delay amounts to unintelligent decision.[24] And not only is judgment urgently time bound ("in the sense" as Dewey put it, "that its subject-matter undergoes reconstitution in attaining the final state of determinate resolution and unification which is the objective that governs judgment"[25]), but it also is enacted. By this Dewey meant that "a proposition must be defined by its *function* . . . [and] finally [a proposition] is deliberately constituted by critical inquiry intended to produce objects that will operate . . . when they are needed."[26] Judgments are always about practices,[27] and there is "no grounded determination without operations of doing and making."[28]

Social and cultural conditions, our "matrix" that creates the language and technologies of our lives, already prefigure the social and scientific problems that we experience and provide the parameters within which our inquiry must be conducted. So although, as we noted, the subject matter of science or math may be "relatively independent" of that of political decisions, it is "never set apart from a social context."[29] This means that although unintelligent inquiry may take science and society to be entirely independent realms with entirely separate goals, Deweyan inquiry recognizes that to clarify an issue we must situate it in the context of a historical and contextual interaction between human purposes and physical conditions. The nineteenth-century obsession with mechanism in science, for example, came more than coincidentally at the same time that industrialization preoccupied society. Dewey thought that society must influence the conduct of science; otherwise science wwill be "intellectually irresponsible" by situating itself as "indifferent to the consequences of its own activities."[30]

But not only does society influence science; the relationship is reciprocal. Science has radically altered the contexts of society and is tied to its purposes. Therefore, we reemphasize the obvious but often ignored fact that the subject matter of science is already political and already of concern to society. As Dewey wrote: "There are no consequences taking place, there are no social events that can be referred to the human factor exclusively. Let desires, skills, purposes, beliefs be what they will, what happens is the product of the interacting intervention of physical conditions like soil, sea, mountains, climate, tools, and machines, in all of their variety, with the human factor. . . . [S]ocial phenomena cannot be understood except as there is prior understanding of physical conditions and the laws of their interactions." But "[s]ocial phenomena cannot be attacked . . . directly," because immediacy with the social problem would require us to ignore its physical dimensions, the "biological" matrices of logic.[31]

Pragmatic bioethics is primarily concerned with selection of emphasis.[32] In particular kinds of inquiry we emphasize different parts of the existential dimension of our problem. If I am hungry, I do not think much about metaphysics. I might eschew McDonalds and make of my meal a political act. But mostly I am satisfying what for me seem to be biological demands by feeding my body. Aesthetic dimensions of that act add richness, obviously. In contrast, when I make my career plans or pledge allegiance to a social structure I emphasize different elements of the experience.

The most important part of bioethics is what I emphasize, not which universal cue card I follow within that emphasis. If I miss the central feeling of a social problem because I am so focused on achieving an abstract state of justice, I am unlikely either to satisfy the demands that led to the problem or to accomplish justice per se. Pragmatism's emphasis on reconstructing institutions stems from the central belief that how we go about solving social problems—through education, the creation of communities, and the sedimentation of personal habits—is much more important than the meta descriptions we use post hoc to label our choices as ethical.

Dewey thought that social inquiry is "existential."[33] So it shares the range of "data" available to any other part of inquiry, including the sciences. In comparison with some of the so-called "pure" sciences, though, social inquiry is "backward,"[34] *i.e.*, human history displays our reluctance to use intelligent inquiry into matters social. The difficulty is in creating a "closed system" for inquiry, already a hard enough task for physical science. But these difficulties should only inspire us to work harder: we *must* solve these problems.[35] What is needed, then, is not a simple method, but an ambitious model.

The model will follow the physical sciences in several important respects. It must find a way to observe and discriminate among data, forming hypotheses. It must also be able to employ these data in ways that allow experimental and gradual testing within social problems rather than committing the whole of society to a radical shift. Of course, it will not be possible to test some matters gradually. The first cloned human child will face heretofore unexamined medical and social risks. As Dewey put it, "social inquiry, *as inquiry*, involves the necessity of operations which existentially modify actual conditions that, as they exist, are the occasions of genuine inquiry and provide its subject matter."[36] The testing of social practices impacts the testers, sometimes in radical ways. But in the main (and even as concerns issues such as genetics and reproduction), gradual and experimental methods must be developed so that we can better control for factors we may not anticipate at the time of the test.

Still, it is worthy of note that one special problem of the social realm is that the test does not even seem to be isolated in the way that a petri dish does. This, though, is an artifact of the long history of seeming objectivity in science, which has been cultivated by long periods of consensus about the method to be used in testing new hypotheses. As Dewey wrote: "Physical inquiry to a considerable extent and mathematics to an even greater extent have now reached the point where problems are mainly set by subject-matter already prepared by the results of prior inquiries, so that further inquiries have a store of scientific data, conceptions, and methods already at hand. This is not the case with the material of social inquiry."[37]

The moment we ask an actuary, "How will you compute data for insurance tables concerning genetic information?" we have asked a question for which there is no ready-made or algorithmic answer. We might expect the actuary to give us numerical options, but the question is essentially a social one, and it requires thinking in a broader way. Social problems are endemically complex. Pragmatism alone among contemporary theories of value both embraces this complexity and attempts to focus on social methods for dealing with complexity.

I have noted that the method of social reconstruction follows the scientific method that Dewey more generally advocates, but that specific methodological precautions are necessary when social and political ends are in view. I have noted that the actions advocated by any social method are always actions that impact the experimenter, and in using the method we will cope with a need for caution within an atmosphere of substantial uncertainty and complexity. Thus social method has been broadly sketched as a careful social articulation of the scientific method. Dewey provided further clarification of the social method by contrasting it with then-current (and still popular) social and political thought in two ways.

First, unlike current methods, Dewey's method does not posit a separation of theory from practice,[38] a split that we have noted is impossible in social policy. This impossibility is often ignored in social theory and ethics, which tend to seek after a body of principles that obtain either from pure reason or from divinity so that these principles might be applied in the field. Bioethics often sees the ethicist as a disinterested expert providing counsel rather than as a community member who is intractably involved and invested and has particular interests.[39]

More important, bioethics usually insists on separating theory from practice, missing the point that theory finds its meaning only in the context of the inquiry. This is not to say, however, that there is not room for a continual immersion in and retreat from the problematic situation, nor to say that contemplation or theory has no value. It is merely to suggest that as part of the effort to solve social problems we must see our activities for what they are. If we bring prefabricated general principles to bear on complex situations ("supply-side" economics comes to mind), we should not be surprised when they fail; after all, such an approach handicaps the diagnostic dimension of social method.

Second, and more interesting, Dewey wanted to resist the temptation to moralize about outcomes or problems. He was at his most vociferous on this point: "[The *Logic*] demands in turn complete abstraction from the qualities of sin and righteousness, of vicious and virtuous motives, that are so readily attributed to individuals, groups, classes, nations. There was a time when desirable and obnoxious physical phenomena were attributed to the benevolence and malevolence of overruling powers. There was a time when diseases were attributed to the machinations of personal enemies."[40] It is all too easy to selectively emphasize one aspect of a problem, to the exclusion (selective exclusion) of other important aspects. When we are making such emphases, which we must inevitably do, we do well to take caution. For instance, we can become convinced, by virtue of emphasizing too little of the complexity of a problem, that "categorical" moral issues are at stake in social life.

In my own experience teaching about abortion issues related to genetic testing, I have found that much of the violent positioning that takes place in bioethics classes is ameliorated when the students see abortion cases as complex cases comprised of interdependent issues of biology and society, cast within difficult decisions made by persons in a society.[41] The simple act of teaching about a specific case of abortion rather than the highly politicized sum total of the issue helps students to interrupt their narrow investments in right and wrong, sin and righteousness. Teaching students to see all of their life as moral life communicates the responsibility of the student (and the teacher, banker, and pilot) to be attentive to the context of decisions, to favor intelligence over prejudice. For some students and teachers, this may not do: Hot-blooded abortion rhetoric attracts crowds of students and creates an electric atmosphere of entertainment. But what is its purpose? Is that purpose morally appropriate to the role of teacher?

The point is that although these issues are indeed moral, they need not be black or white, right or wrong. Dewey found moral investment in the existential context of the social situation itself, not in narrow notions of acceptability and condemnation that we bring to every problematic area. In this way Dewey articulated not a relativism, but a careful and subtly contextual ethics. He believed that our cultural substitution of condemnation for context "is probably the single greatest obstacle now existing to development of competent methods in the field of social subject matter."[42]

Advocating careful observation and evaluation does not mean relegating to the data all moral conclusions. We must not follow the disciplines of sociology and social psychology in their growing tendency to substitute aggregation of statistics from questionnaires for detailed study of how people live. As Dewey said, the truth is not "out there waiting to be catalogued."[43] But neither can we afford to neglect statistics and other related fields as philosophy, perhaps the most recalcitrant of all disciplines, has done.

No finality will be possible in our methods or solutions, because the world is ongoing and because time shifts the playing field. Today's solution may be tomorrow's problem, and we must guard against unrealistic expectations in this regard. To that end, fertile and flexible solutions will be best. To encourage them we can begin sociopolitical discussions of a problem by illustrating the rich variety of options. Dewey believed we also can see each policy or law that we adopt as an experiment rather than as an "isolated policy."[44] There has to be a "tying together" of our efforts in some way, so that we see that the Oregon health plan or the Canadian system could, in fact, inform our larger purposes and expectations for national health care.

Who will enact these methods? What role will philosophers play, if any? Is there a kind of education or art that is appropriate to the task? These are important questions that others in this volume take up at length.

3 Clinical Pragmatism: A Method of Moral Problem Solving

JOSEPH J. FINS, MATTHEW D. BACCHETTA, AND
FRANKLIN G. MILLER

MORAL DECISION MAKING in clinical practice depends on attentiveness both to particular details of cases and to general moral considerations—rules, principles, and virtues. Although casuists tend to stress the former and principlists the latter, there is no fundamental opposition between these two approaches.[1] Both principlists and casuists have concentrated on the modes of reasoning required to arrive at valid judgments about conduct in response to moral dilemmas in clinical practice. Much less attention has been devoted to understanding and guiding the interpersonal process of moral problem solving, involving the interactions of all those concerned with the moral issues posed by particular cases of patient care.[2] In this chapter we propose a method of moral problem solving inspired by the thought of John Dewey[3] that we call "clinical pragmatism."[4] This method, designed to be useful for practitioners, integrates guidance of judgment with guidance of process.

In approaching moral problems, the method of clinical pragmatism seeks solutions that are workable in the real contexts of clinical settings in which clinicians and patients interact. Owing to the negative connotations sometimes associated with "pragmatism," it needs to be stressed that clinical pragmatism is not meant to promote whatever works to serve the agenda of physicians. Pragmatists often have been accused of promoting expediency at the expense of principle, but this is a caricature of pragmatic philosophy and method. Clinical pragmatism embraces principles; however, it understands them as tools for guiding conduct, not as absolute fixed moral laws. The goal of clinical pragmatism is to reach consensus on good outcomes in cases that pose moral problems by a thorough process of inquiry, discussion, negotiation, and reflective evaluation.

The Method of Clinical Pragmatism

Moral problems in clinical practice typically take the form of conflicts about what is the right thing to do in the context of patient care. These conflicts may occur among clinicians or between clinicians and patients or surrogate decision makers, usually family members. The conflicts are resolved by a deliberative process among the parties concerned with the case that arrives at a consensus on how to proceed. Moreno observes ". . . that moral consensus is a natural feature of human affairs, that it manifests itself in and emerges from social practices, and that human experience contains both the conditions that undermine the quality of moral consensus and the resources that enable us to improve it."[5]

We propose clinical pragmatism as a method to assess the relevant facts, diagnose the moral problems, consider the options, set goals and negotiate a decision for an acceptable plan of action, and evaluate the results. It is meant to guide the process with the goal of reaching an ethically acceptable consensus, but it does not guarantee the "right" decision. Clinical pragmatism treats moral rules and principles as hypothetical guides that identify a range of reasonable moral choices for the deliberations of patients, families, and clinicians. In some cases, no consensus can be reached among the clinicians and patients or surrogates concerned with the case, , necessitating ethics consultation, appeal to an ethics committee, or judicial intervention.

A consensus reached in a case may be subject to ethical critique because important moral considerations (rules, principles, or standards) have been neglected in the deliberations or not given adequate weight. In addition to this substantive critique, the interpersonal process of moral problem solving is open to evaluation. In sum, the aim of moral problem solving is to reach a consensus resolution that can withstand moral scrutiny with respect to both the decisions made and the process of reaching and implementing them.

Clinical pragmatism adopts a democratic model of moral problem solving. Moral problems in clinical practice are not to be resolved by expert judgment—whether it be the technical expertise of clinicians or from the ethical expertise of ethicists. Instead, moral problem solving is located within the context of reciprocity,[6] in which all concerned parties are entitled to be heard and work together to arrive at a mutually satisfactory resolution. Clinicians facilitate and guide this process of inquiry without dictating or engineering the outcome.

The method of clinical pragmatism understands moral problem solving as consisting of a series of interconnected steps. Practitioners can engage in this collaborative process of moral problem solving when they (1) assess the patient's medical condition; (2) determine and clarify the clinical diagnosis; (3) assess the patient's decision-making capacity, beliefs, values, preferences, and needs; (4) consider family dynamics and the impact of care on family members and others intimately concerned with the patient's well-being; (5) consider institutional arrangements and broader social norms that may influence patient care; (6) identify the range of moral considerations relevant to the case in a manner analogous to the clinical process of differential diagnosis; (7) suggest provisional goals of care and offer a plan of action, including plausible treatment and care options; (8) negotiate an ethically acceptable plan of action; (9) implement the agreed-upon plan; (10) evaluate the results of the intervention; and (11) undertake periodic review and modify the course of action as the case evolves.[7]

This method is congruent with clinical problem solving in its cultivation of clinical information, hypothesis formation, experimental trials, and generation of operative, but contingent, conclusions that must be validated through experience. In addition to sound clinical skill, moral problem solving in clinical practice requires the ability to take the perspective of others[8], to engage in deliberative dialogue, and to negotiate the goals of care and questions of meaning.

To illustrate the method of clinical pragmatism, we present the following case study in considerable detail.[9] We have opted for this strategy in order to exhibit and analyze the complex reasoning and interactions at work in the unfolding of a single morally problematic case and to do justice to the relevant clinical dynamics and humanly significant narratives that emerge in the care of the patient. In choosing to concentrate on contextual detail and careful delineation of the process of problem solving, we acknowledge that no judgment about the merits of clinical pragmatism can be made by examining a single case analysis. Our goal is to make this method of ethical inquiry explicit to readers so that they may test the validity of clinical pragmatism in their own experience.

Case Presentation

TD is a 91-year-old white male with Parkinson's disease who is currently on the general medical service of an academic medical center following a two-week stay in the intensive care unit for a severe case of aspiration pneumonia that required mechanical ventilation. He is profoundly demented, barely aware of his surroundings, unable to care for himself, and markedly debilitated by his illness and poor nutritional support.

The house staff present Mr. D to the new ward attending physician who has just joined the service at the beginning of the month. On rounds the patient is examined. He is hemodynamically stable, but found to be hypothermic. He is responsive to noxious stimuli, but otherwise nonarousable. Overnight laboratory data reveal that he has a new elevation in his white blood cell count and that his urine is packed with yeast.

After hearing the case presentation and commenting that "a return visit to the ICU would seem futile," the attending inquires about the patient's "code status." The house staff tell him that the patient's eighty-seven-year-old wife, and natural surrogate, has wanted the patient to receive, in their words, all "aggressive measures" including cardiopulmonary resuscitation. The residents also report that they have tried to talk with the patient's wife about the patient's poor prognosis on a number of occasions. Like the previous team in the ICU, they have "tried to get a DNR order" without success. They also report that the patient's wife is demanding and difficult.

Case Evaluation and Analysis

The initial exchange between the new service attending and the house staff is laden with assumptions and intuitions that need to be explored. What occasioned the attending's question about the patient's code status and level of care? His remarks indicate that he felt that more ICU care would be problematic given the patient's cognitive and physiologic state. By inquiring about the patient's code status, the attending implicitly expresses his goals for the patient's care. Although such thinking often is not articulated, this initial question carries with it the attending's assumptions about futility and the risks and benefits associated with the available treatment options. More fundamentally, it betrays his intuitive sense about what the "right thing to do" is.

Ethical analysis is prompted by the perception or anticipation of a moral problem. In this case, the physician's sense of the relevant moral considerations remain in the background although his comments indicate a moral stance. Patients, surrogates, and clinicians may have doubts or moral compunctions about a course of action but fail to articulate them clearly. This is generally the norm and not the exception. These moral compunctions are a rich source of insight and ideally ought to serve as a trigger for a deeper analysis of the ethical issues at stake. Instead of neglecting to examine these feelings and intuitions, clinicians should view them as having an instrumental value that warrants formal cultivation.

A first step, then, in ethical inquiry is to make the moral perceptions more explicit or transparent.[10] In the case of TD, this requires the physician and house staff to engage in a dialogue about the moral dilemma that is brewing. Such an exchange is a necessary prelude to a more formal analysis of the case and prevents the premature closure of all relevant moral considerations. Making the position of the clinical staff transparent also helps to identify and demarcate disagreements that might exist about the appropriate goals of care. In TD's case, the lack of a shared understanding about the proper course of action has resulted in conflict between the clinical staff and the patient's wife. This is the problematic situation and the locus for initiating ethical inquiry.

As a general strategy, the clinicians and the patient's surrogate need to clarify their understandings of the patient's situation and the nature of their disagreement. Such clarification requires that they collectively survey the morally relevant considerations that bear on the case. We believe that this can only be accomplished by maintaining a collaborative discourse that allows for continued discussion and enhanced understanding. Ultimately this negotiation aims at resolving the moral and clinical problems posed by the case in a satisfactory manner. In the process of deliberation and negotiation, alternative courses of action are considered, and their probable consequences are anticipated and evaluated. The agreed upon plan should be adopted experimentally and adjusted depending upon how well it works in practice.

The bedrock of all moral problem solving in clinical practice is the proper assessment of, and concurrence about, the medical facts of the case. Here we observe that the patient has long suffered from Parkinson's disease. Implicit in this biomedical narrative is the trajectory of a chronic and debilitating illness. Mr. D required increasing help with the activities of daily life and eventual admission to a nursing home. The neurologic impairments associated with Parkinson's disease led to difficulty swallowing and repeated bouts of aspiration pneumonia, which necessitated his current hospital admission. Acutely, his hypothermia could portend serious infection, immunocompromise, or impending and rapid hemodynamic instability. It is critically important to be clear about these clinical details because the ethical analysis of a case can often hinge on such clinically relevant information.

Reviewing these data, a clinical picture emerges indicating that the patient has long been afflicted with an irreversible illness and that he may soon become critically ill and require additional ICU care to sustain life. Indeed, given the yeast infection in his bladder and the hypothermia, the patient may be at risk for systemic candidemia and a rapid and precipitous decline. The combination of these chronic and superimposed diagnostic and prognostic possibilities place unavoidable constraints upon the clinical team and the patient's wife. The advanced stage of TD's Parkinson's disease severely limits the patient's potential for functional neurologic recovery regardless of his battle with an acute infection. His more pressing clinical findings of hypothermia and candiduria also suggest that there will be little time for all the stakeholders in the case to make important end of life decisions.

Given these parameters, it is especially critical to speak cogently and compassionately with Mrs. D about her husband's prognosis in a timely fashion. Although we might ideally prefer to prepare her for bad news in a more gradual manner, the medical facts do not make this luxury possible. Failure to respond quickly to these constraints could deprive Mrs. D of the opportunity to participate in important decisions about her husband's care. Excluding her from this decision-making process is ethically inappropriate even if it is not deliberate. If we take seriously the importance of hearing from the patient's surrogate, then we must be attentive to the constraints that could conceivably limit her opportunity to reflect on her husband's illness and their life together.

At this stage in the case, it is necessary to develop an understanding of the medical facts within the broader context of the family's situation, institutional constraints, and social norms. Beginning with the family, we need to understand how Mrs. D will receive the clinician's diagnostic and prognostic assessment. We need to appreciate the basis of her request that her husband receive the most aggressive treatment available. Is this preference motivated by her husband's wishes? Is it based upon her affective state or her own religious, cultural, or fundamental beliefs?

Discussion with Mrs. D reveals that the patient has had Parkinson's disease for more than 15 years. Mrs. D had cared for him at home throughout his illness until just six weeks ago when she had to transfer him to an excellent nursing home in the neighborhood. The patient's decline and Mrs. D's own infirmity had made it increasingly difficult for her to care for him at home. During Mr. D's illness she had been devoted to her husband's care. In her conversation with the doctor, she was tearful about the nursing home transfer and felt that "he had been fine until he went there."

These important narrative details did not come out in prior conversations with the house staff. Institutional factors prevented this important exchange from occurring earlier in the patient's course. A critical assessment of the structure of care giving at the hospital revealed that the patient had been treated by a number of different physician teams since his admission and thus had lacked continuity of care at both the house staff and attending levels. This lack of an ongoing doctor-patient/surrogate relationship was an important barrier to communication. It precipitated anger and frustration between the house staff and TD's wife. Indeed, it presented a nearly insurmountable obstacle to conflict resolution.

Later conversation with Mrs. D revealed that she perceived the house staff as being rushed and too distracted to spend enough time talking with her. She reported that the residents spoke to her in the hallways, holding their clipboards in front of them, and were frequently being paged out of their conversations with her. She acknowledged that they were busy and was sympathetic to their workload. Nonetheless, she felt excluded from participating in decisions about her husband's care despite her long years of fidelity and love. Her disenfranchisement also deprived the clinical team of potentially important information about the patient's prior wishes and the presence or absence of an advance directive and her reasons for objecting to a DNR order.

This split between the house staff and Mrs. D illustrates that clinicians must be attentive to the differing perspectives of each of the stakeholders involved in the case. The breakdown in communication between the residents and Mrs. D was an avoidable error. As has been indicated, Mrs. D was not initially hostile to the house staff. Indeed, she was sensitive to their work load and responsibilities. The house staff, on the other hand, failed to appreciate that from her perspective a decision to write a DNR order for TD was the fateful capstone of a long life together. It was more than just the "end game" for the last 15 minutes of a two-week hospital admission. Furthermore, the anger of the house staff and their description of Mrs. D as difficult and demanding suggests a problem with countertransference,[11] which can often accompany cases that raise the specter of medical futility.[12]

This case illustrates the seemingly obvious, but all too often neglected, point that a fruitful conversation between the clinician and surrogate requires preparation. Because patients and their intimates do not easily engage in discussions about end of life issues, it is important to speak with surrogates in a quieter and less frantic setting than a hospital corridor. Although environmental factors may seem less important than the substance of one's discourse, dialogue can be obstructed when the setting is not conducive to an intimate exchange about a loved one.

When the attending physician took responsibility for coordinating discussions with Mrs. D, neutralized the house staff's anger, and spoke with her in the relative quiet and comfort of a solarium, she began to open up about her feelings and demonstrate her own need to grieve and be healed. Removed from the chaos of the hospital corridor and given proper access to her husband's attending, conversation flourished. Where Mrs. D had been described as being difficult, she now presented herself as a dedicated spouse who had made many sacrifices for her husband over the past years. The attending physician's acknowledgment of her commitment and her prior assumption of responsibility served to solidify their relationship. It also allowed the physician to determine that the patient neither had expressed preferences regarding life-sustaining therapy nor had executed an advance directive.

There was a new level of intimacy to these discussions that permitted the clinician to begin to speculate about some of the reasons why TD's wife was committed to an aggressive course of care. This illustrates that once practitioners have determined the medical facts, orchestrated an inclusive dialogue, and cultivated a requisite amount of trust, they can begin to interpret contextual factors and formulate an ethics differential diagnosis.[13] In creating this process, the clinician considers all the reasonable causes for the moral dilemma presented by the case. This is not a definitive moral appraisal, but a series of tenable and preliminary speculations that follow from an initial review of emerging information. Like the physician who creates a physical differential diagnosis from the details that emerge from a patient's history and physical, the clinician analyzing an ethical dilemma needs to recognize, collect, and organize the clinical and narrative facts into a series of plausible hypotheses that address the ethical issues at stake in the case. These speculations function as reasonably valid hypotheses that can guide the clinician in the process of moral problem solving.

After his discussions with Mrs. D, the physician hypothesized that she felt guilty about her husband's decline following his transfer to the nursing home. The attending interpreted Mrs. D's desire for "aggressive" management as a manifestation of her continued sense of responsibility and obligation to her husband. In a reparative way, she felt obliged to rescue her husband. To Mrs. D, aggressive care was not an intervention approaching medical futility. Instead, the use of medical technology was a means of demonstrating the integrity of their marriage covenant. As she had cared for her husband at home for years, she now would mobilize all of the hospital's resources in the service of her husband. Simply put, she was making amends for a misplaced sense of spousal abandonment. When the clinician suggested to TD's wife that she felt responsible for her husband's situation, she broke down and cried. She confessed that she felt responsible for his current situation because she had not kept him at home.

This psychodynamic interpretation suggested a number of therapeutic interventions that might assist Mrs. D in caring for her husband as his conditioned worsened. It was clear that she needed more information about Parkinson's disease in order to modify her guilt and better understand the nature of her past commitment to her husband and her future obligations to him. Informing the patient's wife of the natural course of Parkinson's disease helped her appreciate that the transfer to the nursing home did not cause his recent and rapid deterioration. Furthermore, once she understood that aspiration and the resultant pneumonia were common complications associated with advanced Parkinson's disease, she was able to distance herself from a sense of culpability.

Remarkably, she said that no one had ever explained the natural history or trajectory of a life with Parkinson's disease to her. This clinical information helped her to appreciate the imminence of her husband's death given the current situation. In this intervention, the doctor is acting in his role as teacher. Without this basic knowledge about the disease's course, Mrs. D could not fully participate in the decisions at hand. It gave her genuine access to the decision-making process by rectifying a fundamental gap in her knowledge about her husband's illness. In this specific case, instruction in the natural history of Parkinson's disease enfranchised Mrs. D, allowed her to overcome some of her guilt about her care of her husband, and helped her to participate more fully in the development of his plan of care. This illustrates that educational interventions by clinicians may be necessary to facilitate lay participation in clinical decision making.

In the context of assuaging her guilt, it was beneficial to affirm the impact that her own caring deeds had had over the past 15 years of her husband's life. Mrs. D found this comforting. It helped her to reconstruct her moral position from one of culpable inattention to one of responsible action. Indeed, against the backdrop of the biomedical and social contexts, she could see her actions as exemplary and not deficient.

After this reconstruction of the case through clinician-surrogate conversation, the setting of new therapeutic and moral goals was collegial and not contentious. The preliminary discussions about TD and his wife's life narrative together, and her felt responsibility, provided the physician with insight into what to recommend to her and what sort of language would be best suited to the task. The physician was able to suggest that there were other ways to demonstrate her fidelity to her husband than to send him to the ICU. He suggested that she could manifest her love by protecting him from harm and by preventing interventions that offered little benefit while posing significant risk or discomfort. By invoking the ethical doctrine of proportionality, the physician was able to help Mrs. D appreciate that the transfer of her husband to the ICU might not achieve the benefits she had hoped for or expected. Her receptivity to this line of thinking made it possible for the physician to suggest an alternative set of goals, which stressed a palliative response to Mr. D's illness.

Offering a plan of action, the physician specifically suggested that TD not go to the ICU and that a do-not-resuscitate order be written for him. When this option was broached with Mrs. D, she remained hesitant but very much open to this treatment plan.

The evolution seen in Mrs. D's responsiveness to a DNR order illustrates the importance of first negotiating treatment goals and then offering treatment plans that cohere with agreed upon goals. This stands in stark contrast to the typical "DNR discussion" where the treatment decision concerning resuscitation is discussed before goals of care are established and agreed upon. This stance may produce avoidable conflict or lead to misguided decisions. In contrast, the decision about resuscitation becomes less contentious once the stakeholders agree on the treatment goals at the end of life.

To assist Mrs. D in reconsidering the plan of care for her husband, the physician encouraged her to think over their conversation and suggested a meeting for the following day. The physician was cognizant of the importance of providing her with the necessary time to incorporate all she had learned about her husband's prognosis and the available treatment options. Any effort to rush the decision could undermine the trust that had been cultivated in prior encounters. Mrs. D appreciated this pause in the process and asked whether she might bring a family friend, who was a clergyman, to the meeting scheduled for the next day.

In the interim, the patient's clinical situation took a turn for the worse. The suspected systemic yeast infection, heralded by the preceding hypothermia, was confirmed by a positive blood culture and new hemodynamic instability despite the use of broad spectrum antibiotics and antifungal agents. This clinical development required that the meeting with Mrs. D and her pastoral care advisor be expedited. To the surprise of the staff, Mrs. D, who was Jewish, brought a Catholic priest to participate in the meeting. The physician briefed the priest about Mr. D's situation and his prior conversations with Mrs. D. The priest subsequently asked the physician to place the specific details of the case into the context of the papal encyclical regarding ordinary and extraordinary means of care. When the technical details of resuscitation and ICU care were described, the priest felt that further aggressive care was disproportionate and extraordinary. With the priest's endorsement, Mrs. D then consented to a DNR order and plans were made to provide only comfort care.

In retrospect, we note that TD's faith was never definitively determined. The staff assumed that he and his wife were co-religionists although the priest's involvement and the fact that the patient had come from a pre-dominantly Catholic nursing home might have suggested other-wise. In the actual narrative of this case, ignorance of Mr. D's religious affiliation did not prove pivotal because the priest's views coincided with the recommendations of the physician with which Mrs. D agreed. However, if the priest's invocation of Catholic moral teachings were used as a rationale to undermine the emerging agreement on the treatment plan, then it would have been incumbent upon the physician to determine definitively TD's faith. For example, if he were a devout Catholic it might have been appropriate to accommodate, as best as possible, the teachings of the Catholic Church and revise the decision plan. On the other hand, if the patient did not subscribe to Catholicism, then the relevance of the priest's moral reasoning might be more akin to that of a close friend trusted by both husband and wife. In either situation, Mrs. D would make a decision based upon the cogency of the priest's argument and her discussions with the clinical staff.

In light of this discussion among the attending, Mrs. D, and the priest, the patient remained on the general medical floor with continued supportive measures including antibiotics and fluids. He died early the next morning. The attending contacted TD's wife by phone and notified her of her husband's death. Mrs. D expressed her appreciation for the staff's efforts on behalf of her husband.

A retrospective evaluation of this case showed that what initially began as a conflict-laden encounter was resolved peacefully through enhanced communication and specific recommendations that followed from a thorough and careful dialogue. The decision to palliate and withhold life-sustaining therapy appeared appropriate given the patient's advanced illness. In this case, an important marker of the success or failure of this intervention was the consensus that emerged among the stakeholders. Although consensus is a valued good, clinical pragmatism should not be construed as a process that inevitably leads to agreement with the clinician's recommendation. This process of moral problem solving can help clinicians, patients, or families to reframe ethical problems in clinical practice and appreciate the contingency of consensus itself.[14]

Mrs. D's acceptance of her husband's condition and her appreciation of the manner in which TD died further testifies to the appropriateness of the decision. The quick resolution of the case obviated the need for additional periodic review. If TD had survived longer and begun to improve, then the stakeholders would have needed to refine the therapeutic goals and plan based upon these developments. This periodic review encourages course corrections that accommodate new data and changes in the perspectives of the stakeholders. Moral problem solving is a dynamic process that is altered by interventions that either disprove or substantiate initial hypotheses.

To summarize, in this case, clinical pragmatism provided a method to assess the patient's situation, evaluate the medical facts, explore the moral issues at stake in the case, and review other relevant contextual details. Following this assessment, it provided a means to negotiate goals between physician and surrogate and determine appropriate treatment plans that followed from these mutually agreed upon goals. Finally, it offered a process for ongoing reassessment of these interventions and a process to revisit these concerns as the disease and illness played itself out. In this case, the structured method of clinical pragmatism led the doctor to undertake authentic communication with the surrogate at a critical moment. In addition, it facilitated decision making concerning appropriate therapeutic interventions at the end of life.

Commentary

The Use of Principles
As this case discussion illustrates, the method of clinical pragmatism is highly inductive. It is a process in which careful attention to clinical and narrative detail helps to elucidate the ethical considerations that may, or may not, guide the resolution of the moral problem involved in a given case. Although Beauchamp and Childress[15] have noted the theoretical importance of specification and balancing in the application of principles, *in practice* clinicians often use principles in a deductive and mechanical way in their approach to moral problem solving.[16] This approach all too often leads to premature moral judgment. In contrast, clinical pragmatism helps clinicians, as well as other stakeholders, to treat principles as hypothetical guides. Their directive force in a given case depends on a careful analysis of the clinical situation. To jump to a conclusion about which, if any, principles are relevant in a specific case would be akin to reaching a diagnosis before all the clinical facts are known and developed. Dewey aptly described this problem of premature judgment as follows:

Imagine a doctor called in to prescribe for a patient. The patient tells him some things that are wrong; his experienced eye at a glance takes in other signs of a certain disease. But if he permits the suggestion of this special disease to take possession prematurely of his mind, to become an accepted conclusion, his scientific thinking is by that much cut short. A large part of his technique, as a skilled practitioner, is to prevent the acceptance of the first suggestions that arise; even, indeed, to postpone the occurrence of any definite suggestion till the trouble—the nature of the problem—has been thoroughly explored. In the case of a physician this proceeding is known as diagnosis, but a similar inspection is required in every novel and complicated situation to prevent rushing to a conclusion. The essence of critical thinking is suspended judgment; and the essence of this suspense is inquiry to determine the nature of the problem before proceeding to attempts at its solution.[17]

The diagnosis and resolution of moral problems in the care of patients also require such a disciplined process of inquiry.

Although invoking one ethical principle or rule may seem to provide structure to a case analysis, this move can actually constrict the emerging ethical discourse at the outset of a case when it most needs to be expansive. At its worst, such a mechanical approach could lead to orchestrated outcomes in which the selected ethical principle predetermines what counts as an important fact or reasonable question. A clinically pragmatic approach, in contrast, seeks to remain open to the range of ethical considerations that might be implicated through a thorough cultivation and appraisal of the details. It is open to the intrinsic ambiguity and uncertainty that inevitably attends complex clinical cases.

In TD's case, this openness helped the attending physician to avoid viewing the dilemma too narrowly. Given the initial profile of this case, it would have been far too easy to stereotype it into a generic moral conflict pitting the rights of a surrogate decision maker acting on behalf of an incapacitated patient against the responsibility of a physician to avoid futile or harmful interventions. However, to view this case narrowly through either the lens of respect for autonomy or that of nonmaleficence obscures the pivotal question about how Mrs. D might continue to demonstrate her fidelity and obligations to her husband even as his medical condition deteriorated. Applying abstract principles mechanically, without due attention to the clinically relevant contextual details of the case, can produce distortion and generate avoidable conflict. Indeed, if the physician brought rigid preconceptions about applicable rules and principles to his analysis, the case might never have been reconstructed into a dynamic that allowed the physician and surrogate to realize the potential for agreement on a course of action. In sum, clinical pragmatism treats rules and principles not as ready made moral arbiters but, in the words of Dewey as "hypotheses to be worked out in practice, and to be rechecked, corrected and expanded as they fail or succeed in giving our present experience the guidance it requires."[18]

Dissolving the Apparent Moral Dilemma: The Importance of Process
By not being tethered to either a preconceived notion of the principles or other morally relevant considerations at stake in a case, practitioners may find that situations that appear to pose an intractable moral dilemma can be reconstructed by a process of creative problem solving that arrives at a plan of action satisfactory to all of the stakeholders. Attention to the narrative details of the case at hand and a concern for interpersonal process revealed that there was no fundamental disagreement about the proper course of action once the physician and Mrs. D engaged together in a reconstruction of the initial dilemma. Although Mrs. D's professed stance of insisting on aggressive treatment to preserve TD's life seemed to be at loggerheads with the physician's sense of proportionality, the pragmatic process of moral problem solving revealed that this was not a "tragic" moral dilemma in the sense that competing values and norms were truly at odds. Rather, it was an operational dilemma that required the clinician to understand and accept the moral worthiness of Mrs. D's sense of obligation even as he questioned the manner in which she demonstrated her felt responsibility to her husband.

We introduced our discussion of clinical pragmatism with this case because we believe, based on our experience, that the apparent moral dilemma it presented is representative of many cases in which an ethics consultation is requested. These cases present the type of challenges that patients and staff confront even though they appear to be indistinguishable from scenarios in which intractable moral conflicts actually exist. Careful and creative problem solving can open avenues of satisfactory accommodation that initially appear to be blocked by fundamental disagreements.

Conclusion

Dewey formulated his theory of moral problem solving based on the experimental method of inquiry, which he called "the construction of good." Clinical pragmatism, inspired by Dewey's philosophy, aims to construct good clinical practice by offering a practical approach to resolving moral problems in the care of patients that integrates ethical and clinical decision making. It equips clinicians with a workable method of ethical inquiry that bridges the gap between ethical theory and clinical practice by focusing attention on the interpersonal process of moral problem solving. This makes clinical pragmatism especially well-suited to the practice and teaching of clinical ethics.

4 Habits of Healing

D. MICAH HESTER

Just in the degree in which a physician is an artist in his work, he uses his science, no matter how extensive and accurate, to furnish him with tools of inquiry into the individual case, and with methods of forecasting a method of dealing with it. Just in the degree in which, no matter how great his learning, he subordinates the individual case to some classification of diseases and some generic rule of treatment, he sinks to the level of the routine mechanic. His intelligence and his action become rigid, dogmatic, instead of free and flexible.[1]
John Dewey

PRACTICE OF ANY SORT is a function of habits, and the activities and attitudes of medical practitioners are no less so. This chapter will explore the idea of habits and how they function in medicine. In particular, I am concerned with those habits of physicians that have stagnated, that make "intelligence and . . . action . . . rigid, dogmatic, instead of free and flexible." These habits I will generally term 'habituations'. Dogmatic physicians—that is, physicians who function out of habituation—miss the fact that patient differences often require the physician to employ sensitive adjudication, if the medical encounter is to be successful. Physicians who practice by rote ignore the desires and interests of their patients as unique individuals, and further, as Edmund Pellegrino points out, they run the risk of developing poor clinical/medical judgments as well.[2] Thus, dogmatic physicians risk not only insensitive/unethical personal interactions but practicing bad medicine as well. Equally dangerous, I argue, are half-reflective habits of so-called "enlightened paternalism," habits that do not adequately account for the changing environment and culture and misunderstand the place of intelligence and community in medical encounters. I suggest that the "science" of medicine, in order to become an "art form," would benefit from an infusion of habits of community that treat patients, in their unique individuality, as members of the health care community.

It may help us, then, to understand what is meant here by 'habit'. Habits are controlled adjustments of individual *and* environment that are readily available within a given situation. They are tendencies to act,

45

tendencies that have been acquired. Note that the breadth of this definition insists that habits can be found anywhere humans reside, infused in anything of human character.[3] We readily accept that many of our physical actions are habits, but beyond this C. S. Peirce, William James, and John Dewey have shown us that beliefs are habits, emotions are habits, and even ideas are habits.[4] For example, the recognition that the back window of my car has been broken causes blood flow to my face, a look at my watch, a realization that some of the electronics in the car are gone, and a brisk movement back toward the house while talking to myself about my misfortune. These activities constitute my idea that something is wrong, my belief that I am the victim of some crime, and my emotional frustration and worry.

But further, these activities occur as functions of habits, as actions waiting in reserve to be mobilized by the circumstances in which I find myself (in this case, violation of property sets in motion my habits of fear, frustration, investigation, and stress). As the American pragmatists have pointed out, *ideas, beliefs,* and *emotions* are general terms applied to biological and cultural habits after these habits have been investigated. We do not believe or emote first, then act. The act is the belief or emotion. Habits are stimulated, and we perform.

However, this may sound as if habits control our activities to the extent that we cannot act intelligently but must act automatically, according to the direction of our habits. Nothing, of course, could be farther from the truth. As Dewey points out, habits and intelligence relate in a number of paradoxical ways.

Habits are a condition of intellectual efficiency. They operate in two ways upon intellect. Obviously, they restrict its reach, they fix its boundaries. . . . All habit-forming involves the beginning of an intellectual speculation which if unchecked ends in thoughtless action. . . .

Habit is however more than a restriction of thought. Habits become negative limits because they are first positive agencies. The more numerous our habits the wider the field of possible observation and foretelling. The more flexible they are, the more refined is perception in its discrimination and the more delicate the presentation evoked by imagination.[5]

Dewey contrasts habits unchecked by intelligence (for which they were initially placed into service) with flexible, productive habits that expand intellectual horizons. I wish to call these productive habits "intelligent" in so far as they serve both in means and ends as thoughtful and flexible, adjusting old habits to the uniqueness of each new situation.

We are always possessed by habits and customs, and this fact signifies that we are always influenced by the inertia and the momentum of forces temporarily outgrown but nevertheless still present with us as a part of our being. . . . [However, i]n its largest sense, . . . remaking of the old through union with the new is precisely what intelligence is.[6]

Opposed to these productive, intelligent habits, are those habits that, though they may provide a kind of efficiency in action, end in thought-less routine that stifles rather than promotes further intelligent activity. I call these thoughtless habits "habituations." They take the environment (at the time) as fixed and uniform; thus "adjustment is just fitting ourselves to this fixity of external conditions"[7] (MW9, 51). Habituations are mechanical and routine. Whereas habits in their fullest sense are readily reflected upon (even if only in small ways), habituations are habit-developed activities that are performed in a relatively unreflective manner. To quote Dewey again:

Habit as *habituation* is indeed something *relatively* passive. . . . Conformity to the environment, a change wrought in the organism without reference to ability to modify surroundings, is a marked trait of . . . habituations. . . . Habituation is . . . *our adjustment to an environment which at the time we are not concerned with modifying.*[8]

Habits are, in the words of Donald Morris, a "double-edged sword." As Morris points out, "By forming habits we restrict the need for conscious consideration of what we are doing. As a result our thoughts are bounded by specific limits, and we may fail to consider all possibilities."[9] Dewey says, "A habit marks an *inclination*—an active preference and choice for the conditions involved in its exercise."[10] As "inclinations," habits "prefer" and "choose" the conditions that call them forth; they do not simply wait in reserve but seek out conditions in which to act. They attempt, at least upon first appearance, to be exercised in particular ways along very restricted lines. The active nature of habits can lead to the "unthinking" exercise of them. Again Dewey:

Routine habits are unthinking habits. . . . [T]he acquiring of habits is due to an original plasticity of our natures: to our ability to vary responses till we find an appropriate and efficient way of acting. Routine habits, and habits that possess us instead of our possessing them, are habits which put an end to plasticity. They mark the close of power to vary.[11]

These routine habits I have termed "habituations," and they are the dangerous side of habits since they lose the ability to be exercised intelligently. Their "rote" nature makes them incapable of working (except by accident) for the benefit of any situation, given that each new situation will require some variation in our habits. To disrupt these patterns takes other habits, habits of reflection and deliberation that must be activated to check habits before they become habituations. Habits like shaving, for example, can be efficient yet dangerous if we are not attentive to the present environment—for instance, the contours of the face with skin blemishes. Habits of depression, as another example, are acceptable in moderation but pathological if they control moods without restriction. Thus, to develop intelligent habits—that is, flexible, adaptive, productive habits—we must first cultivate habits of intelligence.

Intelligence is a complex of habits that work together to produce reflective thought and action. These habits include suspension of judgment, deliberation, experimentation, and, mostly, the courage to act— checked by an acceptance of fallibility. And each of these habits can be broken into still further detailed habits. Suspended judgments rely on habits of patience and prudence. Deliberation takes imagination in the form of dramatic reconstructions of the situation. Experimentation needs habits that help acquire tools and that determine and order their use in the situation. Finally, as Dewey says in *Construction and Criticism*, "The primary prerequisite of critical ability [and activity] is courage. . . . [For] the easy course is always to accept what is handed out."[12] (LW5, 134) Critical reflection requires habits of courage in order to risk enacting intelligent, deliberate judgments that may simply be wrong. All these habits of reflective thinking—namely, intelligence (also known as habits of inquiry or pragmatic logic)—embody an imaginative process that helps make otherwise restricted habits flexible and expansive.

Turning back to medicine, the practices and attitudes of medical professionals are no less functions of habits than any others. Not only do habits undergird medical practices, but the attitudes and activities of most medical personnel are, unfortunately, more often the function of habituations—that is, unreflective approaches to patient care that run on virtually unchecked—than they are functions of intelligent, reflective habits. From the expectations of physicians about their patients (and vice versa) to taking histories to using a stethoscope or palpating the abdomen, habits of medical practice make encounters with patients efficient but dangerous, possibly stifling positive, flexible interactions with unique individuals and situations.

Of course, this general critique is not unique to medicine. Philosophy professors, among others, can also be guilty of simply "going through the paces." However, in medicine two important factors make this problem more acute, pervasive, and problematic. First, medicine often comes into play when individuals grow concerned about their health, and health is typically felt in intimate and sometimes even vital or mortal ways when in the midst of illness or injury. A cough may not simply mean a cold; it may spell pneumonia. A fast heart beat could be the sign of over-exertion or of critical heart problems. Patients come to doctors precisely because they sense troubling possibilities, even when they cannot precisely define them. (Though academicians may wish that their students experienced education in similar vital and even troubling ways, typically they do not.)

Second, the institutions of medicine (from medical education to medical centers to medical insurance to HMOs) provide an environment in which habituations not only thrive but are even encouraged. (Most academics have not yet been forced to deal with formularies). Academic freedom, as it is still defined at most comprehensive universities, still defends the professorial freedom to select materials, define course goals, and emphasize priorities within subject-matter study for the purpose of enlightening students most effectively. Within the health care system at large, the priorities are somewhat different. For example, Columbia/HCA, the nation's largest for-profit HMO, quite recently defined its own business practices primarily in terms of monetary efficiency, not in terms of helping patients.[13] The term "medical-loss ratio,"[14] for instance, refers to any portion of the medical encounter between physician and patient that cannot be itemized from the standpoint of the "business" of medicine. This approach, in turn, demands that health care professionals efficiently spend as little time as possible with patients in order to meet the "bottom line." Of course, this does not bode well for intelligent habits which, admittedly, can be more time consuming than simple habituations. Clearly, the environment into which the institution of medicine is developing works against intelligent habits and in favor of habituations.

The danger of any form of habituation is that it turns the practitioner into an automaton, a machine in both action and attitude. This approach to the practice of medicine has instigated diagnostic computer software to substitute for decision making by the physician. Medical diagnostic applications like INTERNIST and CADUCEUS, developed at the University of Pittsburgh, were designed in the 1980s for just such purposes, and the development of similar programs continues. Simply place certain vital statistics and symptoms into the formula and a flow-chart maps the course of care.[15]

But equal to, if not more problematic than, turning the practitioner into a mechanical functionary are the habituations of the practitioner that translate into treating the patient as a machine also, or at least as a formula-ized member of a standardized grouping—that is, a nonindividual, ignoring the unique content of a patient's life story. Without reflection in activity, medical personnel cannot account for the subtle but important differences among individual patients.

I do not deny that habituation-driven encounters may work on occasion, when during "routine" occasions neither party feels misunderstood or unsuccessful in reaching goals. Stitching up a cut, dealing with the flu, or even setting a broken bone can, depending on the level of disruption in a patient's life, be occasions where rote practice can work to all parties' satisfaction. But danger lies even in these so-called simple cases, where underlying issues can be missed and later develop into ongoing or future health problems. And in more complex cases—head injury, cancer, genetic disorders, AIDS, for instance—the chances of missing the boat both ethically and medically (if these two can be separated) increase if reflective care is not given.

It is clear that this is a moral issue of the first order, for we are talking about how people relate to each other. These issues concern the treatment of others and the responsibility for that treatment. It is important, then, to inquire not only into the issue of habituation in practice but into what kinds of habits and habituations should be developed and perpetuated in medicine to promote helpful, moral encounters between medical professionals and patients.

There is no way, of course, to cover this in full in any chapter, so I will focus on one set of problematic habits that I fear are rampant in medicine and medical activity: habits of "enlightened paternalism"—that is, purposefully providing minimal or inaccurate information for the "good" of the patient. From this analysis I will suggest that two important general habits are currently ignored in medical encounters and should be cultivated; they are habits of recognizing and investigating difference and developing community.

Physicians have long held a position of authority in society at large and in medical encounters in particular. Obviously, there are important reasons for this. Physicians have a kind of knowledge not possessed by most of their patients (which is why patients seek them out), and this fact leads to an imbalance of status and power in medical encounters. As

Richard Zaner points out, a fundamental "asymmetry" exists in physician-patient relationships. He tells us, "[Patients] realize that to be sick is to be disadvantaged and compromised both by the illness and by the relationship to the doctor, who has the edge over the patient in knowledge, skills, resources, and social legitimation and authority."[16] Zaner is pointing to a fundamental "asymmetry" in physician-patient relationships:

[This] asymmetry of power in the helping relationship is marked by the 'peculiarly vulnerable existential state' of the patient and the power of the professed healer(s). . . . From the perspective of the patient, illness or injury forces breaks with the usual flow of daily life.[17]

This disabling "break" forces the patient to place trust in the physician "and obliges the patient to rely on the care of other persons."[18] Meanwhile, the physician, using technical ability and scientific knowledge, is empowered within and by the relationship and, though most likely a stranger to the patient, is implicitly entrusted with a responsibility to help the patient. This imbalance of power, which is prima facie constitutive of physician-patient relationships, acts as a primary obstacle to communication.

Historically, physicians have exercised their authority and power through so-called "paternalistic acts." Particularly before the 1960s, physicians routinely withheld information, performed unexplained procedures, or made unilateral medical decisions claiming that they knew what was best for their patients. Their knowledge and experience gave them the right to reign supreme within the domain of the medical encounter. During the '60s, however, religionists, philosophers, and even some doctors began raising questions about physicians' practices performed ostensibly for the benefit of their all-too-often voiceless patients.[19] By the end of the 1970s, this "ethical" movement culminated in the establishment of four basic principles of biomedical ethics: autonomy, beneficence, nonmaleficence, and justice.[20] In particular, the principle of autonomy was invoked as a safeguard against paternalistic acts by medical professionals. Procedurally, one important way this ethical injunction has manifested itself is in the form of required "informed consent" documentation. Problem solved?

As Dewey has explained, habits are a function of the environment as much as they are of the organism. And in the case of medical habits, as the environment has changed with regard to ethical practice, so too have the activities. The habits themselves did not disappear completely; how could they? They simply became reconstructed in order to accommodate the prevailing attitudes embraced by the social situation. Rather than "overt" acts of paternalism, the habits have become more covert. Still in the name of "doing the best for the patient," physicians fudge the spirit of "informed consent" in favor of following its legal letter. Physicians have become habituated to reading the form, accepting the signature, and moving on. But even more dangerous are the half-reflective habits performed under the guise of "good medicine." It is not uncommon for physicians to tell just half the story, to explain the information only in the "best possible light," or skew the information in a particular way to get a desired result.[21] A personal story might help illustrate.

In 1996 I spent several weeknights at a local hospital as a participant in a seminar for health professionals on end-of-life issues. Each evening consisted of reading articles, listening to a presentation by a physician, and taking part in discussion. One night the topic focused on the "four principles" of bioethics, which the presenter listed on a whiteboard and pointed to as *the* basis for ethical practice. Without debate all but two of us nodded in agreement. The discussion that followed was led by an internist who claimed to accept the notion of autonomy readily, yet who also knew that sometimes sharing everything about a condition would simply frighten the patient. Medical knowledge on the physician's level may simply be too scary for the layperson. He went on to say that because illness is a time of difficulty and compromise for the patient, his moral duty required making many decisions for the patient and directing the tone and tenor of the conversations to relieve the patient and his or her family of stress. His term for this practice was "enlightened paternalism" since he felt he had learned the lessons of the principle of autonomy and applied it consistently to his encounters with patients. Quickly and almost unanimously, the medical professionals in the room agreed and supported his position with similar confessions of their own.

Clearly, situations like these offer challenges for moral interaction in medicine. This story, in particular, raises at least two questions: First, why is medical knowledge too frightening for some but does not overwhelm physicians themselves, and if it does frighten physicians, even a little, why sell patients short on their ability to handle frightening, difficult information?[22] Second, what understanding of "autonomy" is at work here that allows physicians to see their "enlightened" paternalistic actions as ethically acceptable without argument?[23] These questions go to the heart of medical practice, for they raise questions about the way physicians actually interact with their patients and about the attitudes displayed by these interactions.

What is crucially important is the institution (both its culture and purposes) in which these attitudes arise. And yet, the experiences that bring patients to see doctors and the needs from which the very institution of medicine itself arises are rarely adequately examined.The institution of medicine arises from a human need to be healthy; it develops through the education of medical professionals and reaches patients during medical encounters in hospitals, clinics, and private offices. In response to the need for healthy living, our very being seeks connections within our culture to other experiences that we enjoy or from which we grow. The biological phenomenon of disease or injury creates social disjunctions in and around the individual. As Zaner notes, "Any sort of affliction, trivial or grievous, effectively breaks into the usual textures of daily life with its taken-for-granted network of concerns, interests, preoccupations, activities, and involvements."[24] When biological disturbances within the body manifest themselves in human experience, the results are felt as disconnections from the "taken-for-granted" (or "everyday") quality of our experiences. The habits we so often rely upon, fail us. On those occasions when social, physical, and mental faculties are not enough to overcome the biological forces of injury or disease, we seek the aid of professionals trained in the science of medicine. We want to become reconnected with the world we once knew—the everyday experiences we so often take for granted. Our illness thwarts our attempts to move along our accustomed paths. We turn to physicians to find ourselves again.

This phenomenological description, however, implies certain expectations in the physician's approach to our health problems. If illness is experienced as disconnection from our everyday world, then health implies connectedness. If illness is loss of self, then health is living with a sense of self. But all this entails that those working toward health and away from illness have some sense of self (no matter how malleable this sense might be) toward which to work. Further, this implies that physicians who ignore the patient's self in all its many connections (and for that matter disconnections) ignore the very nature of health and healing. As many have argued, this is clearly one problem that grows out of medical education today. An overwhelming focus in medical schools on science, biochemical manipulation, and disease has resulted in physicians who treat patients as merely biological processes and material objects. It can lead to habits that distinguish the patient according to disease or injury and not in terms of the experience of that affliction. Social and personal aspects of the human patient are lost altogether.

Unfortunately, medicine has long equated the "technically, scientifically competent physician" with the "good physician." However,

we need to recover from the impression, now wide-spread, that the essential problem is solved when chemical, immunological, physiological and anatomical knowledge is sufficiently obtained. We cannot understand and employ this knowledge until it is placed integrally in the context of what human beings do to one another in the vast variety of their contacts and associations.[25]

This is not to say that technical ability and medical/scientific knowledge are superfluous. On the contrary, technical ability and sound medical knowledge are necessary habits to cultivate, but they are not sufficient conditions for good doctoring. As John McDermott has said,

[A]ny situation which cripples or enervates the human organism, however unusual or vague it roots, is a pathological condition. The task of medicine conceived as a social science (which is not exclusive of medicine as a natural science) is to build into its diagnostic procedures a sensitivity to this dimension of contemporary human experience.[26]

To understand healthy living in the context of a particular patient, physicians must not only account for biological/physiological conditions and modifications—that is, the "scientific pathology"—they must investigate how these conditions play themselves out in a particular patient's experience.

The paternalistic physician, however enlightened, assumes a great deal of similarity between the desires, obligations, and values of the physician, on the one hand, and those of the patient, on the other. This "certain human blindness," in William James's words, ignores difference, irradicates individuality, and runs the risk of "stupidity and injustice . . . , so far as [our opinions] deal with the significance of alien lives . . . [and] falsity . . . , so far as [our judgments] presume to decide in an absolute way on the value of other persons' conditions or ideals."[27] But unlike autonomy theorists of the Enlightenment traditions who believe society to be an impediment to true individuality, James and the other pragmatists recognize that difference and diversity of individuals arise *within* community, not prior to and separate from it. Thus, in order to tolerate, respect, and understand the desires, interests, and values of others, we must account for the communal/social aspects of their differing characters. We must take the self, not as atomic and isolated, but as mediating and situated. For the physician, then, a thorough exploration and recognition of the patient as an individual in community is not only useful but necessary if the physician does not wish to run the risk of "stupidity," "injustice," and "falsity." To do this takes new habits of communication that culminate in new attitudes toward patient care, attitudes that go beyond self-concerned paternalism and narrow-minded biochemical investigations:

What is relied upon is personal contact and communication, while personal attitudes, going deeper than the mere asking of questions, are needed in order to establish the confidence which is a condition for the patient's telling the story of his past. . . . [O]rganic modification is there—it is indispensable. . . . But this is not enough. The physical fact has to be taken up into the context of personal relations between human being and human being before it becomes a fact of the living present.[28]

Ultimately, what is misunderstood by both autonomy theorists and physicians, I want to argue, is that a self is both individual and communal. Theories based on the principle of autonomy do not do justice to actual human experience, particularly the experiences of physicians and patients. Successful physicians cannot function in a vacuum because, for one thing, medical practice assumes that other human beings need the aid of physicians. Also, patients rarely desire to be "left alone" and treated as "insulated," "atomic," or "separate"; often the very experience of isolation that is brought on by illness—indeed, that characterizes most illnesses—urges the patient into the medical encounter in the first place.

An individual self is a social product both created by and creating the communities of which it is a part, and healthy living is characterized primarily by strong connections within those communities. Physicians who practice "enlightened paternalism" have misunderstood or misappropriated *autonomy* and lost contact with any useful meaning the term once may have had. An understanding of self, and thereby a healthy self, demands that we explore each individual's interests within the human environment (both biological and cultural). And if Zaner is correct that illness is characterized, at least in part, by disconnections from everyday experience and community, it follows that the investigation and development of community is essential to healthy living and, therefore, to medical practice. Thus, the remainder of this chapter will focus on habits of community within the context of medicine—that is, on the idea of "community as healing."[29]

What is the meaning of *community* employed here? One example of my meaning comes from Dewey when he says, "The parts of a machine work with a maximum of coöperativeness for a common result, but they do not form a community. If, however, they were all cognizant of the common end and all interested in it so that they regulate their specific activity in view of it, then they would form a community."[30] The contrast highlighted by Dewey's illustration is that between a mere gathering of individuals and a community. The individual members of a gathering work toward their own ends which, by either chance or external construction of the situation, may or may not fit well with the ends of others in the group. The workers on the line at in industrial plant, for instance, can easily find themselves members of a "mere" social group in their work, to the extent that their activities are mechanized and their pursuit of ends is limited to their individual tasks. These bonds are strengthened to form a community, however, when individuals become aware of the ends of others, take others' ends as common and shared, and recognize that satisfying the interests of others in the community is of value to themselves. While attempting to fulfill their own interests, members of a community take note of others' desires, adjust and regulate their activities, and employ means appropriate to the mutual fulfillment of common ends. This awareness of mutually fulfilling interests manifests itself through a sharing of activities—through truly shared experiences that forge a common perspective—and responsibilities in order to consummate the desires of all members of the community.[31]

This is most important because an integration of interests and the awareness of this integration ("awareness," here, being an active process of regulating and adjusting activity) yields the very experience *of* community. Culturally, this means satisfying individual and social interests simultaneously; that is, our activities satisfy both our individual desires and community interests, and vice versa.

For an example, following G. H. Mead,[32] we can turn to baseball: the shortstop has certain tasks to perform on the field, ends he desires to satisfy, like fielding the ball between second and third or covering "the bag" or throwing a runner out. But these tasks are regulated by the actions of the other team members and by the shortstop's own understanding of how others' actions affect his own—as when the shortstop must cover third on a bunt down the line with a runner on second. As a matter of fact, his very position exists only within the complex of the game, the other players, and the rules they all follow. It must be clearly noted, though, that regulating individual activity according to community demands need not mean wholly subsuming individual interests under those of the community.

[E]very individual is in his own way unique. Each one experiences life from a different angle than anybody else, and consequently has something distinctive to give others. . . . Each individual . . . is a new beginning; the universe itself is, as it were, taking a fresh start in him and trying to do something, even if on a small scale, that it has never done before.[33]

Each person, then, contributes uniquely to the community in a way that would be altogether lost to the community if that particular individual were not present.

The key in positive, progressive human interaction, it would seem, is to balance individual and social interests by finding ways to retain individual desires and values (in their vast multiplicity and diversity) while making them work within the context of the social good.[34] As Dewey points out, this is an idea as old as Plato, but unlike the ancient Greek view that divided humans into only three categories, Dewey stresses that there are as many categories as there are humans:

We cannot better Plato's conviction that an individual is happy and society well organized when each individual engages in those activities for which he has a natural equipment. . . . But progress in knowledge has made us aware of the superficiality of Plato's lumping of individuals and their original powers into a few sharply marked-off classes; it has taught us that original capacities are indefinitely numerous and variable.[35]

To develop Deweyan democratic community in this radical plurality requires "utilization of the specific and variable qualities of individuals," an emphasis that promotes individual intelligence within an existing and ever-changing biological and cultural matrix.[36] But still further, it takes an educated ability to locate oneself continuously within a community of one's choosing. The ideal here, as we have seen in the above examples, is a community of individual interests that work together so that individual and social ends are contemporaneous (or coincident) and inclusive of each other.

Of course, the ideal is difficult to attain. Communal associations take complex negotiations. These are not always pleasant and are rarely neat or clean. But so long as those negotiations both account for the interest of all participants and accomplish some end that envelops those interests to the highest degree possible given the circumstances, a community of shared experience will arise. Community is found in a "society which makes provision for participation in its good of all its members on equal terms and which secures flexible readjustments of its institutions through interaction of the different forms of associated life."[37] And members of such a community will find that their own "[s]ocial perceptions and interests can be developed only in a genuinely social medium—one where there is give and take in the building up of a common experience."[38]

Habits of community, then, develop both to retain individuality while reaching for common ends within a group and to become aware of others' ends in our common reachings. They include habits of reflective thinking that help put into perspective the needs of all individuals involved, the institutional features at play, and the ends to be achieved. They are habits of discipline, intelligence, courage, tolerance, togetherness, perseverance, acceptance, curiosity, communication, and hope. It takes genuine interest in others to build community. It takes the ability and willingness to communicate one's own desires and to accommodate others' desires as well. And most importantly, it takes a realization that atomic individuals simply do not exist, that insular autonomy is a misnomer, and that individuals and communities, far from being in fundamental opposition, are implicitly integral to each other.

"Enlightened" paternalism misses the boat, not simply because it trods on the "autonomy" of another, but because it ignores the place of the patient as a member of the health care community. As we have noted above, paternalism of any kind relies on self-concerned habits that run counter to habits of genuine community. And even if decisions made by the physician about the patient could be called "technically correct," they fail to account for and take advantage of a most important resource within the encounter, namely, the intelligence and cooperation of the patient. Paternalistic acts misunderstand healthy living, relying primarily on biochemical factors as the only factors truly important to health, while personal-social aspects are taken as superfluous. Paternalism forces the patient to rely on a physician's choices while restricting the patient to under-informed and, thereby, unintelligent activities. And mentioned above, Pellegrino has shown that this is not only bad ethical practice; it is bad clinical practice as well. The paternalistic physician says, "I will heal you on my terms, for it is beyond question that my terms should be your own." However, recalling the fundamental asymmetry of the relationship, how can this be? Physicians in their "authoritative" roles are the paradigms of health—well connected in the social order of medicine—whereas patients are by definition struggling to find this connection for themselves within their own culture and experience. Clearly, forging a "healthy" relationship between these parties is perilous. It is my belief that good habits of community will help here.

We have been talking here about changing or modifying attitudes and practices—that is, changing fundamental habits of mind and body, of culture and biology. This is no small order. Recall that I have already acknowledged that these habits and habituations have arisen in response to the medical environment, the institutions of medicine that enculturate the practitioner. And as habits are the result not only of biological factors and prior socialization but of the environment in which they are currently at play, much needs to change to complete any modification of fundamental habits. Everything—including social attitudes toward doctors, government, industry, medical education, and so forth—will have to be at least reevaluated if not completely overhauled. Such an undertaking would be unprecedented in our history and is, likely, "pie in the sky."

Clearly, though, such changes begin in simple ways, with at least one voice speaking out. They can eventually grow into a pedagogy that fosters new kinds of learning. Such an approach would require that some practices change in direct response, if not direct opposition, to the prevailing environment. We must focus on contradictions and inconsistencies in the desires of medical professionals. And most importantly we must remember that medicine is a human profession developed for humane purposes. It exists to reach patients in all their humanity, with their affections and in their biological conditions, meeting their desires as much as possible. This takes communication, of course, but further, I believe, it requires a new attitude of community infused into medicine that demands consideration of the patient as integral to its operations, a member with full standing and voice, recognizing the patient's intelligent individuality. It takes all parties' awareness of others' goals and objectives; it requires appropriately adapting one's own habits in light of the demands of the environment while working to adapt the environment to one's own interests and desires. A "healthy" interplay between diverse individuality and pluralist community needs to be achieved, and nowhere is this more evident than in the encounters between patients and medical professionals.

5 The Bioethics Committee: A Consensus-Recommendation Model

KELLY A. PARKER

THE IN-HOUSE bioethics committee has become an established fixture in medical institutions of every sort, but one still encounters a variety of negative or simply inaccurate impressions concerning the nature and function of such a committee. Some committees no doubt have been established as mere window dressing, public relations vehicles designed to project an image of institutional concern and integrity where such virtues may not actually exist. Others have been established merely to satisfy an external mandate. Even where an ethics committee genuinely does contribute to providing quality health care, it can be difficult to communicate the nature and significance of that contribution. An ethics committee does not, after all, directly engage in saving lives, effecting cures, or alleviating physical pain. Nor is it directly responsible for personnel, administration, finances, legal representation, or any of the other obviously necessary nonmedical concerns of an institution. Even in the best circumstances, an ethics committee may remain somewhat mysterious to many persons whom its actions can affect.

In spite of such possible failings and misconceptions, however, an ethics committee can fulfill a genuine need for any community involved in the morally complex practice of medicine. The nature of that need—and the particular suitability of the ethics committee for meeting it effectively—are not readily assimilated under traditional ethical theories. The problem is that these theories, which tend to base the practice of ethics on the application of moral rules, would endow the ethics committee with a degree of moral authority that such groups almost never assume.

The nature and function of an ethics committee may be better explained if *ethics* is understood in terms drawn from pragmatist philosophy. Pragmatism takes the transiency and fluidity of human experience, including moral experience, as a given fact. Moreover, pragmatist ethics acknowledges and works with the pluralism of real communities and the diverse values their members uphold. Pragmatism regards the practice of ethics as a response to the concrete need for melioration in the problematic, potentially disruptive situations that any community must occasionally face.[1]

The role of the ethics committee in this context is not to render decisions or judgments based on authoritative deliberations. Such an approach might be called the judicial decision model practice of ethics. Pragmatism instead suggests what can be called a consensus-recommendation model practice of ethics. Under this model the ethics committee provides a forum for nonadversarial discussions aimed at hearing and mediating among various relevant (and often conflicting) perspectives. When a consensus develops out of such discussion, the committee may articulate that consensus as a recommended resolution for the problem at hand.

A working model of the nature and function of a bioethics committee will help clarify the mission of such a group, enabling both committee members and the persons they serve to better understand how the committee's work contributes to providing quality health care. The consensus-recommendation model appears promising for several reasons. First, it conforms to the nature and function of many existing ethics committees. Second, the model affords a perspective from which ethical deliberation—and the practice of ethics itself—can be understood as integral to the practice of medicine. Finally, the consensus-recommendation model allows us to delimit the authority of such a committee in at least one respect that is important for understanding—and perhaps for preserving—its most constructive function: to carry forth an ongoing discussion of the basic nature and conduct of the medical practice itself.

The Nature and Function of a Bioethics Committee

Ethics committee membership typically represents a variety of perspectives and interests, drawing members both from inside an institution and from the broader community it serves. Medical personnel, administrators, legal counsel, client advocates, social workers, clergy, academics, and others may all be regular committee members. Clients and others involved in specific cases may also be included in a committee's deliberations. Rotation of membership is a common means of maximizing the sense of democratic pluralism. A diverse membership is desirable, because no single perspective is authoritative for arriving at solutions to the variety of issues that are likely to be addressed by the committee, especially where their resolution will affect a number of constituencies.

The following mission statement, developed by the ethics committee of Visiting Nurse Association (VNA) of West Michigan (a home health care agency), identifies the typical functions of a committee operating under the consensus-recommendation model:

It is inevitable that ethical issues will arise in the operation of a home health care provider. We, therefore, establish an ethics committee with this mission: to develop and implement a formal process to identify, report, evaluate, and resolve the ethical issues encountered in our practice. We will accomplish this through staff education, the formulation of procedures and policies, and the review of specific cases. As appropriate, clients, families, and all involved parties will participate in the consideration of the ethical issues that concern them. All information will be kept confidential. We further recognize that ethical issues can cause much stress for the staff and we are committed to provide support for them.[2]

Perhaps the most important function identified here is implicit: merely by virtue of its existence, and through its direct efforts at staff education, the committee both legitimates concern about broadly defined "ethical issues" and provides a forum in which such issues can be addressed properly. The issues may include anything that does not clearly come under the purview of existing technical, administrative, or legal resources within the organization, or is not likely to be handled satisfactorily with such resources alone. Without a forum for consideration such as that provided by an ethics committee, these concerns might be dismissed as irrelevant or merely "personal" problems. The difficulty is that the issues involved are usually at least interpersonal, and failure to address them can affect the well-being of all involved in the practice. The ethics committee provides a resource for handling ethically problematic situations before they escalate into conflicts requiring administrative or legal resolution.

Staff support and education may be seen as general components of an ethics committee's mission: Almost any committee activity might be seen as fulfilling these functions in some respect. The specific regular tasks identified in the VNA mission statement involve either reviewing specific cases or formulating and reviewing institutional policies and procedures.[3] Both kinds of tasks involve a process of discussion, mediation, and search for consensus, and problems are often resolved by articulating a consensus in the form of recommendations.

One form of case review involves responding to an immediate ethical crisis or conflict; such a review aims at "putting out a fire." When an issue has developed to the point where a staff member finds it difficult to perform his or her duties effectively, for example, the ethics committee provides an impartial and safe forum in which all sides can be heard fairly. The committee is in a position, unavailable to the involved parties individually, from which mediation may be possible. The conflict may be resolved simply by engaging multiple perspectives in frank dialogue. Short of this kind of resolution, a consensus may emerge within the committee that some specific course of action would be an appropriate response to the conflict. A similar process of mediation can occur where conflict is not yet serious enough to constitute an immediate problem, but threatens to intensify. Often the staff member with such a concern seeks no resolution or advice per se, but merely feels the need to make his or her situation known to colleagues and to elicit support. Such a review of an imminent crisis can often avert its further development.

Staff support and education are prominent features of both the "immediate" and "imminent crisis" case reviews. Airing concerns and considering the diverse responses they elicit from committee members is educational in the truest sense of the word: All involved in the dialogue are pressed to consider and clarify the validity of their own views as well as those of others, and to seek together the best understanding of the matter at hand. When dialogue arrives at that best understanding in a given case, consensus has been achieved and provides a basis on which to proceed.

The ethics committee is involved in the task of formulating and reviewing institutional policies and procedures for several reasons. First, committee members are familiar with the kinds of problematic situations that arise often enough to warrant establishing a policy for handling them, and they are presumably familiar with the considerations behind precedents set in previous cases. Second, committee members have some experience, and perhaps formal training, in identifying and discussing the ethical issues addressed by or involved in the policy being considered. Moreover, they are familiar with the various perspectives of those who will be affected by the policy. Finally, the committee can employ the same deliberative process it uses in specific case reviews (discussion, mediation of conflicting views, search for consensus, and articulation of recommendations) when formulating or reviewing institutional policies.

This overview of the functions of a bioethics committee operating under the consensus-recommendation model suggests a generic statement of its role: The ethics committee (1) provides a pluralistic and non-adversarial forum for ongoing dialogue about ethical issues broadly defined as ambiguous, uncertain, or controversial situations that arise for caregivers, clients, families, or others involved in or affected by an organization's health care practice; (2) is often able to discover or develop consensus about the best resolution for such issues; and (3) may offer advice or recommendations, including policy recommendations, for resolving those issues, based on its consensus. This account of the function of an ethics committee introduces language specifically intended to link the practice of ethics on a biomedical ethics committee to a pragmatist conception of ethics in medicine.

Mediation and Consensus in Communities of Medical Practice

A full appreciation of an ethics committee's work under the consensus-recommendation model requires an account of how ethical conflict arises and of how the activities of discussion, mediation, search for consensus, and recommendation can meliorate and even prevent such conflict. Central to the following account is the view that health care, like any other complex activity, is carried out by individuals who together constitute a pluralistic community of practice. The consensus-recommendation model's emphasis on the idea of community challenges medical professionals to think of their relationships with one another—and with those they serve—in a way that may appear at odds with much in the tradition of medicine.

However, the "community of practice" view suggested here seems to describe medical practice more accurately than the traditional individualistic view—and from this view ethics assumes a place of crucial importance. Seen as the community's ongoing examination, criticism, and adjustment of its basic purposes—and of what is expected from individuals in light of those purposes—ethical deliberation is a primary means of adjustment and improvement within any practice. In medicine, where practitioners encounter new developments daily and the ethical stakes are high, these mechanisms must function effectively indeed.

The cherished image of the lone nurse or physician treating a grateful "patient" lies at the heart of medical practice.[4] It is a commonplace, however, that even the most routine care often requires the contributions of a whole team of professionals; it is also increasingly recognized that in many cases complete and effective treatment may involve providing some form of care to people other than the client.

The early pragmatists Charles S. Peirce and Josiah Royce made the concept of community central to their understanding of human knowledge and action. Individual knowledge and efforts of any sort generally require complex social organizations that provide the resources, information, and support to make them possible. Medical practice could not occur in its familiar form without that vast network of scientific, techno-logical, educational, political, and economic institutions known as the medical sector. Beyond this rather obvious fact, though, pragmatism points out that an individual's knowledge and activities are meaningful only within a community of people who consciously share similar aims, knowledge, and efforts.

Royce defined *community* as the relationship that exists among indi-viduals who consciously understand themselves and their actions in the context of common past experiences or expectations for the future. As he wrote: "[W]hen these interests of each self lead it to accept any part or item of the same past or the same future which another self accepts as its own,—then pluralism of the selves is perfectly consistent with their form-ing a community, either of memory or of hope."[5]

The community of medical practice, then, includes the immediate group of professionals who are involved in a particular case or work within a particular institution, but it also includes any other involved persons who share relevant past experiences (such as training or direct knowledge of the case) or expectations for the future (such as hope for successful treatment). All such persons are united by some degree of interest in and loyalty to the community of medical practice: They gener-ally believe in and promote not only its aims, but also its established methods and its body of acquired knowledge, and they generally support the other individuals who are its members.

Royce observed that our activities are experienced as meaningful when there is reciprocal loyalty within communities devoted to worthy causes. However, the element of loyalty is precisely what gives rise to ethical conflict. Royce wrote: "As a fact, that cause, which in any sense unifies a life as complex as my human life is, must of course be no simple cause. By virtue of my nature and my social training, I belong to a fam-ily, to a community, to a calling, to a state, to humanity."[6] Wherever there is loyalty to more than one community, there is potential conflict among loyalties. When such conflict arises, the individual faces a problem that can be resolved (if it can be resolved at all) only by consulting the various relevant communities in the hope of reconciling their respective demands.

Ethical conflict consists in genuine uncertainty about what should be done when individual loyalties to different communities appear to require different actions, and when these requirements cannot be easily reconciled. What will be done, what possible future reality will become actual, is for the moment genuinely indeterminate. Both the individual and the communities presumably desire that the best possible course of action be followed. The crux of the matter, though, is that in a given problematic situation the answer to the question What is best? is simply ambiguous. This ambiguity does not arise from any misunderstanding of the various separate demands, but rather from the novelty of the situation created when these demands are taken together. In order to allow a meaningful answer to be given to the ethical question, the demands of the situation must be clarified and rendered less ambiguous in concert.

This process of clarification may be accomplished in several ways. One common approach is to arbitrarily strengthen the demands of loyalty on one side so that they become irresistible: A community might simply compel individual members to conform to certain existing expectations of loyalty. There may be no examination of those expectations in light of the unique features of the present situation, and no exploration of whether fulfilling those expectations will in fact contribute to the unifying aims of the community.

Consider the familiar ethics case in which a nurse is torn between a client's request for information, on the one hand, and a superior's directive not to disclose full information on the other. The nurse seeking guidance may be given an ultimatum: To disobey the directive will be considered contrary to the best medical interests of the client, and the nurse will be disciplined accordingly. A certain loyalty (to the institution) is declared to be the highest concern, at the expense of other important loyalties (in this case, to the client) operative within the same community. This method of "clarifying" the ethical demands of the situation overlooks two important facts: There is more than one important form of loyalty involved, and any form of loyalty is ultimately valuable only if it helps the community achieve worthy ends.

Alternatively, the ambiguous situation might be rendered more clear by reinterpreting the various demands of loyalty in light of the present situation so as to seek a reconciliation among these demands. Not only would the ambiguous features of the situation be clarified in this process, but so would the community's understanding of its own demands and the purposes they serve.

In our nurse's case, an ethics committee would provide a forum in which the value of loyalty to the client could be weighed against the value of loyalty to authority; it is through just such discussions that medical communities have lately given higher priority to "the client's right to know." Such discussions address the central question of how best to provide quality care. An ethics committee can safely ask whether such characteristics as paternalism and obedience to authority are genuinely in the best interests of the client and the medical community, and the answers will come from a variety of perspectives. Pragmatist ethical and political philosophy stresses the point that the consensus of an informed and pluralistic group is usually a far better guide to determining what is right for the community than is the opinion of any isolated faction.

Both ways of clarifying the intrinsically ambiguous situation—and so rendering moral action possible—involve the involvement of a third party. The ethics committee's greatest strength lies in its recognized role as such a mediator. Following Peirce, we can identify this role as being characterized by its "Thirdness." The committee's function is interpretive: It not only sorts out the feelings ("Firstness") and facts ("Secondness") of an ambiguous situation, but in the process it discovers the more general objective meaning and value of these components of the situation.

The judicial decision model and the consensus-recommendation model, briefly illustrated in the two responses to the nurse's conflict, describe alternative approaches to an ethics committee's interpretive task. The first resolves the situation by supporting one of the opposing sides in a conflict. The only "mediation" involved consists in the fact that a third party is brought in to deliver a decision to the original two conflicting parties. Royce named this adversarial approach forensic mediation, and emphasized that it poses dangers of alienation and estrangement within the community. The consensus-recommendation model is designed to facilitate the nonadversarial approach to conflict resolution that Royce called nonforensic mediation.[7] Here the mediator maintains a sympathy for all perspectives in a conflict and looks for a resolution that not only will provide a basis for moral action, but will simultaneously protect or promote the relationship of community among those involved. Royce considered this latter function essential. As he wrote: "Without some form of institution that embodies such offices [of mediation or agency] civilization could not exist."[8] By enlisting opposing parties themselves in the process of finding an appropriate resolution to conflict, an ethics committee engages in one of the most effective means known for building community.

The suggestion that a bioethics committee should promote such characteristics as inclusiveness, democratic pluralism, mediation, and interpretation within the community of medical practice runs against medicine's well-established tradition of individualism, paternalism, authoritarian action, and reliance on established knowledge.[9] The traditional image of medicine is undergoing radical reform, however, perhaps because the traditional circumstances of medicine are changing. As noted earlier, the norm is no longer that isolated doctors treat poorly informed "patients" for maladies thought to be caused entirely by external agents. The emerging conception of medicine emphasizes client rights and autonomy, a holistic understanding of health and disease, and partnership in treatment.

It is in many respects unclear exactly where the practice of medicine is going, or what features ought to characterize it in the future. Members of the medical community therefore need to practice ethical deliberation, and not just medicine. All need to be able to examine, criticize, and adjust their conceptions of basic purposes in light of new developments, and continually revisit the question of individual obligations in light of those purposes. An ethics committee operating under the consensus-recommendation model is an indispensable resource for negotiating the ongoing transformation of medicine as a practice.

Adversarial Mediation: Beyond the Consensus-Recommendation Model

The consensus-recommendation model is proposed both to facilitate and to protect the ethics committee's role as an advisory or consultative body. At present its typical main functions are staff support and education, individual case review, and formulation and review of institutional policies and procedures. We may expect that the kinds of tasks entrusted to ethics committees will expand, however, as confidence in their value and effectiveness increases. With an expansion in duties may come an increase in authority as well. In particular, it seems likely that many committees will at some point face the prospect of assuming decision-making authority, which would suggest adopting the judicial decision model for at least some of the committee's tasks. Although it would be foolish to rule out in advance any potentially useful role for the ethics committee, care must be taken to ensure that any changes to its nature and function do not undermine its ability to provide a forum for nonadversarial (nonforensic) mediation within the community.

Sigrid Fry-Revere points out three ways in which the ethics committee's authority might expand to include decision-making rather than advisory power. First, such authority might simply accrue over time. As Fry-Revere points out, "The burden of showing why a committee or consultant's advice should not be followed may become very great as society's confidence in bioethics consultation grows."[10] Second, institutional administrators or professional organizations may grant ethics committees decision-making authority in mediating certain kinds of conflict. Finally, legislation may mandate that certain decisions or actions be remanded to institutional ethics committees. Fry-Revere expresses legitimate concern over potential abuses and side effects that might arise should an ethics committee hold such authority, and suggests ways to ensure due process and accountability for its exercise.

Although such measures would certainly be needed to protect members of the community from misuse of such authority where it existed, they would do nothing to protect the fragile process of ethical deliberation and consensus building that is perhaps the ethics committee's most important function. One thing that distinguishes the practice of ethics from practices such as law is that ethics favors the nonadversarial approach to mediation (the consensus-recommendation model) wherever possible, and resorts to adversarial mediation (the judicial decision model) only when absolutely necessary. Institutionalized communities always have some formal means to render decisions based on established policies and rules. Formal mechanisms for ethical deliberation, such as the bioethics committee, are less common. Although the processes of ethical deliberation and judicial decision making clearly must inform one another at many points, we run the risk of bypassing ethical deliberation—and consequently of overusing judicial decision making—when the two are intermingled.

The process of ethical deliberation presented here aims to mediate conflict by developing nonbinding recommendations based on open discussion and consensus. The process of judicial decision making, on the other hand, mediates conflict by issuing directives based on established rules and policies. Ethical deliberation may be regarded as a distinct process that often raises fundamental questions about the validity of established policies and rules themselves. Although the judicial decision process can also raise fundamental questions, its resolutions tend to be binding in a way that forecloses further general discussion: Its preferred way to alter an established policy is to establish a new one in its place. This is desirable in cases in which resolution itself has a high value. It is inappropriate, though, when the aims of the practice, and the validity of established methods and knowledge—the touchstones of loyalty themselves—are in question. In such cases ongoing experimentation and reflection on various alternatives are likely to lead to greater overall improvement in the practice.

Ethical deliberation tolerates ambiguity, whereas judicial decision making does not. The willingness to experiment with guides to action—and to tolerate ambiguity and uncertainty concerning fundamental questions in doing so—are virtues when a community finds itself functioning in complex and rapidly changing circumstances. New conceptions of what is right emerge slowly within a practice, and gradually they introduce new expectations of individual practitioners. Only after these conceptions and expectations have developed and been critically examined does a community possess the shared and certain knowledge (literally, the "conscience") needed to enforce valid policies. During their development, the guidance of more transient and fallible recommendations is usually preferable. Recommendations express a shared sense ("consensus") about what is right in a given situation. Consensus may develop into more certain knowledge if given time and the kind of deliberative forum in which it can be tested. An ethics committee is often characterized as the "institutional conscience"; it should perhaps be regarded as an incubator for consensus, the precursor of institutional policies and conscience.

TWO

Current Debates and

American Philosophers

6 Collaboration and Casuistry

MARY B. MAHOWALD

ALTHOUGH Charles Sanders Peirce never addressed the issues of contemporary medical ethics or clinical decision making, his insights are relevant to the methods and assumptions of the clinical setting. In particular, his concepts of fallibilism, community, belief, truth, and science, all embodied in his view of pragmatism, are descriptive and instructive regarding clinical and ethical decision making in medicine.

In this chapter I use these Peircean concepts to provide a fuller critical account of two activities persistently observed in the clinical setting: collaboration and casuistry. *Collaboration* describes the manner in which individual physicians address the complex questions of modern health care; it also represents an antidote to paternalist and instrumental models of the physician's role.[1] *Casuistry*, a term revived recently by Albert Jonsen and Stephen Toulmin, describes the case-based method through which physicians learn and practice their profession.[2] A Peircean account acknowledges the validity of this approach while pointing to its pitfalls and suggesting ways of overcoming them. Just as Peirce invoked the method of science as a paradigm for pragmatism, ethical decision making in health care follows the clinical model. However, my critique of decision making extends to both contexts. Peirce's concepts are the foundation of that critique.

Collaboration

More than other academic professions, modern medicine is practiced collaboratively. This is so by necessity, and sometimes for questionable reasons; it is nonetheless a desirable state of affairs. The collaborative approach is not incompatible with the independence or autonomy that also characterizes the physician as a professional. Neither does it imply an altruistic motive, since the physician's own best interests as a professional are generally best served through collaborative interactions with colleagues and patients. From a Peircean perspective, physicians recognize that it is illogical to be antisocial.[3] Peirce thought that the illogicality of antisociality occurs because of its inconsistency with the goal of science. For physicians the result is inconsistency with the goal of successful practice and its concomitant rewards.

The demand that medical research and clinical practice be practiced collaboratively is clearly greater in an age of specialization than it was in Peirce's own day. From my own vantage point in a humanistic discipline I have observed that some philosophers seem to succeed academically with little interaction with other philosophers. Such individuals remain in ivory towers that seal them off not only from the lay world, but also from their colleagues. Still, even they have books and articles whose authors communicate to them through the printed word, and they communicate to those authors through their own publications. Thus, even in the recondite world of philosophy, good research is accomplished collaboratively.

Scientists are less prone to insularity than are philosophers because they work in laboratories where many hands as well as many heads are needed in order to carry experimental projects to successful completion. Traditional distinctions between scientific disciplines, embodied in separate departments of biochemistry, anatomy, molecular biology, and the like, have broken down in recent years. Although individual researchers pursue specialized projects, the expertise required for their pursuit generally draws on many disciplines, necessitating collaboration.

Similarly, because health and disease affect the whole person, clinicians trained in narrow specialties depend on other specialists to ensure that their treatment takes account of other patient needs, and generalists depend on specialists for diagnosis and treatment of more complex diseases. In short, given the limitations of human nature, even those belonging to brilliant doctors, the effectiveness of modern medicine can be maximized only through collaboration.

Having worked in a hospital and medical research environment for the past seventeen years, I have been impressed by the extent to which collaboration is routinized in this setting. Consults with specialists are a commonplace of clinical practice. Interdisciplinary management conferences are convened on an ad hoc basis when such discussion is expected to prove helpful; at times these take the form of ethics review committee meetings.[4] Journal clubs and reports of individual and group research are regularly (e.g., weekly) presented and subjected to peer criticism. Continuing education programs for health professionals (physicians, nurses, and social workers) are required and facilitated by institutions and professional organizations. Didactic presentations and formal case reviews (e.g., in clinical rounds or staff conferences) are scheduled at least weekly in most clinical departments, as well as in the clinical subdivisions of major departments in large hospitals.

Casuistry

The teaching and learning of medicine is often based on cases. In ethics a case-based method has traditionally been called casuistry. Although the historically developed method of casuistry has generally been repudiated, Jonsen and Toulmin have recently attempted to revive it, describing the repudiated approach as an "abuse of casuistry."[5] They concur with the *Oxford English Dictionary* (*OED*) definition of *casuistry* as "that part of ethics which resolves cases of conscience, applying the general rules of religion and morality to particular instances in which circumstances alter cases or in which there appears to be a conflict of duties."[6] However, they further cite a reference (also from the *OED*) that alludes to corruption caused by casuistry: "Casuistry destroys by distinctions and exceptions all morality and effaces the essential difference between right and wrong."[7] In other words, the cost of apparent resolution of moral conflicts is a denial of the very basis of those conflicts.

If Jonsen and Toulmin are to succeed in the rejuvenation of casuistry, they obviously need to avoid the pitfalls to which it has succumbed in the past. Peirce's concepts of truth, belief, fallibilism, and pragmatism provide a stronger defense than Jonsen and Toulmin offer for the validity and usefulness of casuistry as a method for resolving moral conflicts. From Peirce's point of view the "case of conscience" is comparable to the genuine doubt that irritates the moral agent, prodding him or her to examine the consequences of alternative clarifications so that a plan of action (belief) may be determined. Such a belief remains mixed with doubt (fallibilism), because the goal of absolute objective Truth is not yet achievable. It is (ultimately) achievable only by a community of inquirers indefinitely and collaboratively pursuing it.

In the clinical setting, Peirce's method of pragmatism as well as the first definition of casuistry are commonly utilized. For example, a patient presents in the emergency unit with a certain set of symptoms. The medical team, uncertain (doubtful) about what the symptoms imply, attempt to specify the possible diseases through differential diagnoses (cf. general rules) that may explain the symptoms. By considering possible consequences of alternative treatments, they then determine a plan of action (or belief) expected to confirm a correct diagnosis through its success in ameliorating the presenting symptoms. Caregivers are never certain that a given treatment will be successful, because knowledge of the patient as a dynamic entity is inevitably limited (fallibilism).

Jonsen and Toulmin have formulated the legitimate practice of casuistry as embodying six steps: "the reliance on paradigms and analogies, the appeal to maxims, the analysis of circumstances, degrees of probability, the use of cumulative arguments, and the presentation of a final resolution."[8] All of these are evident in clinical decision making, and they are generally incorporated into ethical decision making, whether advertently or not. Although Peirce did not literally emphasize reliance on paradigms or analogies and appeal to maxims, he generally exemplified the pragmatic idea that theory (concepts) and actions (consequences) are inseparable, which suggests that the governing principle through which one moves from doubt to belief ("look to the consequences") necessarily entails consideration of paradigms and maxims. Although both accounts are consistent with medical and ethical decision making as observed, I believe they merit further consideration and critique. In the next section, therefore, I wish to review the key Peircean concepts that are applicable to the clinical-ethical context.

Key Peircean Concepts

Fallibilism, according to Peirce, is "the doctrine that our knowledge is never absolute but always swims, as it were, in a continuum of uncertainty and of indeterminacy."[9] The continuity on which the doctrine rests is an essential characteristic of all of reality. To the extent that we recognize the evolving nature of reality, we realize that knowledge is always incomplete. Infallibilists, for Peirce, are those who ignore evolution, pretending that nothing ever changes substantially. They therefore deny, either implicitly or explicitly, the habit-taking function of human intelligence. By *habit-taking* Peirce meant generalization or thirdness; it is at once inevitable and useful, as well as fallible. The spirit of science animates those who support the doctrine of fallibilism; such persons contribute to social progress through their willingness to take risks.[10]

Peirce viewed community as both present and future or as real and ideal. Real communities, modeled on the best practice of science, consist of individuals united in collaborative pursuit of knowledge or truth. It would be inefficient, illogical, and anti-intellectual to pursue such a goal atomistically or individualistically, because community within the context of inquiry reduces the inevitable incompleteness of knowledge, and thereby avoids erroneous judgments. The concept of community is thus linked to the doctrine of fallibilism.

Peirce's ideal of community is necessitated by the logic of scientific method applied to all of our human affairs. "We are driven to this," he maintained,

that logicality inexorably requires that our interests shall *not* be limited. They must not stop at our own fate, but must enhance the whole community. This community, again, must not be limited, but must extend to all races of beings with whom we can come into immediate or mediate intellectual relation. It must reach, however vaguely, beyond this geological epoch, beyond all bounds. He who would not sacrifice his own soul to save the whole world, is as it seems to me, illogical in all his inferences, collectively. Logic is rooted in the social principle.[11]

Not only is this ideal of an indefinite community logical; it is also methodological and epistemological. In the context of Peirce's idealism, however, the ideal may further be construed as ontological. Peirce even hinted at the applicability of the ideal of community to moral and social issues. For example, he appeared to endorse the moral reasoning exhibited by those who transcend personal interest out of concern for the destiny of their nation or the welfare of future generations.

Peirce thought that truth is also present and future, or real and ideal. Truths as we currently come to know them are partial and plural; the ideal of Truth is one and complete. With regard to the former, Peirce subscribed to a correspondence theory: "Truth," he said, "consists in the existence of a real fact corresponding to the true proposition."[12] His epistemological realism was grounded in the independent status he attributed to such truth. However, "truth's independence of individual opinions is due (so far as there is any 'truth') to its being the predestined result to which sufficient inquiry would ultimately lead."[13]

Peirce believed that the ideal of Truth is pursued both by individuals and by communities of inquiry. Although reality is independent of our opinions, it "affects our senses according to regular laws, and, though our sensations are as different as our own relations to the objects [i.e., the "Reals"], yet, by taking advantage of the laws of perception, we can ascertain by reasoning how things really and truly are."[14] Ultimately, when the process is conducted over an indefinite period of time by a community of inquiry, it leads to ascertainment of Truth in its entirety, and this is identical with the full unfolding of Reality.

Peirce thought that belief is related to doubt. Although doubt triggers the process of inquiry, it is belief rather than knowledge that resolves the unsettlement of doubt through a plan or habit of action. Peirce proposed his pragmatic maxim of "looking to the effects"[15] as a means of resolving doubt, but he realized that the belief or disposition for action remains provisional, and therefore mixed with doubt, because of the ongoing nature of experience from which doubt, belief, and knowledge all derive.

Probability and chance influence one's degree of belief. Although belief itself is more than feeling, "there is a feeling of believing, and this feeling does and ought to vary with the chance of the thing believed. . . . [W]hen there is a very great chance, the feeling of belief ought to be very intense. . . . When the chance becomes less, then a contrary belief should spring up and should increase in integrity as the chance diminishes."[16] Absolute certainty, according to Peirce, can never be attained by mortals. Peirce saw science as a kind of religion. It is necessarily based on belief in the service of Truth.[17]

Science consists not so much "in *knowing*, nor even 'organized knowledge,' as it does in diligent inquiry into truth for truth's sake, without any sort of axe to grind, nor for the sake of the delight of contemplating it, but from an impulse to penetrate into the reason of things."[18] Science as inquiry is a process that entails imagination as well as reason and commitment. It stands opposed to conservative morality because of its willingness to take risks.

Despite his proposal of pragmatism as scientific method, Peirce claimed that true science is not oriented toward useful knowledge. Because useful things can and will be studied without the aid of scientists, it would be wasteful to employ scientific minds in pursuit of useful knowledge. The serendipitous discoveries of those whose sole purpose is knowledge regardless of its usefulness are the source of radically new understandings that could not otherwise be obtained. In the long run, then, it is esoteric rather than utilitarian research that accounts for scientific progress.

Peirce's Concepts in the Clinical-Ethical Context

Each of the preceding concepts (as well as others) developed by Peirce seems particularly applicable to the clinical setting.[19] The doctrine of continuity on which fallibilism is based reflects the dynamic aspect of patient diagnosis and treatment. Unlike the cadavers from which medical students may learn a great deal, living patients change. They respond or do not respond to treatment; they get better or worse, go home or die. Physicians tend to think that whenever a patient gets better the physician's own decisions produced that result. In fact, the reason for improvement may have been quite different. Only an infallibilist physician would deny this, and the denial would close off possibilities for acquiring more medical knowledge.

In clinical ethics there are no empirical proofs of the correctness of moral judgments, but the nonempirical nature of moral values makes us less prone to pretend certainty. For the modern doctor as well as for Peirce, fallibilism promotes the experience of doubt, which stimulates inquiry. Physicians as medical scientists are anxious to know what illness or malady explains a certain set of symptoms. By examining the empirical symptoms through inspection and tests, they formulate differential diagnoses. They then pick the diagnosis that seems most probable in terms of its expected consequences, and affirm this as their belief by prescribing a certain plan of action. That the belief is mixed with doubt is evident in their ongoing check of the patient's condition. If subsequent experience does not confirm the diagnosis, another one is tried. And so on. All this is done in search of the true answer to the real questions the doctor is asking: What is my patient's problem, and how might I best treat it?

On the way to answering these questions, most doctors attempt to reduce their inevitable intellectual limitations by joining a community of inquirers—the community of medical researchers who are also committed to pursuit of medical truths. In fact, that commitment is a kind of religious dedication. Devotion to the religion of (medical) science, as Peirce put it, may even supplant devotion to the individual patient. The altruism that Peirce imputed to the scientific inquirer is clearly a commitment to ultimate absolute Truth rather than to partial truths, beliefs, or even persons. Thus, a Peircean framework may exacerbate the conflict experienced by physician investigators who attempt to heal patients while also acquiring scientific knowledge. For Peirce, the latter goal appears to have been paramount. For physicians, according to the code of their profession, the patient's interest must never be sacrificed for the sake of scientific progress.

Obviously, physicians do not always adhere to this ethic. However, their service to patients is usually enhanced through their collaborative pursuit of scientific knowledge. Ideally, of course, Peirce and others would deny that science and clinical practice are ever at odds; they would say that the truth pursued is also the Truth that heals. Patients are also attracted to the scientific dedication of physicians. In an age in which traditional religions have receded in popularity, physicians who work "miracles" by creating, saving, and prolonging life are seen as gods within the context of the new religion of medical science.

Assessment

From Peirce's point of view, the new casuistry described by Jonsen and Toulmin is only partially useful in the clinical setting. Its usefulness arises from the fact that the method succeeds in resolving conflicts in which traditional theoretical approaches have failed. A problem that remains has to do with whether the resolution reflects a true state of affairs or, in Peirce's terms, whether the belief that follows analysis of the case is a true belief. There clearly is no way within the context of even a renovated casuistry of determining the truth of clinical or ethical decisions or the maxims that guide the process of decision making. Peirce thought the criterion for determining such truth was entirely empirical: Look to the consequences. But the beliefs that result from that process are at best only partial truths: The entire Truth remains the ultimate goal of the community of inquiry. Thus, Peirce's pragmatic method, unlike casuistry, is essentially linked to the community of inquirers, and so to a collaborative method.

In clinical practice physicians recurrently confront dilemmas that their categorical knowledge of diseases, symptoms, and treatment modalities are incapable of resolving. Consultations may or may not ameliorate the difficulty—because the conceptual armament of consultants is also limited. In such cases a frequently heard maxim is "When in doubt, look at the patient." Obviously this maxim is more like Peirce's pragmatic criterion than the moral maxims of casuistry, which are generally developed over time by consensus.

A certain ambiguity remains within casuistry regarding what maxims should govern consideration of particular cases. Although Peirce's single criterion refers only to empirical consequences, casuistic maxims often reflect nonempirical moral values. However, the epistemology on which that method rests defines the content of concepts in terms of anticipated empirical effects. This applies to abstract terms as well as concrete concepts. On that account casuistry's nonempirical maxims are subsumed under Peirce's pragmatic criterion. His pragmatism therefore applies to ethical decision making as well as to clinical decision making, but only if there is no essential dichotomy between thought and action.

Charges of anti-intellectualism and relativism have been directed against both pragmatism and casuistry. The charges were easily refuted by Peirce in his account of pragmatism, but not by Jonsen and Toulmin in their account of casuistry. Peirce's doctrine of truth as well as his concept of scientific method necessarily involves a metaphysical realism that assumes the objective status of reality and of truth as ascertainment of reality.

In contrast, casuistry operates only as a method of resolving conflicts, without alluding to the possibility that resolution may be superficial rather than real. Decisions are apparently acceptable solely on the basis of their fitting one paradigm more closely than another, governed by maxims that apply to the paradigm as well as to the case or issue at hand. Moreover, cases apparently become paradigmatic solely on the basis of their having evoked a long-standing consensus about their resolution. Peirce thought that a decision is based on perception of objective consequences and is necessarily provisional; each decision is a belief mixed with doubt that serves as a continuing provocation to further critical inquiry.

Jonsen and Toulmin have proposed a case-based method of teaching as well as practicing medical ethics. The analogue for this in Peirce is his concept of doubt that triggers pragmatic inquiry . This doubt, he maintained, is genuine rather than contrived.[20] As such, it is not the doubt induced in a student in a large lecture hall who is asked to imagine a case in which she is called upon to make a decision. Genuine doubt occurs when the student confronts an actual patient whose condition she is asked to determine on the basis of physical examination and history.

A case-based method of teaching is often pedagogically effective because its appeal to imagination stimulates the student to think more carefully and critically. There is nonetheless a danger that case-based teaching remains anecdotal, entertaining students and sometimes inspiring them, but leaving them with no conceptual tools to bring to future experience. Peirce, of course, would consider such a method of teaching regretfully inadequate: he insisted on the reality and practicality of "generals"[21] even while maintaining an openness to change and to clarification of ideas through application of the pragmatic maxim.

Jonsen and Toulmin have proposed casuistry as a means of settling ethical dilemmas that arise either as issues or as cases involving particular patients. For example, Jonsen used the method in developing his view on the issue of fetal tissue transplantation.[22] But a view on an issue implies a view on cases that exemplify that issue. This relationship suggests a type of deductive reasoning that Toulmin and Jonsen generally reject in their critique of traditional "reductionist" ethics. Through his concept of doubt as well as his concept of thirdness, which he identified with reality, Peirce provided a better means of relating general issues to particular cases. So long as doubt is real it can apply to either context. It is real so long as the inquirer is irritated by the realization that she does not know what she wants to know.

A collaborative model of medicine may apply either to the physician-patient encounter or to medical research. The latter most resembles Peirce's notion of a community of inquiry. Altruism in the service of truth, however, which Peirce considered essential to a true scientific spirit, is often lacking among egoistic researchers, who use rather than collaborate with some of their colleagues, pursuing their own prestige or profit rather than truth.

The collaboration I have generally observed in medical practice occurs mainly among physicians, and sometimes between them and other caregivers (nurses, social workers, etc.), but rarely between physicians and patients. Obviously the latter type of collaboration may sometimes be impossible—for instance, when patients are unable to communicate because of disability, disease, or the effects of medication. Physicians still reflect the paternalistic imperative of Hippocrates—"to do good or at least to do no harm."[23] In some situations, however, paternalism is reversed and physicians purport to be only instruments of patients' wishes. Obstetrician-gynecologists are especially attracted to the latter model because it affords them a way of avoiding the particularly thorny and controversial issues raised in their specialty.

The Peircean concepts of science and community, on which a collaborative model is appropriately based, is one that supports different competencies and insights on both sides of the relationship, eschewing both paternalist and patient autonomy models if they neglect one side or the other. Unfortunately, Peirce did not explicitly address the key ethical principle that may be betrayed by either of those modes—respect for autonomy. If may be argued, however, that this principle was assumed in his notion of pragmatism as a scientific method.

The collaborative method of clinical decision making has recently been extended to ethical decision making.[24] Ethics consultations and ethics review committees are the mechanisms through which the extension has occurred. For the same reasons that prompt clinical consults, physicians seek advice from those who have greater knowledge or expertise than they regarding ethical dilemmas. Shared responsibility and more enlightened judgments result, despite the fact that the recommendations from ethics consults or committees are generally advisory rather than mandatory. The benefits of these means of addressing ethical issues are the same as the benefits of clinical collaborations and Peirce's community of inquiry: the reduction of human error through rational interaction. Accordingly, ethical decision making ought to follow the clinical model.

This chapter breaks no new ground in Peircean exegesis, nor does it attempt to do so. As someone who "grew up" in philosophy and who early on found Peirce's philosophy both sound and appealing, I have explicitly applied some of his core insights to the practical context in which I have worked for many years. In doing so I have considered casuistry and collaboration as central themes of clinical and ethical decision making. The correlations with Peirce are, I believe, valid and educative. Both theoretically and practically, as befits a pragmatist, Peirce provided a rich resource for clinical ethics.

7 The Medical Covenant: A Roycean Perspective

C. GRIFFIN TROTTER

IF EVERYTHING went smoothly in clinical medicine, there would not be much talk about models or paradigms of the patient-physician relationship. Entering the clinic or the hospital would be like taking a warm bath—purely satisfying. But the halls of medicine are not so placid. There are many troubled parties and as many ways of classifying the patient-physician relationship as there are perceived difficulties.

In this chapter I will use the term *model* to designate a detailed, tentative framework or plan. Models are elaborate hypotheses about how things should or might be worked out. I will use *paradigm* to mean a comprehensive model that integrates several other models. William F. May has referred to covenant as an *image* of the physician-patient relationship.[1] Images are in many respects like models. Nevertheless, I prefer to use *image* in a manner that accentuates the sensual nature of visual images. Images—such as the image of parent, technician, teacher, warrior, etc.—are useful because of their visceral appeal. In this regard, models and paradigms are enhanced by images.

Differing medical taxonomies reflect differing perspectives on what is crucial. At one end of the spectrum are children, who characteristically employ two concretely unambiguous models of the patient-physician relationship—the "boring" model, in which they must sit still during history-taking and physical examination, and the "horrific" model, in which boredom is punctuated by some form of torture, usually a "shot." At the other end are philosophers, whose concerns are, on occasion, so abstract as to seem irrelevant to nonphilosophers.

It is with trepidation, then, that I introduce the thought of philosopher Josiah Royce, to address some of the difficulties that regularly beset patients and physicians. My plan is to develop the notion of a medical covenant, using Royce as a guide. In so doing, I hope to make progress toward the construction of a Roycean paradigm for the patient-physician relationship (let us call it the "clinical relationship").

The project of constructing such a paradigm demands that theorists examine the clinical relationship from a multiplicity of angles. Ultimately, every locus of concern should be surveyed. My aim here is more modest. I will examine the clinical relationship primarily from two perspectives: what I will call the "philosophical" and "strategic" perspectives.

From the philosophical perspective, I ask: what are the central moral principles and commitments that should pertain to patient-physician relationships? The goal is to develop a conceptual framework for understanding patient-physician interactions and also, hopefully, to enrich clinical relationships by molding this framework along the contours of human experience. In other words, I aim at practical relevance as well as conceptual soundness. Among pragmatists, Royce is especially qualified for the topic of clinical relationships, not merely by virtue of his intellect but because of his intimate experience with human illness and suffering.[2]

The strategic perspective is where philosophical commitments are wielded in the face of hard economic and social reality. For the pragmatist, all philosophy is applied philosophy. However, at the strategic level applications are somewhat more direct and concrete than they are in abstract philosophical discussions. Strategic questions focus on how clinical relationships ought to be structured by larger social arrangements. At this level, developing a model of the clinical relationship is often a matter of selective emphasis. Is the relationship between patient and physician primarily a market arrangement? Or is it more a matter of complying with laws, guidelines, and regulations?

Both the philosophical and strategic levels offer varieties of distinct models. At the philosophical level, several models of the clinical relationship compete for preeminence. These include contractarian,[3] transcendentalist,[4] intuitionist,[5] deontological[6] and virtue models,[7] among others. From the strategic perspective, there are three dominant types: (1) economic models, which view the clinical relationship as a market arrangement, (2) legalistic models, which hold that it is primarily an affair of adhering to directives, and (3) covenantal models, which view the clinical relationship as the centerpiece of a moral community. In this chapter I will characterize and argue for a Roycean version of a covenantal-virtue model of the physician-patient relationship.

General Features of Roycean Ethics

I classify Royce as a pragmatist, for at least one reason that should already be apparent. Royce, like the classical pragmatists Peirce, James, and Dewey, begins and ends his philosophical quest in the realm of human experience. His philosophical preoccupations always consciously derive from human concerns, and his solutions are aimed at the goal of human flourishing. Further, Royce's mature method and metaphysics both employ Peircean doctrines of interpretation and fallibilism.[8] Like Dewey, Royce strongly emphasizes harmony and moral growth as ethical ideals and, consequently, seeks to cultivate the virtue of tolerance.[9]

But perhaps the most central feature of Royce's ethics that binds him to the pragmatists—especially to William James—is his voluntarism. Pragmatism is, at its core, the view that ideas are potential plans of action. Royce, like James, and perhaps more than Dewey, conceives moral life as the endeavor of creating a life plan. Though he is careful to weigh the impact of inheritance, nature, and culture on human behavior, Royce insists that human beings are defined by moral commitments that are freely made.[10] Like the pragmatists, Royce views these commitments, and the moral principles that undergird them, as action plans.

Royce's personalism is another characteristic he shares with many pragmatists, especially Dewey. Personalism, in the sense used here, is a twofold doctrine holding (1) that there is an ethical imperative to becoming a person and (2) that persons are, in an important sense, metaphysically and ethically constituted by voluntary commitments to various communities.[11] Royce defines a person as "a human life lived according to a plan."[12] Thus, the first of the above claims is linked to Royce's position that moral life is the endeavor of creating a life plan. The second claim is a fundamental tenet of Royce's social ethics, exemplified in his doctrine of loyalty.[13]

Royce does not believe in moral recipes. Formulating an adequate life plan, in his view, requires practical wisdom.[14] Practical wisdom involves an ability to perceive diverse, sometimes incompatible, personal and social needs, and to fashion workable moral ideals that fulfill these needs in a maximally integrated manner. This process requires more than mere application of moral rules. In some situations, no clearly satisfactory course of action appears. Royce illustrates this problem with his discussion of Robert E. Lee's decision to lead the Confederate Army.[15]

For Royce, as for other virtue ethicists, human activity is evaluated primarily in terms of the interplay between moral virtues and meaningful human ends, rather than by dissecting actions into discrete intentions, acts, and consequences. Thus, the moral significance of Lee's leadership at Gettysburg is constituted neither by his tactical decisions nor by their result (the Confederate defeat). Royce evaluates Lee in terms of his fidelity to central moral commitments and according to the integrity of the process by which these commitments have been undertaken.

Unlike some of his pragmatist colleagues, Royce is deeply committed to a theology of human moral imperfection, struggle, and hope for spiritual redemption through divine grace. Through grace, Royce believes the great community of all humanity becomes an eternal, beloved community. Through grace, the human psyche, with its will to interpret, is assisted in the quest for meaning and truth. To develop a Roycean notion of covenant, we will need to tap the wellspring of Royce's natural theology.

Loyalty and Covenant

Royce's provisional definition of loyalty in *The Philosophy of Loyalty* is "the willing and practical and thoroughgoing devotion of a person to a cause."[16] With this formulation, Royce hoped to emphasize several points. First, loyalty is a voluntary orientation. We choose our causes; they cannot be thrust upon us wholly without our consent. Second, loyalty is a nuts-and-bolts affair, manifested in our daily routines as well as in our finest hours. It is not constituted by intellectual assent to a bloodless collection of abstract moral principles. Instead, it propels us to action. Third, loyalty is internalized. It is thoroughgoing in the sense that it permeates our lives to the point of constituting our personal identities. Loyalists are not content merely to pursue a cause; they breathe it.

Another aspect of loyalty, especially relevant to medicine, is its psychological basis in the need to serve. The loyalist is one who has answered humanity's call for help. This aspect of loyalty is perhaps best summarized in Royce's letter to Elizabeth Randolph:

Suppose I come to see, or even just to imagine, that there is some good to be done in the world that nobody but myself can do. Suppose I learn that there is something or somebody who needs just me to give aid for worthy ends of some sort. Suppose that this world of people, all so needy, needs my help. Well then the question, Why must I live? begins to get its answer. I must live because my help is needed. . . . But of course that first answer does not of itself tell you what it is which you are needed to do to help the other people. . . . The help which my friends really most want of me, is help in living "in the unity of the spirit," as lovers and faithful friends, and patriots, and all those who together are devoted to . . . whatever binds the souls of men in the common ties of the spirit. . . . Now thus to live,— to live for the sake of the "unity of the spirit," to live for some "cause that binds many lives in one," to live thus is to possess what I call Loyalty.[17]

When loyalists aim at binding "the souls of men in the common ties of the spirit," they aim for an eternal community. The cause of the Roycean loyalist is more than a momentary need or desire. It is a fragment of the comprehensive harmony of human activities that Royce foresees as our ideal destiny.

In light of comments about the intensely practical nature of loyalty, reference to comprehensive unity and eternal quests may seem far-flung. To the contrary, this marriage of the practical with the eternal is the essence of genuine loyalty. The cause of the loyalist is always an ideal that animates, nurtures, and helps define a human community.

But causes, just as human communities, can be good or bad. Good causes, in Royce's view, are determined by their relation to the comprehensive goal of human unity and harmony in a "great community." In the great community, loyalties no longer destroy one another. Instead, they cohere. Royce has equated loyalty to the great community with "loyalty to loyalty" just because the great community is where everyone lives in the spirit of loyalty, and every loyalty exists in symbiosis with others. A good cause is one that helps us progress toward the ideal of a great community. To function in this capacity, the cause must be tangible. It must have a place in the contemporary, imperfect world. Otherwise, loyalty will not be psychologically compelling, nor will it be efficacious. At the same time, if they are to be genuine, naturally occurring loyalties must be transformed by the sense of a common human destiny.

This deep sense of connectedness is also the essence of covenant. In fact, the central feature of covenantal relationships is that they require members' mutual loyalty to a cause that eclipses the personal interests of any member alone. Royce holds that genuine communities are constituted by such covenantal relationships.[18]

The general characteristics of covenants naturally reflect the aforementioned characteristics of loyalty. Covenants are relationships that define and sustain communities by: (1) promoting ideals that are willingly shared by each community member (covenantor), (2) transforming the personal identity and practical life of each covenantor in accordance with these ideals, and (3) instilling an attitude of kinship and trust between covenantors. We will now examine the patient-physician relationship in light of these features.

The Patient-Physician Covenant

"If you are able to quit, please do." Such advice has issued from a number of older clinicians in response to young colleagues who grumble about the hardships of medicine. This advice reflects a traditional view about the practice of medicine that has, perhaps, gone out of vogue. It is the view that medicine is a calling. It amounts to a belief that, through a covenantal relationship with patients, physicians find an answer to the crucial question that Royce posed for Elizabeth Randolph. "In what specific respect should I serve?" To answer this question is to discover something essential about oneself—and to undertake a relationship with something larger than oneself.

The medical covenant is identity-transforming for patients as well as physicians. For patients, it provides a crucial structure through which illnesses are reinterpreted. Illness, threat of illness, and beliefs about the proper management of illness all exert potent effects on our self-images.[19] These beliefs are manifested by our proclivity to visit physicians when we are sick, and by our financial and emotional support for arrangements that guarantee medical help will be available should we or the ones we care about become ill. We enter into relationships with our physicians when we make such provisions. These relationships become more determinant when illness threatens and we visit the clinic or hospital.

If the patient-physician relationship is a covenant, then it will engender an attitude of loyalty. That is, in a covenantal view, patients are expected to support the medical community they wish to appropriate, not merely as an act of prudent self-interest but also out of a sense of dedication to community well-being. Recall that in the Old Testament, *covenant* expressed a relationship between individual Hebrews, as well as between the Hebrews and God. Likewise, the patient's covenant is not merely with physicians or with corporate health care. It is also a relationship with other patients.[20]

For physicians, the medical covenant provides a more expansive criterion of personal identity. This covenant is the basis for a moral community, and service to this community is the life work of physicians. The community that arises from the medical covenant may be called "the greater medical community" (GMC). It can be defined as the community of persons who are committed to utilizing and advancing the knowledge, customs, and methods that have emerged during the history of clinical medicine, with the aim of furthering the health and alleviating or mitigating the suffering of human beings.[21] Membership in the GMC is not exclusive. It is open to patients, potential patients, clinicians, ancillary health-care personnel, politicians—to anyone with an interest in health care.

The physician's dedication to the GMC must of needs be more thoroughgoing than the patient's. For the patient, loyalty to the GMC is a small part of loyalty to a larger human community, just because treating illness and promoting physical health are only limited aspects of human flourishing. For physicians, loyalty to the GMC is a chosen path. The values or ideals animating the GMC are internalized and embodied by physicians. That is to say, physicians work to express these values in their personal characters. Such is the covenantor's view of virtuous physicians. If this view is accurate, then the profession of medicine will be radically self-transforming. We can understand this transformation better if we delve a little deeper into the clinical relationship.

The clinical relationship is the centerpiece of medicine. This status, however, does not make it the locus of all medical authority. Like any dyadic relationship, the patient-physician relationship, taken in isolation, is unstable.[22] This instability reflects the moral, physical, and intellectual limitations of human individuals. Physicians are fallible; therefore, patients are naturally apt to question their advice. Physicians are prone to selfishness; therefore, their motives will be questioned. Patients are also prone to undue selfishness or to erroneous judgments; physicians, therefore, will feel at times that they must oppose their patients' wishes.

Conflict within the clinical relationship requires the same solution we apply to other conflicts—mediation. The manifold ways of mediating conflicts boil down to two general categories: (1) by an appeal to ideals or standards or (2) by an appeal to a mediating body, generally called upon to interpret a set of ideals or standards. In the clinical relationship, there are a variety of ideals and standards that may be invoked in times of trouble. Among them are the technical conclusions of medical science—for instance, knowledge that chewing an aspirin can increase the chances of surviving a heart attack. There are ethical standards, such as the principle of non-maleficence, legal standards, and general conventions about the practice of medicine.

When a mutual appeal to such standards does not resolve a controversy within the clinical relationship, the second form of mediation must be utilized. We tend to think of the courts as fulfilling this role. More frequently, an appeal is made to other physicians (the well-known "second opinion"), to hospital administrators, to insurance organizations, to hospital ethics committees, to former patients, or to the person on the next gurney. Royce would hold that standards guiding the decisions or recommendations of mediating bodies should reflect the ideals of communities that give those bodies their authority. In the case of mediators for the clinical relationship, these ideals are the ones that characterize the GMC. The GMC, then, is a locus of authority for the patient-physician relationship. Mediators such as legislatures, courts, hospital administrators, or physician consultants have genuine moral authority for the clinical relationship insofar as they fairly represent the ideals of the GMC. The GMC, in turn, must promote the great community if it is to bear the requisite moral authority. In sum, a Roycean view requires that medical care be structured by the ideals of a moral community—the GMC—whose membership extends to everyone (patients and professionals inclusive) with an interest in health care. These ideals, in turn, ought to be structured by the members' loyalty to the goal of universal human flourishing.

The authority of the GMC should not be interpreted as an illegitimate threat to patient or physician autonomy. Royce argues consistently that human health and moral growth are maximized by encouraging a broad range of human liberties and by the cultivation of human diversity. In health care, it is paramount that patients be allowed to infuse clinical goals with the personal aims that characterize their unique perspectives and life plans. This task requires a sensitivity to ethnic and gender differences, as well as to patients' specific personal characteristics.[23] Liberty and autonomy thus become central ideals of the GMC. However, respect for autonomy is justified not because liberty is a self sufficient or wholly complete human end, but because it is an aspect of human flourishing. Liberty may be good in itself, but it is not the comprehensive human good.

The centrality of the patient's role in determining the goals of therapy derives from the fact that medicine originates in the patient's perception of illness and culminates successfully in the patient's perception of restored health. Just as the general ideals of the GMC arise out of general characteristics of illness, suffering, and recovery within the community, the working ideals of the clinical relationship should reflect the particular characteristics of the patient's life plan and experience.[24]

The advantage of a covenantal model of the clinical relationship over economic or legalistic models derives from its ability to integrate these general and working ideals and is embodied in three principles. I will call them the principles of therapeutic alliance, beneficence, and community service.

Therapeutic Alliance

Francis Peabody claimed that the bond between physician and patient constitutes "the greatest satisfaction of the practice of medicine."[25] Undoubtedly, much of the disquiet about health-care reform centers around worries that the companionship celebrated by Peabody will be disrupted. This concern derives not only from a desire to retain the indisputable therapeutic benefits of close patient-physician relationships, but also from respect for the concrete good of human fellowship. That a personal bond between physicians and patients should be a goal of the clinical relationship is a tenet of covenantal medicine. Economic and legal models, on the other hand, do not provide for this ideal.[26]

Economic models of the clinical relationship transform physicians and patients into providers and consumers (or customers). Several consequences of this transformation work against the ideal of therapeutic alliance. First, it is unlikely that providers who view their clinical relationships primarily as market arrangements will develop the depth of commitment found in physicians who view these relationships primarily as covenants. Second, if patients are customers, then the comprehensiveness and continuity of medical care are not central issues for corporate medicine. Instead of attending to the whole range of human suffering, economically motivated health care offers only those services that are profitable. "Providers" are evaluated in terms of "productivity," which is often measured by parameters that have little to do with the cultivation of a therapeutic alliance. Further, whenever employees change jobs or their employers change health plans or their health-plan restructures, they are apt to be forced into changing physicians. This discontinuity seems to go hand in hand with the economic model.

Legalistic models do not address the therapeutic bond. Instead, they view clinical medicine as an affair of following rules or guidelines, or of demanding one's rights. When courts, regulatory commissions, and legislatures are viewed as the primary source of medical values, the clinical relationship is apt to take a viciously forensic turn. Patients and physicians become antagonists rather than friends. Even more benign legalistic models, such as those structured by nonjudicial notions of a "standard of care," provide too little guidance or inspiration to nurture a genuine therapeutic alliance.[27] It is quite possible to supplement a covenantal framework with a system of rules, guidelines, or standards, overseen by professional, judicial, legislative, or regulatory authorities. But the medical community will not thrive, at least in Royce's view, when adherence to such directives is taken as the essence of good medicine.

Beneficence

The principle of beneficence in health care holds that physicians are obligated to do good for their patients. In the day-to-day practice of medicine, this principle is paramount. Loyalty to the great community and its corollary, loyalty to the GMC, are more authoritative; but they are also more abstract. The higher principles point the way to beneficence and in the fast-paced, concrete world of clinical medicine, it is by concentrating on serving individual patients that physicians are best able to fulfill their duty to the greater medical community.

In an address to Vassar College, Royce commented:

A newspaper once asked me to contribute to a so-called symposium whose problem was to be this: What characteristics will the ideal man of the future possess? As I only knew about the ideal future man this, that when he comes, he will, as in him lies, adequately attend to his own business, I felt unable to contribute anything original to the proposed discussion.[28]

The task of medicine is taking care of patients. Thus, for Royce, the ideal physician is one who, as in him lies, attends to the needs of his patients. Philosophical abstractions can be useful, also inspiring, insofar as they help us understand the greater meaning of our work. Within the workplace, however, one must concentrate on the job at hand.

Though beneficence is often regarded as antagonistic to the principle of autonomy, this antagonism is not conceptually necessary. If doing good for the patient corresponds to respecting the patient's will, then beneficence and respect for autonomy are the same. In one sense, Royce holds that this correspondence is guaranteed. Let us examine how.

To respect a person's autonomy is to respect that person's will. For Royce, "will" denotes the purposive aspect of thought, and has two usages.[29] In the wide usage, will includes all of an individual's purposes—even the neglected, unrecognized, or unarticulated ones. In the narrow usage, will includes only purposes that are attentively selected, over and against other purposes. Royce believes that each person wills, in the wide sense, to be a loyal member of the great community and that the only viable means of integrating other purposes is to bring them under the authority of this unifying purpose. This will to loyalty, however, may not be recognized. Many of us do not consciously aim at being genuinely loyal.

Now the principle of autonomy can be interpreted to require a respect for either of the aforementioned versions of a person's will. Usually the narrow sense is used. Otherwise the autonomous desires of any given individual would remain too nebulous or open for interpretation. But if autonomy is understood in light of the wider notion of will, then, for Royce, beneficence and respect for autonomy are the same thing.

This equation reflects Royce's belief that all of us realize our best interests and the deepest object of our will only through loyalty to the great community.

Whether we subscribe to the narrow or to the wide version of will, we should recognize that the best estimates of any individual's well-being—including estimates about the person's loyalties—generally come from the individual. Further, as stated earlier, loyalty is always the result of a conscious decision. Loyalists must choose their proximate causes, and they must personally develop the manner in which they will integrate and serve these causes. On the basis of such considerations, Royce would insist that the principle of beneficence implies a high degree of regard for patient autonomy (even as conceived in accordance with the narrow version of will). At the same time, he would reject any principle of autonomy that views persons as isolated decision makers, unencumbered by ties or obligations to communities.

Since beneficence is doing good, and Royce understands human good in terms of the realization of a life plan, Roycean ethics holds that physicians can best honor the principle of beneficence by helping patients live out their life plans. It is through such a plan that each person gradually works out a unique, personal, living form of loyalty. When patients present to physicians, it is usually because their plans have been disrupted by illness or the threat thereof. If we are to serve our patients, we need to offer help that is specifically aimed at helping them to alleviate or smooth out these disruptions. Curing disease is secondary (and complementary) to this goal.[30]

The customer service orientation of the economic model shows promise in this regard, since it attends to patient preferences. However, once again we find several problems with this model. First, if we define "quality" in terms of meeting patient expectations, as some managerial consultants do,[31] then we are apt to injure patients by accommodating unrealistic or unschooled expectations. It would not be proper to treat viral pharyngitis with antibiotics, or to operate on a bruised kidney, even in patients who wrongly insist that these treatments are effective. Second, the economic model tends to view patients as one among a number of "customers." Often, the patient is less important, in this view, than employers or insurance companies that hold a lot of economic clout. Finally, to view patients as customers is to overlook some fundamental differences between medicine and other goods and services. When they enter the hospital, "customers" are more vulnerable than they are when they purchase new shoes or hail a taxi. They are vulnerable because they are sick. And they are vulnerable because they are unfamiliar with the vast array of information and technology that is pertinent to their problem. This vulnerability requires that health-care "providers" be committed to higher ends than enhancing the bottom line.[32] In the same vein, "meeting the standard of care" or abiding by current laws is also insufficient.

Community Service

When students enter a karate class, they bow. When sparring or addressing others, mutual bowing is much in evidence. These gestures are designed to nurture an attitude of respect for the martial discipline and for the values it embodies. Due in part to a background in martial arts, I often feel inclined to bow as I enter the hospital or approach a patient at the bedside. This inclination does not restrain me from being a critic of hospitals or of medicine. To the contrary, deep respect for medicine is not consistent with slavish obedience to convention. It begets a tendency to critique and revise the medical tradition.

Royce cautions against uncritical worship or obedience to public leadership or cultural convention. Our moral communities are flawed, and we are tasked with the labor of overcoming these flaws. Nevertheless, the Roycean contrarian is never a cynic. Like the traditional Japanese masters, Royce believed that genuine loyalty involves an attitude of reverence toward the community one serves. This attitude is reflected in his advice about cultivating communities of memory and hope. Loyalty is feasible just because of loyalists' high regard for the community ideals they uphold.

Thus, while it is true that beneficence to individual patients is a physician's working maxim, love for the community and its ideals is apt to be the clarion call inspiring physicians to persevere through the trials of medical training and practice.[33] While the economic model offers profit, and the legal model offers impunity, a covenantal model of the clinical relationship offers the prospect of living for a purpose.

When a narrow view of beneficence leads to a conflict with loyalty to the GMC, it is the broader, higher loyalty that must win. Physicians do not prescribe flouroquinolones to everyone with diarrhea—the potential benefit is overridden by the specter of community-wide antibiotic resistance. When a patient arrives in the ER with gunshot wounds, the physician is expected to report it, even if that means that the patient will ultimately be incarcerated as a result. And, occasionally, physicians must leave a patient's bedside to attend a mass casualty. In each case, loyalty may demand that physicians act against the immediate preferences of established patients. When faced with a conflict between patient prefer-ence and community interest, physicians should act in the spirit of loy-alty. They should acknowledge their primary role as beneficiaries and advocates for individual patients. This function can be trumped only for compelling reasons, derived from the ideals of the GMC. In these situa-tions, the art of loyalty requires more than applying a formula.

Beyond the formation of individual personal identity, Roycean loy-alty begets the sense of being member and creator of a superpersonal reality.[34] Loyalty is the devotion to such a superpersonal reality—mani-fested in the love of a community.[35] Ultimately, the medical covenant is valid only insofar as it anticipates the greater medical community, and effective only to the degree that it is inspired by reverence for the ideals that animate the greater medical community—compassion for the suffer-ing and hope of human flourishing. A Roycean perspective of the patient-physician covenant is grounded in this compassion and hope.

8 On "Tame" and "Untamed" Death: Jamesian Reflections

WILLIAM J. GAVIN

It is high time for the basis of discussion in these questions to be broadened and thickened up.
A Pluralistic Universe

Not unfortunately the universe is wild—game-flavored as a hawk's wing.
Preface, The Will to Believe and Other Essays on Popular Philosophy

It is . . . the re-instatement of the vague and inarticulate to its proper place in our mental life which I am so anxious to press on the attention.
Psychology Briefer Course

Life is in the transitions as much as in the terms connected; often, indeed, it seems to be there more emphatically.
Essays in Radical Empiricism

I find myself willing to take the universe to be really dangerous, without therefore backing out and crying "no play."
Pragmatism

THE ABOVE QUOTES from William James are all well known, but they are usually employed to refer to being, reality, or life in general. In this chapter I do something a bit different. Using these quotes from the Jamesian corpus as a jumping-off point, I want to offer a few reflections on the topic of death. My thesis is that the subject is once again becoming too "tame" in our everyday conversation and that if James were present, he would caution us against considering a too-proper, too-"dignified" view of death as the only "acceptable" one.

Death As Pornographic

Earlier in this century death was viewed as a rather pornographic topic, one to be kept out of polite everyday conversation. As Geoffrey Gorer had put it, "[T]he natural processes of corruption and decay have become disgusting, as disgusting as the natural processes of birth and copulation were a century ago; preoccupation about such matters is (or was) morbid and unhealthy, to be discouraged in all and punished in the young."[1] One result was that embalming had as its goal the production of a beautiful—that is, lifelike—corpse, one that masked the reality of death. Extensive mourning was discouraged; the widow was to act as if nothing out of the ordinary had happened—if she wished to return to society at large.

Gorer warns us that such a posture will have harmful results: "If we dislike the modern pornography of death, then we must give back to death—natural death—its parade and publicity, readmit grief and mourning. If we make death unmentionable in polite society—'not before the children'—we almost ensure the continuation of the 'horror comic.' No censorship has ever been really effective."[2] Gorer's point here may indeed be acknowledged; but doing so should not prevent us from asking whether there is a purely "uncensored" manner in which death may appear. Differently stated, a particular view of death as supposedly uncensored and natural may well already include some form of repression. We must be careful that the death that is allowed to publicly appear at the table has not already undergone some more subtle form of policing.

Death as Acceptable

More recently there have been significant—and, one must say, highly successful—attempts not to sweep death under the table. The most noteworthy of these has been represented by the work of Elisabeth Kübler-Ross, who has presented us with a phenomenology of dying as occurring in five stages: denial, anger, bargaining, depression, and acceptance.[3] Denial is the stage in which one says, "No, not me. You have mixed up my chart with another patient's." Although Kübler-Ross admits that this stage is a "healthy way of dealing with the uncomfortable and painful situation," ultimately, she says, the stage is temporary and very rarely maintained (35). It is replaced by anger, the stage of rage and envy. In this stage the patient asks "Why me? Why not the person next to me, or the one down the street?" This stage is a difficult one for those around the patient to deal with, since the anger is displaced in all directions in a random fashion. The third stage, bargaining, is one in which the patient enters into a sort of pact with God, saying, for example, something like, "Okay, okay, I have cancer, but let me live long enough to see my daughter married." However, patients tend not to keep their original promises, but try rather to renegotiate initial bargains entered into.

The fourth stage, depression, has two parts. The terminally ill patient initially undergoes a "reactive" depression in which he or she grieves over the loss of some thing or item once enjoyed in the past, such as good looks or a full head of hair. The second type of depression is "preparatory" and consists in a patient's grieving over impending losses, such as the loss of all love objects in the near future.

These two types of depression are different. The first type can be alleviated via suggestions, for example, concerning available breast prosthesis for a cancer patient. However, over-encouraging the patient to continue to think that she will get well in the second instance "hinders [the patient's] emotional preparation rather than enhances it."[4] This second type of depression is usually silent and is a tool to facilitate the fifth and final stage, acceptance, about which Kübler-Ross writes: "If a patient has had enough time (i.e., not a sudden, unexpected death) and has been given some help in working through the previously accepted stages, he will reach a stage during which he is neither depressed nor angry about his 'fate.'"[5] This is the stage of acceptance; it is a stage almost devoid of feelings.

Dignified Acceptance versus Rebellious Hope

At this stage (pun intended) of our cultural development, one would think that the alarm raised by Gorer has been answered. Death is no longer repressed. A move from considering death to looking at dying and a concrete description of the process of the latter has made death an everyday—that is, "normal"—topic. Death has, in short, come out of the closet.

In spite of the attractiveness of such a view—and, indeed, the real comfort offered by it—there are reasons why we should remain suspicious of it. Death may have come out of the closet, but we have been rather "puritanical" in deciding exactly what clothes she has to wear. Specifically, the messy process involved in dying has been reduced to a neat set of stages. Secondly, one of those stages is viewed as more "natural" than the others. A connection has been made between a dignified death and one involving acceptance. Finally, when death does come out of the closet, she is usually required to wear the gray conservative suit of a legal definition, not the ratty attire of narrative clothing.

The scenario offered by Kübler-Ross is a recipe for making death acceptable or tame—as opposed to pornographic or repressed. But is it either inevitable or desirable that all patients arrive at the stage of acceptance? Some indication that a problem has been covered over can be gleaned by turning to the chapter on hope in *On Death and Dying*. There Kübler-Ross states that "the one thing that usually persists through all these stages is hope,"[6] which, she agrees, at least for some patients, "remains a form of temporary but needed denial."[7] As Kübler-Ross indicates here, hope seems to require some form of nonacceptance; indeed, it appears as a form of rebellion against one's condition. And if, as she notes, "all our patients [maintain] a little bit of it and [are] nourished by it in especially difficult times,"[8] this raises serious questions concerning the overall desirability—or even the availability—of the acceptance stage.

A second problem with this progression toward the "closure" of stage five concerns the supposed neutrality—or lack thereof—of Kübler-Ross's analysis. She states at the beginning of her text that "this book is in no way meant to be judgmental,"[9] but indeed it sounds as if arrival at stage five is optimal. This impression is only strengthened when Kübler-Ross says, in a later text: "I think most of our patients would reach the stage of acceptance if it were not for the members of the helping professions, especially the physicians, who cannot accept the death of a patient. If we as physicians have the need to prolong life unnecessarily and to postpone death, the patient often regresses [from acceptance] into the stage of depression and anger again and is unable to die in peace and acceptance."[10]

The language of regression employed by Kübler-Ross is clearly normative or "policing" in tone and is in conflict with claims of neutrality. When challenged about this, Kübler-Ross responded by saying that "it's a matter of semantics. The ideal would be if both the dying patient and the patient's family could reach the stage of acceptance before death occurs. . . . It is not our goal, however, to push people from one stage to another."[11] Even while acknowledging that patients will tend to die as they have lived—that is, in anger or depression or rebellion—she continued to speak of stage five as the ideal one: "Patients who are in the stage of acceptance show a very outstanding feeling of equanimity and peace. There is something very dignified about these patients."[12] The subtext here, indeed, seems to indicate that there is a form of policing still going on—a form of prescription rather than description. Perhaps pure description is impossible. As James has noted: "Every way of classifying a thing is but a way of handling it for some particular purpose."[13] But if this is so, prescriptions alleging to be descriptions constitute doubly dangerous forms of imposition.

Death as Tame

The sociologist Philippe Ariès has presented us with a historical analysis of attitudes toward death that is somewhat parallel to that of Geoffrey Gorer. In *Western Attitudes Toward Death* and other works, Ariès too argues for the importance of context in approaching the subject of death. In his account of the changing attitudes toward death, which he sees as having both "disjunctive" and "conjunctive" transitions, he alludes to "tame death," "my death," "thy death," and "forbidden death."[14] The first of these was seen during the first millennium A.D. Most people were forewarned of their death; diseases were, in general, fatal, and if persons did not recognize their impending lot, others had the obligation to inform them. The dying person prepared for death, asked others for forgiveness, forgave others in turn, and in general presided over the ritual of his or her dying in a public fashion. There was, in short, an appropriate, correct way to die, an *ars moriendi*. Death was familiar— and was allowed to sit at the table, so to speak.

The attitude toward death as tame began to modify in the eleventh and twelfth centuries, with more emphasis placed on the individual self and his or her struggle for salvation at the moment of death, which was now seen as the occasion for the "last judgment." The moment of death could be the climax of one's self-realization or, on the other hand, the time when one succumbed to the temptation of pride in one's accomplishments or despair over one's failures. As such, the moment of death itself began to take on the aspect of an enemy, of something to be overcome.

By the eighteenth century a third change had occurred; it was the death of another ("thy death") that had become unacceptable to the survivors. The family was no longer passive, but rather assumed the dominant role. The dying person was to be "discrete"—that is, dignified. Even if the person knew about his or her illness, he or she was not to be too emotional about it—or, on the other hand, too indifferent to the efforts of those around him or her.

In the twentieth century, according to Ariès, death is denied. Effaced, death disappears as shameful or "forbidden"; it is displaced from the home to the hospital. Death in the hospital is no longer the occasion for a ritual ceremony over which the dying person presides amidst his or her assembled relatives and friends. Death, as a technical phenomenon, "has been dissected, cut into bits by a series of little steps, which finally makes it impossible to know which step was the real death, the one in which consciousness was lost, or the one in which breathing stopped. All these little silent deaths have replaced and erased the great dramatic act of death, and no one any longer has the strength or patience to wait over a period of weeks for a moment which has lost a part of its meaning."[15]

Here Ariès has insightfully indicated that death has evolved from an event to a process—though he seems unhappy about this. Second, he has portrayed death as the occasion for self-awareness, ignoring, it seems, his own identification of that self-awareness with a view of death as a challenge or battle—as opposed to something we should simply accept. Indeed, he has gone so far as to draw the opposite conclusion—that is, that our refusal to accept death will result in the loss of our individuality: "The clear correspondence between the triumph over death and the triumph of individuality during the late Middle Ages invites us to ask whether a similar but inverse relationship might not exist today between the 'crisis of death' and the crisis of individuality."[16]

Ariès' presentation here, although insightful, makes death in the twentieth century sound more like a triumph over individuality, linked with acceptance, than it does a triumph of individuality. If death has moved from event to process and we "can't go home again" (as Ariès himself would admit), this change in context requires a new, more Jamesian view of the self as a fragile yet ongoing process—one that perhaps interacts with the process of dying rather than trying either to completely accept it or, on the other hand, to completely rebel against or deny its obduracy.

Tame Death versus Peaceful Death

Daniel Callahan believes that Ariès' portrayal of the changing attitudes toward death is "essentially correct," though he has been "surprised at the resistance many people have to the idea of tame death in the past, as if it simply could not have been that way."[17] For Callahan, "tame" death has been lost; it did not survive. But although he finds Ariès' account correct, Callahan also thinks that it is incomplete:

It does not pay attention to the pain that marked many earlier deaths, unrelieved by narcotics or analgesics. There were no respirators to relieve the suffocation induced by collapsing lungs, or drugs to control the erratic beat of a heart out of control, or antibiotics to stem gangrene or the torture of spreading bedsores. If the course of dying was usually shorter, it could be and often was more intense in its agonies. A tame death was, it seems, possible and common, but by no means certain; luck and chance played their part. . . . The price, moreover, of the tame death brought on by the rapid death of an epidemic, common and widespread in earlier centuries, was the devastation of entire families. . . . There are no good reasons to want to return to these earlier social and medical conditions that made a certain kind of tame death possible but also allowed death that could, with some frequency, be anything but tame.[18]

Callahan warns us against viewing tame death—as defined by Ariès—as a state to which we might nostalgically wish to return—even if it did not exist as completely painless in the first place. Going further, not only is it not desirable to return, it is also not possible. We have made a bargain with medical technology that cannot be undone. However, although we cannot go home again, Callahan argues that there are elements of a tame death that we can try to retain, so as to die what he calls a "peaceful" death if not a tame one.[19] In a peaceful death one accepts the fact that one will lose control over one's fate; one dies an alert, conscious death, supported by loving friends and family.

Callahan admits, however, that most people fear that these conditions will prove extremely elusive. Toward the end of his insightful text, *The Troubled Dream of Life: Living With Mortality*, he seems even more unsure of this possibility, telling the reader that "not everything that has meaning need be acceptable" and describing himself as "watching and waiting"—that is, trying to accept a "hard truth" that "requires of us a view of the human condition broader than that of our own fate and gives us a common stake in the ongoing enterprise of human life—even if, inescapably, that enterprise must grind us down as individuals."[20]

More than any of the earlier accounts, Callahan's position does not explain death by explaining it away. He realizes the attractiveness of some aspects of a "tame" death while also indicating, though perhaps underestimating, the difficulty of attaining these. The price of giving them up seems to be, to some significant degree, loss of the sense of self as embodied and efficacious. This raises the issue that is of most importance—that is, what should be an individual's basic posture toward death, acceptance or rebellion?

Further reflection would not just view these as mutually exclusive alternatives, but would raise the issue as to whether both alternatives are not to be found internalized, but not reconciled in each human being. The result would be a rather fragile human self, idiosyncratic in nature, striving for a modicum of self-realization concerning a process (dying) whose existence has to be acknowledged but not necessarily accepted whole. Ironically, as discussed below, only if the vagueness of dying is preserved can the dying person participate in his or her own death.

Unfortunately, this basic human issue often does not receive the attention it deserves because it is masked by much tamer technical versions of the problematic.

"Tame" Death by Another Name

The real problem about death is, in a sense, that death is not a problem at all—and attempts to view it as such constitute a new form of denial or policing. As an extreme formulation, keeping in mind James's warning about the importance of the inarticulate, the very attempt to name death constitutes a form of denial. As James so eloquently noted, "[N]amelessness is compatible with existence."[21] A less extreme formulation of the issue would be one that warned of the possibility that the form of death now coming out of the closet is indeed in danger of becoming a new iteration of "tame" death.

As Callahan himself has put it, "Death has not come out of the closet; only its foot is showing. . . . The debate has mainly been about law, regulation, moral rules, and medical practice, and about making legal, or ethical, or medical choices about dying. It has not been about death itself, about how we should think it through in our lives."[22] Or again: "Death was, in a sense, taken out of the closet. But instead of being put forward for common thought and probing, it was put into the courtroom, turned into a matter of grand human rights. That is not altogether inappropriate, but is it enough?"[23]

Two things occurred in the 1950s that rendered death more wild, opaque, or vague: medicine acquired the ability to employ respirators and to engage in organ transplants. These technological achievements, together with other advances in medicine, have come together to render death less easy to identify, "unnamable" at a specific moment in time. They have called into question the traditional biological definition of death as respiratory-circulatory failure, and suggested, via the Harvard Ad Hoc Committee to Examine the Definition of Brain Death, assembled to consider the issue, that it be replaced by a new definition of death, so-called whole-brain death.[24]

Initially there was confusion—and indeed it continues to exist—as to whether there are actually two different concepts of death vying against each other or whether there is one concept and two different criteria to employ to indicate that death has occurred.[25] The issue was further complicated by a third group of thinkers who suggested yet another biological definition of death, neocortical failure.[26] The pluralist upshot of these events unfortunately resulted in a backlash—a demand for closure as to which definition of death is the "correct" one.

But, at least from a Jamesian perspective, pluralism may well be a good thing. Besides, the decision as to which definition of death to employ is a "sentimental" one, perhaps even one involving "the will to believe." In America the current debate is over whole-brain death versus neocortical failure as the two possible definitions of death. However, in Japan, hardly a country that can be labeled technologically backward, the debate is over whole-brain death versus respiratory-circulatory failure.[27] In either case the decision as to which definition to employ will involve an irrational or nonrational dimension. It will be, in short, a decision involving some personal risk—and one that cannot be made by legislative fiat.

Pluralism as Wild

Robert Veatch is a thinker who has argued, correctly in my opinion, that no biological definition of death is neutral—or exists without prior philosophical commitments.[28] He himself prefers neocortical failure as the most adequate definition, believing that a person is no longer present when he or she has lost the ability to engage in social interaction. However, realizing that different people have different preferences, and trying to preserve a thick context, Veatch suggests that we adopt a sort of "legal pluralism" in our public policy about death:

When dealing with a philosophical conflict so basic that it is literally a matter of life and death, the best solution may be individual freedom to choose between different philosophical concepts within the range of what is tolerable to all interests involved. . . . There must . . . [however] be limits on individual freedom. At this moment in history the reasonable choices for a concept of death are those focusing on respiration and circulation, on the body's integrating capacities, and on consciousness and related social interactions. Allowing individual choice among these viable alternatives, but not beyond them, may be the only way out of this social policy impasse.[29]

Here death is not simply "in the eye of the beholder," but neither is the ambiguity of the situation legislated out of existence—that is, tamed, covered up, or policed by a refusal to allow for pluralism.

A few states have indeed enacted legislation that included some very minor version of Veatch's proposal. New Jersey, for example, created a statute that recognizes a personal religion exemption (a conscience clause) to application of the whole-brain definition of death. Those who wish to do so for religious reasons may select a heart-based definition. However, pluralism in the other direction was not condoned; that is, objectors to the whole-brain definition of death may not opt for a higher-brain (neocortical) formulation of the issue.[30] Most states, however, have not (yet) gone in this direction, opting instead for closure—that is, a non-pluralistic formulation that does not view death as vague.

Several years ago the ethicist Han Jonas warned against this fascination with an exclusive definition. In "Against the Stream: Comments on the Definition and Redefinition of Death," Jonas argues that what the Harvard Ad Hoc Committee really defined was "not death, the ultimate state, itself, but a criterion for permitting it to take place unopposed— e.g., by turning off the respirator."[31] Although the report of the committee purported to be neutral, the desire to save lives through organ transplants renders any definition less than purely theoretical in nature. In Jonas's opinion, an attempt has been made to turn an essentially vague situation into a nonvague or clear one through linguistic or legalistic leg-erdemain.

In opposition, in a very Jamesian manner Jonas argues for the impor-tance of the vague. He says, "Mine is an argument—a precise argument I believe—*about* vagueness, viz., the vagueness of a condition. Giving intrinsic vagueness its due is not being vague."[32] And again, "We do not know with certainty the borderline between life and death, and a defini-tion cannot substitute for knowledge."[33] If Jonas is correct, the whole attempt to update the definition of death is essentially flawed; that is, it is by no means neutral or merely epistemic, regardless of which defini-tion is selected. Going further than Jonas does on this matter, however, we would argue that the recognition of vagueness results in the need for personal selection rather than passive acceptance—much as is the case in James's description of consciousness in *The Principles of Psychology*.

A similar concern about the need to preserve the vague or the ambiguous concerning death—that is, not to let the law exclusively police the issue—is voiced by Patricia D. White, herself a lawyer and a professor:

It seems to me mistaken . . . to *assume* that there is a specific point of division between life and death and that all hard cases must fall on one side or the other.

. . . The Commission [The President's Commission for the Study of Ethical Problems in Medicine and Biomedical and Behavioral Research, which issued its report, *Defining Death*, in 1981] was operating in a context within which (1) there were (and still are) explicit and specific legal standards for determining death and (2) the clear expectation was that a proposal or proposals would issue which undertook to update and make more uniform the various formulations of those standards. It is not surprising, therefore, that the report which accompanies its proposed Uniform Determination of Death Act shows little evidence that it considered seriously the possibility that it should instead have fashioned a systematic retreat of the law from the business of defining death.[34]

As described earlier, Veatch has opted for legal pluralism, but White has gone even further, questioning whether death should be forced to assume primarily or exclusively legal clothing if it is to be allowed to sit at the table in polite society. Going further, case studies that are exclusively legal or even biological in nature may be illuminating, but at a price. They may reveal, but they also conceal. They are "amplification-reduction"[35] structures, highlighting particular aspects of the situation at hand while marginalizing others. Such procedures, if not constantly watched, result in loss of the richness of the original context, which is replaced by a model.

Differently stated, case studies can be looked at in both a "thin" and a "thick" fashion. Thinly viewed, they tend to be evaluated almost exclusively in terms of legal outcomes and technological instrumentation. This narrowing of the problematic results in the focusing of discussion on gradations of change occurring within a very confined conceptual space. It is another version of what Whitehead has called "the fallacy of misplaced concreteness."[36]

Thickly viewed, case studies strive to preserve incompatible—perhaps even incommensurable—dimensions. Idiosyncrasies are not eliminated; final closure, to the extent that it is achieved at all, is not stated in exclusively algorithmic terms. There is no one "ideal" textbook case—or, if there is, it is ideal because it contains this very richness and ambiguity. As Dena Davis has put it: "We need thick description to allow cases to remain open to different interpretations over time, and also to enable cases to ground an ethics of care. The thicker the case, the more contextual the response. . . . People relate to narrative, and thick description allows for true psychological empathy, more powerful than the more abstract claims of shared humanity. Finally, *life* isn't as simple as thinly described cases would have us believe."[37]

Wild Stories over Tame Stages

The emphasis on personal narrative referred to earlier suggests that personal stories have "moral primacy" over essentialist stages, that pluralistic stories have priority over linear, policed inevitability. This position is seen in its most sustained form in Larry Churchill's critique of Kübler-Ross.[38] While acknowledging that the "stages" of Kübler-Ross have benefited the health community immensely, he charges that there is a "progressivist" bias to her presentation, wherein only the fifth stage is viewed as "aesthetically pleasing"—that is, fit for polite company. But, for Churchill, "to put the dying into stages is to control them and to deny them the needed opportunity to tell us what dying means to them."[39] In this sense the dying become victims of the stages and are not allowed to interpret their own deaths.

Churchill's alternative emphasizes personal narratives—unpoliced by legal or biological officials. Only individual dying patients are able to tell their particular stories, because only they know how the story line goes. To use stages as replacements for stories, therefore, constitutes a form of "moral hubris," or, in our terms, it is a puritanical way of making sure that death appears as acceptable and tame. "The point at issue here," according to Churchill, "is that 'story' is a category of interpretation for the experience of dying which is logically prior to 'stage.' The stories of dying persons are the primary data: stages are formal abstractions created by professionals who attend the dying. Stories are the primary texts; categorizations into stages are best seen as commentaries on these texts."[40]

For Churchill, then, each person is best viewed as a narrator or storyteller, and the story of each cannot be generalized without significant loss of meaning. Going further, stories—as opposed to stages—may or may not be progressive in nature; they may well proceed in zigzag fashion, and may contain contradictions. Stories are not always fully logical or consistent. As Churchill writes, "The narration of the meaning of death does not follow a catenarian, or chain-like sequence, but follows the story line, with inconsistencies, sudden turns, and proleptic movements."[41]

Advocating "acceptance," then, is insufficient precisely because it is too acontextual. One needs to ask, rather, "What does *this* particular acceptance mean?" That is, the binary seemingly contained in the logical exclusiveness of the stages approach is to be rejected. "Many persons combine acceptance of terminal illness with defiance toward both the disease and, in some instances, God. We do these persons a disservice if we try to describe their responses solely in terms of anger."[42]

Churchill calls for a "thick sense of narrative"—one where everything is not tamed by the rules of either logic or propriety; where idiosyncratic space is not only tolerated, but nurtured; and where the dying assume a teaching role as opposed to existing as prisoners being policed. "What the dying have to teach the living," he writes, "is not that they all uniformly cope with dying in stages, but that each is as unique an individual in dying as in living. Nobody dies by the book."[43]

The Indignity of "Death with Dignity"

One of the first thinkers to stress the importance of *only* caring for the dying—that is, of avoiding a good deal of seemingly necessary medical intervention—Paul Ramsey more recently worried that too many people were not only agreeing with his position, but were actually generalizing it into an all-too-bland statement about death with dignity or "calisthenic dying."[44] In opposition, Ramsey argues that "there is nobility in caring for the dying, but not in dying itself."[45] We cannot hand dignity to the dying person like it was a billiard ball; rather the most we might be able to do is to remove some obstacles and then manage to get out of the way.

Ramsey's point is actually twofold. First, death itself is not dignified, "whether accepted or raged against";[46] second, talk about death as dignified constitutes a further indignity—a sort of police assault. To drive home his point Ramsey turns to and proceeds to refute a series of arguments offered by death-with-dignity advocates. For instance, some would argue that death is simply a part of life. But for Ramsey this is unpersuasive, since they do not tell us whether it is a good or bad part of life. Disease is also a part of life; that does not necessarily make it dignified—or acceptable. As for the argument that death is a part of the evolutionary process and, as such, a necessity, Ramsey responds that "the man who is dying happens not to be in evolution."[47]

The suggestion that only "untimely" death is unnatural, that there is "a time to die," fares no better. As Ramsey writes: "We know better how to specify an untimely death than to define or describe a 'timely' one."[48] Opinions to the contrary run the risk of descending the "slippery slope" to the stage where one makes suggestions concerning the departure of old people. Statements that death, like birth, is (or can be) beautiful are merely attempts to attain "innocence by association."

Ramsey is more sympathetic to the approach of Pascal, whom he quotes as saying that "man is but a reed, the feeblest in nature, but he is a thinking reed. . . . Were the universe to crush him, man would still be nobler than that which kills him, for *he knows that he dies*, while the universe knows nothing of the advantage it has over him. Thus our whole dignity consists in thought."[49] Here we see, for Ramsey, the greatness of the human being fused with his or her misery in the experience of death. It follows that death cannot be viewed as completely acceptable. "To deny the indignity of death," he says, "requires that the dignity of man be refused also."[50]

If death is as undignified as Ramsey would have us believe, if a "newly dead" body arriving at a hospital emergency room still awakens feelings of awe and dread, then why is it that we tend to dignify death—or to wholeheartedly accept an acceptance model? For Ramsey, there are two ways in which the dreadful picture of death is policed or masked. One way is to view bodily life as unimportant. Ramsey points to Plato's Socrates in the *Phaedo* as representative of this position. The second way to repress the problem is to hold to a philosophy or view of human life that sees the uniqueness of the individual person as transient or interchangeable. Ramsey offers Aristotle's philosophy as an example. Here the form/matter distinction is primary, the individual secondary.

These, then, are the two main ways of working oneself into accepting the acceptance model by denying the fear of death. As Ramsey writes:

Whenever these two escapes are simultaneously rejected—i.e., if the 'bodily' life is neither an ornament nor a drag but a part of man's very nature; and if the 'personal life' of an individual in his unique life-span is accorded unrepeatable, noninterchangeable value—then it is that Death the Enemy again comes into view. A true humanism and the dread of death seem to be dependent variables. I suggest that it is better to have the indignity of death on our hands and in our outlooks than to 'dignify' it in either of these two possible ways.[51]

In contrast to the two philosophers alluded to by Ramsey, James saw the self as both personal and embodied. In *The Principles of Psychology* he described consciousness as "personal" and noted that "every thought . . . [is] *owned*."[52] In *Essays in Radical Empiricism* he went much further, telling the reader, "The individualized self, which I believe to be the only thing properly called self, is a part of the content of the world experienced. The world experienced . . . comes at all times with our body as its center. . . . The body is the storm center, the origin of co-ordinates. . . . Everything circles around it, and is felt from its point of view. The word 'I,' then, is primarily a noun of position, just like 'this' and 'here.'"[53] Ramsey's attack on Platonism and Aristotleanism has its parallel in James's constant fight against the "block universe" of monistic idealism, which explained pluralism and particularity by explaining them *away*. Given this similarity between James and Ramsey, a Jamesian approach to death and dying might well find itself agreeing with Ramsey's warning against our "accepting an acceptance model" too quickly by substituting a "tame" illusion for the real thing.

Conclusion

The old debate over whether death was an event or a process has been replaced by the realization that, in our times at least, death has evolved or devolved from an event to a process, and that, at least in some significant way, we can't go home again. This loss of certainty or arrival of the vague has not been fully accepted; it causes some discomfort and anxiety. There have been some cautious attempts, such as Callahan's above, to recover at least some aspects of the tame death that once was. But, more generally, we have set out to "to tame death anew," thereby making it supposedly more acceptable, more natural. Attempts to do this have included reducing the vague process of dying to a set of stages and concentrating on achieving a single correct legal definition of death.

But, from a Jamesian perspective, death—or, more *non*-precisely speaking, dying—remains at least somewhat wild-game flavored. It is indeed the case that we need to "accept" the fact that death is vague, as Hans Jonas maintains. But that very vagueness may serve as the occasion for choice, for selection, for acting efficaciously. Differently stated, the very vagueness of the topic of dying—and when it is actually over—perhaps may be brought to closure only by our exercising "the will to believe." Here, truly, we may be confronted with a situation in which the options are "forced, living, and momentous."

The various biological definitions of death (respiratory-circulatory failure, whole-brain death, and neocortical failure) can be viewed as three paradigms that are equally coherent and that have some empirical data to which they correspond. Even if these were to change somewhat, the issue of choice would remain the same as long as the problem remained pluralistic in nature.[54] We cannot await—that is, accept—death itself, but we can—and should—choose a particular form of death to await. There is no absolute guarantee that the form of death we choose will actually show up, as Sartre has noted,[55] but that is not sufficient reason for not taking a chance. The ending quote from James's "The Will to Believe" can be applied to the topic of dying itself:

In all important transactions of life we have to take a leap in the dark. . . . [W]hatever choice we make we make it at our peril. . . . We stand on a mountain pass in the midst of whirling snow and blinding mist, through which we get glimpses now and then of paths which may be deceptive. If we stand still we shall be frozen to death. If we take the wrong road we shall be dashed to pieces. We do not certainly know whether there is any right one. What must we do? "Be strong and of good courage." Act for the best, hope for the best, and take what comes. . . . If death ends all, we cannot meet death better.[56]

9 Significance at the End of Life

D. MICAH HESTER

I WISH to explore in this chapter three aspects of the dying process and our attitudes toward meaningful acts of dying through suicide, assisted suicide, and euthanasia: (1) how death comes to many of us, (2) why and how some of us might wish to die differently, and (3) why and how those of us involved with dying persons might help in their dying processes.

Quite simply, though controversially, I believe that because many people who are left to the ravages of disease and bodily decline die horrible, painful, lonely, undignified deaths, some of these individuals would understandably wish to have some control over these final acts of living. Furthermore, significant and meaningful acts of living, as pragmatist William James has explained, consist of the fusion of personal ideals and the fortitude to attempt carrying them out, and this is no less true for dying persons than it is for those in the full bloom of health. Uniquely meaningful creative acts can occur even here at the end of life. These acts occur in a complex web of relationships that affect and implicate many people. In the dying process, family, friends, lawyers, insurance companies, and medical professionals all play important roles, accounting for and participating in the acts of the dying person. On those occasions when thoughtful, reflective individuals make decisions to end their lives on their own terms through suicide, assisted suicide, or euthanasia, we who are involved with these patients run the risk of true moral peril if we simply ignore or deny their wishes, condemning them to die alone in meaningless acts of biology and medicine. Instead I suggest that we often have within our powers the ability to help these people end their lives in the bosom of a loving community through significant activities of their own making, and under particular circumstances I believe that this is the morally right thing to do.

How We Die

That we *live* should be obvious; *that* we *die* is not in question either, regardless of the promises of some geneticists or even some cryogenicists. However, these two facts taken together often lead to stress and frustration concerning our futures. Death is inevitable while living is actual. Living is what we know; death is obscure. Eventually, though, it is possible to come to grips with one important fact: Even though death is the end point of our living embodiment, dying is itself a process within embodied living itself; that is, dying is part of our on-going life-stories. When this realization occurs, the focus can shift from *that* we die to *how* we die.

Illustrating what she calls the "cinematic" myth of the "Good American Death," Nancy Dubler writes, "[The death scene often] includes the patient: lucid, composed, hungering for blissful release—and the family gathers in grief to mourn the passing of a beloved life. The murmurs of sad good-byes, the cadence of quiet tears shroud the scene in dignity."[1] Unfortunately for many of us, our deaths will not be the spiritual, peaceful "passing" that we might envision or desire. As physician Sherwin Nuland explains, "To most people, death remains a hidden secret. . . . [T]he belief in the probability of death with dignity is our, and society's, attempt to deal with the reality of what is all too frequently a series of destructive events that involve by their very nature the disintegration of the dying person's humanity."[2] For many the hope is that they will die surrounded by loved ones (or quietly in the night), slipping away without pain after tying up all loose ends. The reality for the great majority of us, however, is that we will find ourselves ravaged by disease, struck down by illness; we will be hooked up to machines, ingesting drugs. Nurses and physicians, strangers to us really, will be our most consistent contacts with humanity. Family and friends will find themselves without resort and at a loss to help, if for no other reason than because we will rarely give a clear account of our desires before it is too late to give any account at all. We would like to think that these situations are at the margins; if so, the margins are awfully wide and cannot be ignored. Death, as William Gavin has argued, is a complex of historical and cultural as well as biological factors that do not present themselves for tidy packaging.[3] Crudeness and vagueness, frustration and mutilation are at play as much as scientific, technological precision in diagnosis and prognosis. Loneliness, pain, and bitterness are more common than peace and joy.

The complications involved in how we die might best be illustrated through accounts of dying persons.

Approximately forty years ago, then-medical-student Sherwin Nuland on his first night in the hospital encountered a dying patient, James McCarty. Recalling the situation, Nuland writes:

James McCarty was a powerfully built construction executive whose business success had seduced him into patterns of living that we now know are suicidal. But the events of his illness took place [at a time] . . . when smoking, red meat, and great slabs of bacon, butter, and belly were thought to be the risk-free rewards of achievement. He had let himself become flabby, and sedentary as well. . . .

McCarty arrived in the hospital's emergency room at about 8:00 P.M. on a hot and humid evening in early September, complaining of a constricting pressure behind his breastbone that seemed to radiate up into his throat and down his left arm. . . . The intern who saw McCarty in the emergency room noted that he looked ashen and sweaty and had an irregular pulse. . . . The electrocardiographic tracing . . . revealed that an infarction had occurred, meaning that a small area of the wall of the heart had been damaged. . . .

McCarty reached the medical floor at 11:00 P.M., and I arrived with him. . . . As I walked onto the division, the intern, Dave Bascom, took my arm as though he was relieved to see me. ". . . I need you to do the admission workup on this new coronary that's just going into 507—okay?" . . .

McCarty greeted me with a thin, forced smile. . . . As I sat down at his bedside, he suddenly threw his head back and bellowed out a wordless roar that seemed to rise up out of his throat from somewhere deep within his stricken heart. He hit his balled fist with startling force against the front of his chest in a single synchronous thump, just as his face and neck, in the flash of an instant, turned swollen and purple. His eyes seemed to have pushed themselves forward in one bulging thrust, as though they were trying to leap out of his head. He took one immensely long, gurgling breath, and died.[4]

In another story, James Buchanan discusses the circumstances surrounding Alzheimer's victim Murray Wasserman.

The third stage of Alzheimer's is surely the most benevolent, the most understanding and merciful, of death's trimesters. All the confusion, embarrassment, and agony of self-observation are forfeited in favor of grateful amnesia. Family and friends become strangers while the familiar and foreign lose the elasticity of their boundaries and become one. . . .

For survival, only simple tools are needed: air, food, water. Life at its most basic and most elementary level has no need for anything unnecessary and burdensome.

Murray simplified all that he had become for the purpose of concentrating what little he had on that which remained. Indeed, he was a child again. His bowels and bladder were liberated from social customs. . . . Rules and regulations . . . were abandoned in favor of more immediate concerns. He had become a child again.

Of course, his friends and family saw none of this. Rather, they saw an old, emaciated man who wore diapers and wept to himself alone, and sometimes cried in grateful acceptance of the slightest things. . . .

Murray was engaged in a desperate struggle for his life, for his existence, for some shred of solidity against the possibilities of death and nothingness. . . . [E]very minute, every hour, every day was a desperate struggle to remain something against forces that sought to make him nothing. . . .

In the end, all death comes from anoxia. . . . One tries not to breathe, to end it all quickly, but the body is too desperate to obey such intellectual suicide. It wants to live even if the brain desires to die. And so like a heaving straining animal, the frightened lungs continue again and again their futile effort until coma and unconsciousness discontinue this malice of self-observation and self-torture.

Murray died in such a way; he died wrapped about himself—actually holding on to himself for dear life—in a fetal position. Were it not for the gray hair, the wasted six-foot body, the wrinkled and puffy face, one might have thought him a child who died of crib death. . . . But Murray Wasserman was not a child but rather an old—very old—man who died before his time and looked far more ancient than his sixty years could ever foretell.[5]

Finally, author and physician Richard Selzer tells of his encounter with an AIDS patient and his partner in 1990.

At precisely 4 P.M., as arranged, I knock on the door. It is opened by . . . let him be Lionel, a handsome man in his late thirties. . . . He is an ordained minister. . . . In the living room Ramon is sitting in an invalid's cushion on the sofa, a short delicate man, also in his thirties. Ramon is a doctor specializing in public health—women's problems, birth control, family planning, AIDS. He is surprisingly unwasted, although pale as a blank sheet of paper. . . . He and Lionel have been lovers for six years. . . .

For a few minutes we step warily around the reason I have come there. All at once, we are engaged. I ask him about his symptoms. He tells me of his profound fatigue, the mental depression, the intractable diarrhea, his ulcerated hemorrhoids. He has Kaposi's sarcoma. Only yesterday a new lesion appeared in the left naso-orbital region. He points to it. Through his beard I see another, larger black tumor. His mouth is dry, encrusted from the dehydration. He clutches his abdomen, grimaces. There is the odor of stool.

"I want to die," he announces calmly without the least emotion.[6]

The common thread among these stories is simply that death is rarely clean, hardly ideal. Also, the character of each death is shaped by the person's history and community. Furthermore, these cases illustrate a continuum present among specific acts of dying—from where there is no control to where controlled manipulation is not only possible but preferable.

James McCarty killed himself through his own extravagant living, an "unintended suicide" as Nuland put it. He died in one powerful instant, virtually alone, tended only by an inexperienced medical student. In an important sense, we can also say that his death could not have been otherwise. Though he may have had control over his eating and living habits before his heart gave out, once McCarty found himself in the hospital, it was simply too late. Control over his death was clearly not at issue.

Murray Wasserman, on the other hand, reveals the very real distance between one's situation and the perceptions of others. An old man dies like a child while his relatives find him pathetic and decrepit. Fighting for a self he long ago lost, however, Murray dies as alone as McCarty, lost in a world of his own. And here one could argue that so much more could have been done. The progressive nature of Murray's disease allowed for the possibility of proactive measures aimed at determining the dying process, on a personal level. Advanced directives and communication among health care professionals, family, friends, and of course Murray himself during the early stages of the disease may have helped with care in the later stages.

Finally, Ramon's situation expresses a desire to avoid the emptiness of the previously described deaths. Influenced by the nature of his profession and the character of his relationships, Ramon was keenly aware of the issues involved in his own disease. Committed to a loving relationship, his desire to die also was concerned with his partner, the burdens involved in care, and the embarrassment of continued existence in his condition. Ramon seized the opportunity to exercise his agency, wishing to participate in his own dying process.

Why and How We Might Wish to Die on Our Own Terms[7]

Death is the end of living, but as I have already noted, dying is a process within living. As such, we can easily move from thinking of how most of us die to asking if we might die "better." Most often death is not pretty; it is uncontrolled and unwanted. It seems reasonable, then, for us (like Ramon) to desire to have a hand in our deaths, to the extent that we shape our deaths to our liking and to the liking of those around us.

Attempts at shaping the dying process are "meaningful" in so far as they mirror other acts of living that we consider significant and meaningful. I want to suggest, therefore, that a meaningful death is neither insensible nor impossible.

Following William James, I believe that we create meaning in our own lives every time we couple some personally and intelligently conceived goal or ideal with the courage and labor necessary to achieve it. A life gains significance through intelligence and fortitude. "The significance of life," [8] James explains,

is the offspring of a marriage of two different parents, either of whom alone is barren. The ideals taken by themselves give no reality, the virtues by themselves no novelty. . . . [T]he thing of deepest—or at any rate, of comparatively deepest— significance in life does seem to be its character of *progress*, or that strange union of reality with ideal novelty which it continues from one moment to another to present.[9]

Individuals progress in life whenever they can develop an end and deploy means to attain it within their lived experience. For example, a student's pursuit of a medical degree gives meaning to life as the student progresses through medical school to become a physician. The activity is meaningful precisely for the reason that it entails a personal ideal (becoming a physician) and the wherewithal to achieve the ideal (the strength of character to succeed at the four year grind through medical school).

Of course, simpler, less time-consuming, nonprofessional ideals and labors (such as desiring to eat and then preparing a meal) are in their own ways instances of meaningful progress. Our everyday labors develop the character of our grander schemes, while grander schemes help to shape the development of everyday pursuits. Our daily ideals often become part of the means to yet further ideals, while remaining, themselves, ends to be enjoyed without recourse to their function in our higher goals. Building a house, for example, takes many individual labors that come together to form the finished structure, and each activity—laying brick, framing walls, or painting trim—can be satisfying and enjoyable in its own right, quite independent of the connections to the whole.

Every person at any stage of life can have ideals. For James, ideals are both "intellectually conceived" and have "novelty at least for him whom the ideal grasps." Ideals must reside in reflective consciousness and take hold of individuals uniquely. James further claims, "[T]here is nothing absolutely ideal: ideals are relative to the lives that entertain them."[10] Meaning in life is highly individualized. For James, there simply is no over-arching meaning to life; there are only the particular instances of meaning created by a particular person. And this process of meaning begins when the "novelty" of an "intellectually conceived" goal takes hold of the attention and calls forth available habits and abilities into action.

"Novelty" denotes the quality of uniqueness exemplified by possible ends as they are experienced by an individual. Ideals that "grasp" an individual take hold of the attention and move the individual to action. The idealizer finds in the ideal the possibility for the unique expression of talents. And even though some goals may seem mundane to others, for the person who is "grasped," a sense of engagement is felt where an individual's abilities and creativity are called forth. "Sodden routine is incompatible with ideality, although *what is sodden routine for one person may be ideal novelty for another*."[11] The ideal itself is further shaped by a person's individualized approach to it. Take as an example the activity of flying an airplane. Some individuals (my father in-law, to name one) find a joy, a "freedom," a "rush" in being up in the sky in control of an airplane. For you or me, there may be no great novelty or enjoyment in flight school, ground checks, and aerobatics, but individuals like Chuck Yeager as well as my father in-law and other enthusiasts find the act of controlled soaring through clouds an outlet for their individual and unique talents. Furthermore, moments of historic novelty arise when particular individuals idealize an activity for an entire epoch (becoming "ideals" themselves)—obvious examples include Charles Lindberg and Amelia Earhardt. More common, however, are the daily engagements by any one of us pursuing desirable ends—like my father-in-law in love with flight.

"Intellectually conceived," on the other hand, takes us beyond mere novelty; it signifies that ends need to be reflected upon in light of means available before they are pursued. Intelligent ideals are those that help create an acceptable, coherent story; they "fit" within the means available and other ends that have been put forth in the situation. As John Dewey noted in his statement on the continuum between means and ends, James points out that reflection takes mere valued objects and makes them valu*able*; that is, intelligently conceived ideals are not only desired as ends in themselves but are discovered to be desir*able*—worthy of our desire—upon investigation of costs and consequences. For example, I may want to take flying lessons, but the desire alone is not enough to make it worthy of my pursuit. I must investigate economic factors, availability, time constraints, family obligations, my own abilities and fears, and so on. Only after having followed out this inquiry can I move from a mere "whimsical" ideal, to something determined to be either valuable or not. "Whimsical" desires without reflection rarely come to fruition and make for the possibility of unforeseen conflict down the line. Intelligence helps us to sort through various ends-in-view and to consider the means available to achieve them in order to determine those "worth the effort."

These requirements of "novelty" and "intelligence" imply that ideals do not reside beyond experience as formal or absolute ends; they are created within and by our daily lives; that is, they arise out of our ongoing stories as well as the stories of those with whom we come into contact. As both intellectually conceived and novel, ideals must touch us and come to fruition in our experiences as they guide us in employing means available and accounting for others' ends as well. Admittedly, according to James, "[T]aken nakedly, abstractly, and immediately, you see that mere ideals are the cheapest things in life. Everybody has them in some shape or other, personal or general, sound or mistaken, low or high."[12] However, significance in life cannot stop with "cheap" ideals. As James insists, the means employed are of equal importance to the ends, and the means also arise out of our experience. An ideal must be not only immediately and abstractly desired but wedded to the discipline and courage to pursue it; ideals, to become meaningful, must be found to be desir*able*. If personal ends are to become fulfilled (within experience), we must back our "ideal visions with what the laborers have, the sterner stuff of . . . virtue; we must multiply [the ideals'] sentimental surface by the dimension of the active will, if we are to have *depth*, if we are to have anything cubical and solid in the way of character."[13] Again, we see that a continuum of means and ends exists such that the means employed give otherwise empty, flighty ideals content and character. Significance, then, comes from this active striving to actualize our personal goals.

Taken in this way, "significance" develops from personal, particular ideals fusing with courage, strength, and intelligence—that is, the virtues that drive people to embody these ideals in their daily lives. James's term for this is 'progress', and progress incorporates the intellectual ability to create goals and the actional fortitude to fulfill them, regardless of our current location on the timeline between birth and death. Also, whereas fortitude and strength are sometimes difficult to muster, ideals arise everywhere, part and parcel of our daily lives, "the cheapest things in life."[14]

Why Someone Might Wish to Die

With this understanding of *meaning*, we should begin to see that potential significance through the development of ideals and their achievement (whether "grandiose" and long-term or everyday and more immediate) can arise out of any of life's situations. Opportunities for significance, James reminds us, are "with us really under every disguise."[15] As a matter of fact, we might find that "vital significance . . . blossoms sometimes from out of the very grave wherein we imagine that our happiness was buried."[16] Even in the depths of despair, ideals can come to us; our "sick-rooms have their special revelations."[17] Echoing this insight when speaking of the courage of some chronically and terminally ill patients, psychiatrist Arthur Kleinman states that "it [is] precisely situations of utter despair and terminality that [are] essential to create authentic meaning."[18] He continues later, "Meaning is created out of the context of serious illness. . . . The meaning of illness need not be self-defeating; it can be—even if often it is not—an occasion for growth, a point of departure for something deeper and finer."[19] In other words, in the face of the abyss of death itself, we might just find some last meaningful, progressive ["growth" enhancing] moments.

But here we may find ourselves taken aback by a collection of terms that seem paradoxical: *terminal, ill, death, abyss,* and *progress*. If death is the final event of life (the end of possible futures) and the meaning of one's life is found in progress (which implies a future), how can we possibly relate death and progress? To make this connection, we must return to my earlier thesis that our focus on "death" should refocus on "dying." This shift places emphasis on an active process, not a singular moment or event. As William Gavin has pointed out, "[J]ust as one would not identify a melody with the last note in the score, so too one should not focus on the last moment of dying, that is death, at the expense of the entire process of dying."[20] Emphasis on the process of dying brings to light the potential for meaning that dying affords at the end of life. As a process, dying has its movement not only toward a final end—death—but it can have a movement toward a goal—namely, dying well, a movement that can be manipulated by us through our determined activities and technologies. Given the nature of the process, this can be our final opportunity for meaning in life, and our control over the means to the end shapes the very character of the end itself. Further, we must recognize that these processes go on in the world of living social beings; others, not only ourselves, become implicated in our activities and changed by them. Therefore, when death comes to our bodies, a part of us continues, to the extent that others participated in the meanings of our lives and carry those meanings forth in their own after our bodies are gone.[21]

Dying with meaning, then, is transformative. It reshapes the lives of others that are left behind. Our dying gives to others new groundings for considering their own lives and dyings by engaging them in the meaning that our own dying has for us.

Even further, and maybe more importantly for the dying patient, however, dying with meaning empowers the patient during the final stages of living. It makes the patient a participant in the activities that surround the dying process. Meaningful dying explicitly treats the self as connected to meaning in life by giving patients control of their personal narratives. Meaningful acts of dying take the seemingly formless void of the abyss of death and give it a significant purpose while making it a meaningful achievement in the last stages of life itself; such acts turn potential nothingness into actual significance.

How Someone Might Wish to Die

How does this definition of life's significance—progress—take shape for patients who are in the process of dying? For some patients, a significant dying process may involve specifically controlled means of securing death through suicide, assisted suicide, or euthanasia. These acts of acquiring death, by the hands of patients themselves or of those deputized by them, can empower patients and help to make their lives significant up to the moment that biological death occurs. For many who consider euthanasia, the alternative to a controlled death is meaningless existence, both created by and culminating in depression, suffering, and death.

To focus particularly on medical situations, it becomes important, then, to discuss the kinds of patients who find themselves dealing with (or involved in) end-of-life issues, and I am concerned here with a particular group of adult patients—namely, the mentally lucid, yet terminally ill.[22] The issues of control, participation, agency, and empowerment are central to a medical encounter. A patient with an illness already lacks a certain power and control in his or her life. In the case of a terminally ill patient, however, the issue of control is magnified by the gravity of the situation. To be characterized as terminally ill is to be, in most respects, thrown into the category of medical futility, to be placed in a position outside the reach of medical ability.

A terminally ill patient with decision-making ability can be keenly aware of the abyss of death that is marked by a complete lack of control; a terminally ill condition is itself a condition of diminishing control and a loss of self. While staring into this void, the patient often is fighting to retain health, control, and dignity—that is, to retain *self*. Rarely is this abyss immediately desired, but the alternative—continued living—may hold a complete lack of significance or meaning, heightened by pain and suffering and the inevitability of the nearing end. As our earlier discussions of meaning and dying show, however, dying can be a positively transformative process that changes the abyss of death into an idealized end to be controlled, manipulated, and achieved on terms that terminally ill patients develop for themselves. The character of the activities of patients who chooses suicide, assisted suicide, or euthanasia takes on a purpose and direction when they know when and how death will come. Therefore, some terminally ill patients take the opportunity to shape the end of their lives by creating a meaningful death, one which embodies an ideal to be realized through courage and discipline. For a few patients, acts of suicide, assisted suicide, or euthanasia make the process of dying a vital part of their life-stories. The process thus constitutes a controlled choice and activity that helps complete life on their own terms.

Cultivating a character that adjusts desir*able* ends to the means available and, at the same time, summoning up the fortitude necessary to fulfill goals in a life nearing its own end open up the possibility for a vast variety of satisfaction in the everyday things of life. Terminally ill patients who are capable of setting their sights on daily activities and personal contact while courageously accepting, yet looking beyond, their terminal condition find meaning in living during the process of dying. However, when most all means and abilities are exhausted by disease or severe trauma and daily ends fade from view, little possibility for meaning is left. For patients in these conditions, then, the *choice* to die and the ability to control the dying process can become a last act of significance, a way to end their stories on personal terms. They might wish to be progressive *in* their dying, transforming the abyss of death by giving meaning to the end of their lives.

For these patients several options present themselves—suicide, assisted suicide, or euthanasia[23]—however, it is often the case that the means of exercising these options is unavailable. This leads to the need for others to participate in the act of dying.

Why and How We Might Help the Dying

A common saying is that we die alone. But in several important ways for many people, nothing could (or, at least, should) be farther from the truth. Death of a loved one affects others in a variety of ways. Certainly, at one end of the spectrum, there are dying people with few if any ties to other individuals in society, but even their deaths affect government workers, hospital personnel, acquaintances. Small ripples from a small pebble, perhaps, but any ripple affects the surrounding waters. At the other end of the spectrum are the deaths of well-connected individuals who have made contributions not only to their own immediate circle of friends and family but beyond. Some say, for example, that when John F. Kennedy died a part of the United States died with him. The deaths of prominent individuals act in this way as waves rather than ripples. More common, though, are the deaths of average persons who have good friends and relate well enough with their families; their deaths create holes in the communal space they once occupied.

However, most tragic, it seems to me, are those "connected" individuals who still die alone. I am thinking particularly of those situations when a dying individual asks for help from family, friends, or physicians in controlling the patient's dying process, only to be ignored and denied this last wish. A terminally ill individual reaches out to a loved one or medical professional for aid, requesting that this life be completed in a personally meaningful manner; instead of helpful response the other turns away, frightened by or confused concerning or simply axiologically against the plea. However, *if we outsiders do not aid in a competent patient's intelligent request to die, we needlessly leave that fellow human alone at a time when our support is most important.* More critically, if life's significance comes from the development of ideals and the ability to achieve them, *when we turn away, we condemn the patient desirous of a "noble" or, at least, "controlled" death to end life facing a complete lack of significance*; in turning away we cripple the ability of the patient to reach his or her final ideals. If *human dignity* has any meaning, it comes from the personal participation in and intelligent development of one's life by responsibly setting goals and meeting them through appropriate means at one's disposal. Meaningful living while dying can only come through recognizing and acting in such a way that we treat the dying as agents in life and participants *in* the community with love and support *from* the community. Those who would turn their backs on the cries of the dying do so at the expense of positively helping to shape the meaning of that person's final stages of life.

At least two possible objections to my stance arise immediately.[24] One objection states that the ending of life through human manipulation is wrong regardless of the dying person's desires. This is a position explicitly taken by a variety of religious institutions within the Judeo-Christian tradition, such as the Roman Catholic Church and others.[25] This objection to euthanasia is based on the idea that human life, regardless of its quality, is an unquestionable good that cannot be begged, borrowed, or stolen, as its value transcends mere human existence on earth. James's (and my own) account of significance in life, however, is not directly affected by this position, since he is committed to issues in "lived experience" and not issues that transcend it (unless those transcendent issues can be shown to affect positively lived experience). His discussion stems directly from the question of how we might live better lives in our experience. But this is not the place for theological debate, and I shall have to pass over any further comments on this difference in ideology concerning human nature.

The second objection, however, does not go quite so far as the first but may be more prevalent in society. To some it may be acceptable for reflective, terminally ill people to take their own lives; the moral prohibitions arise when others are asked to aid in carrying out this desire. This objection is illustrated, for example, by ethicist Daniel Callahan in his essay entitled "Self-Determination Run Amok." Space does not permit rebuttal in full, but I shall sketch a reply in brief before I conclude this section.

Callahan's central question concerning assisted suicide and euthanasia is, "How are we to make the moral move from my right of self-determination to some doctor's [or other individual's] right to kill me—from *my* right to *his* right?"[26] Callahan's focus is on the problem of moving from a personal right to die according to one's wishes to allowing a physician or any other person to take the life of a patient who requests it. As he explains, "voluntary euthanasia . . . can only be called 'consenting adult killing.' By that term I mean the killing of one person by another in the name of their mutual right to be killer and killed if they freely agree to play those roles."[27]

Although Callahan's view seems oddly expressed—moving from my right to die to another's right to kill—I take his position to be that it is never morally acceptable for a person to help a patient die, even when that desire is expressed and adjudicated. It is clear that any particular person may decline to assist, but should it be allowable for someone, anyone, to accept the responsibility?[28]

Terminally ill patients often find themselves in highly compromised situations that demand the aid of others. The question here is not one of "rights," as Callahan portrays it, but instead, What should we do when a dying patient asks for our help? Particularly in cases of assisted suicide and euthanasia, others are asked to participate in securing the means to the patient's desired ends since the patient is unable to carry out the task alone. Of course, these requests can simply be ignored; however, that neither makes the requests go away nor rules out complicity of others, because the expressed desires of the patient now exist within a situation obligating others to adjudicate these claims, over and against other concrete claims and obligations. John Dewey describes this situation quite well:

Some activity proceeds from a man; then it sets up reactions in the surroundings. Others approve, disapprove, protest, encourage, share and resist. Even letting a man alone is a definite response. Envy, admiration and imitation are complicities. Neutrality is non-existent. Conduct is always shared. . . . It is not an ethical "ought" that conduct *should* be social. It *is* social, whether good or bad.[29]

As James has said also, "[T]*here is some obligation wherever there is a claim.* . . . [E]very *de facto* claim creates in so far forth an obligation."[30] Constitutive of a personal claim is a corresponding request that this claim be satisfied in the social context in which it arises; quite simply, this implicates others.

Of course, it is important to realize that I am *not* here using the term 'obligation' to denote the *outcome* of an adjudication of claims. That is, I am not saying that simply because I request a car and you have one, you *must* give it to me. The outcome of moral inquiry is Dewey's "ethical 'ought'," which is deeper and richer than James's use of the term 'obligation'. Dewey's "ethical ought" results only from the reflective process of weighing competing claims by the moral artist—as when such scrutiny focuses on my desire for a car versus your desire to keep your money or car. What James is saying, however, is that a much more basic kind of obligation weighs on us with the manifestation of each new claim. Every expressed claim demands that we recognize and react to it. This is not an insistence springing from a right; it is, instead, a constitutive part of communicating interests. When some actual person, perhaps a woman dying of debilitating and irreversible disease, tries to give meaning to her life through active participation in her own dying, others are *de facto* implicated—that is, *prima facie* obligated. It is not always easy to adjudicate these claims. Work like this requires courageous intelligence, artistically pursued. The question at that point is, How am I to evaluate the obligation raised by this desire to die in light of other existing obligations? To the extent that no overriding obligations trump this one, I will find myself "ethically" obligated in the deeper sense of that term.

Quite opposed to Callahan's implications, there is nothing magical in a move from rights to duty, from one's claim to another's obligation. This connection between claims and obligations is simply part and parcel of social interaction when individuals express their desires to and with others. This is certainly no less true in the medical arena at the bedside of a terminally ill patient. Space does not permit nor does the present argument require consideration of the many other issues that could be addressed in this matter, such as the role of physicians and the medical establishment in aiding the dying process. But given contemporary technology, given the horrific suffering, given the lack of physical abilities in this patient, given a "terminal" diagnosis, given this patient's voice asking to die, what are we to do? We are, it seems clear, to assess her claim reasonably and in the complex of her personal, medical situation and our own standing obligations. And given the vast number of different patient situations, it will not be surprising to find that we are not only initially but reflectively—that is, "ethically"—obligated to help some particular terminally ill patients die.

Choices surrounding dying processes are based, no doubt, on grim options, and they may come down to trying to provide for the terminally ill what Margaret Battin calls "the least worst death."[31] I, however, have attempted to put a more positive spin on human interactions concerning issues of death and dying. I believe that real occasions arise making it not only possible but morally demanding the decision to aid the dying on their own terms when their desires are "intelligently conceived" and wed to appropriate means at our disposal. This aid provides the opportunity for a significant death—dying meaningfully. Avoiding this realization and ignoring the pleas of the dying can be morally tragic indeed.

Conclusion

As human beings, we will die, but *how* we die is yet to be determined for each one of us. That we might wish to have some control over the dying process, then, is neither unusual nor inappropriate. Desiring to live a meaningful life, guided by intelligent activity, a life that includes the process of dying, is understandable and laudable. For some terminally ill patients, human dignity and significant living cannot continue when the body becomes only a biological apparatus that can, through mechanical measures, be kept alive. For them the meaning of life comes from the activity of fusing virtues with ideals, adjusting means and ends to each other in order to shape the outcome of their participations in the world.

Within a consistently significant life, problems concerning death rarely arise. At the end of significance is the abyss facing the terminally ill patient. It is up to the patient, then, whether to progress toward death or to resist it. The argument in this chapter attempts to make clear that no legitimate reasons, a priori, exist to condemn all acts of euthanasia and assisted suicide. In very real, deeply painful, tragic, and even loving situations, we who merely look on as others suffer and request to die do so at great cost to them, to ourselves, and to society. I believe that through genuine, sincere, and thorough reflection we will find that moral justification exists for these acts, and that through them we will help provide meaning to a dying person's last living moments.

10 William James, Black Elk, and the Healing Act

BRUCE WILSHIRE

THESE ARE tumultuous times for the institution of medicine. It is not only the health maintenance organization (HMO) revolution that has disrupted traditional practices and standards. The very concepts of health and healing are undergoing radical shifts and extensions. Traditional "mainstream" medical education is criticized for its alleged narrowness, its unquestioned acceptance of "hard science" as the only approach to healing—for example, its insistence on double-blind experiments as the only way to truth. Alternative medicine is no longer automatically stigmatized and safely marginalized as "crackpot," but in places is moving into the margins of the threatened medical establishment itself.

These developments are all the more significant because of great strides being taken in hard science. Genetic studies detect and isolate more and more genes, and brain science does likewise with neurotransmitters, to take but two examples. Nevertheless, alternative approaches—psychological or spiritual ways of healing—are gaining momentum. This suggests the massiveness of the paradigm shifts underway in bedrock conceptions of health, self, group, and world. However, new capacities—for example, capacities to alter humans genetically—still leave fundamental questions concerning what is good for human beings and what our capacities are as imagining, thinking, knowing, aspiring beings.

To get a handle on what is happening, we must rethink the most fundamental philosophical questions. Some of this is already underway in widely read books by doctors of medicine themselves. For example, Larry Dossey has written recently of the power of prayer in healing. Andrew Weil discourses on spontaneous healing, and Bernie Siegel on self-healing. Earlier Carl Simonton published a book on the power of imaging in treating cancer. Patients are informed of the precise locations and natures of the cancers and of the workings of the immune system and the healing power of white blood cells. He counsels them to form vivid images of these cells eating up the cancer. He describes cases in which this technique very probably eliminated cancerous tumors.[1]

I propose an even more radical approach. To understand how these alternatives methods sometimes work, I think most of us in America— mainly European in our roots—must completely rethink what mind and body are, must rework our thought at the most fundamental level conceivable. This was best begun, I believe, by William James between 1892 and 1910. More thoroughly than ever before, James exploded mind-body dualism, the ingrained view that mind is a nonphysical, nonextended, noninertial domain or substance that can somehow affect the body. But how? How could such disparate entities as the mind and the body possibly interface or interact in any way? James proposed to eliminate the imagined dualism and to replace it with one level of reality made up of fundamental properties of energy that can be experienced in the most immediate possible way, with certain sorts of linkages between the properties characterizing what we call mind, other sorts characterizing what we call matter. Mind is minding, something the body does. The question is, How is it possible for our imaging and thinking *not* to affect the rest of our bodies?

I will sketch James's view and see how well it accounts for a classic case of alternative healing, which was recounted in 1931 by Black Elk, an indigenous American shaman or healer, who described a cure that had been effected fifty years earlier. Black Elk's account, reported to John Neihardt, is a precious connection to a world almost totally destroyed by European incursion—that is, the introduction into indigenous populations of our world-girdling science and technology, with all their incredible power, arrogance, and blindness (not to mention European diseases introduced into populations with no immunity to them). I will try to reconstruct the manifold concrete details that formed Black Elk's world and that of his people, at least to the extent of imagining how James's revolutionary reconfiguring of our place in the world might begin to account for the cure Black Elk described. I will try to do it in a way that is understandable (with effort) to European eyes and ears.

William James's monumental work *The Principles of Psychology* (1890) was supposed to be a natural scientific study, the grand objective of which was the lawful correlation of brain states and mental states. James realized from the beginning that there were philosophical problems involved, particularly those related to how anybody can know anything, or how anything ever gets "known into" any mental state. But he thought that for his purposes these problems could safely be suspended, left in limbo. Through twelve years of effort and fourteen hundred pages of print he discovered that he was mistaken. He could not specify mental states in such a way that they could be correlated to brain states.

James thought that the only way initially to take hold of a mental state is to grasp what it is *of*, its object. But this is no particular thing thought of, but the whole sweep of the experienced world, the context within which any particular thing gains its emphasis and meaning (James calls this the Object). Surely there is thinking of this thought of, something mental going on. But when James looked closely, all he could find was more in the Object, particularly movements in his head and throat and alterations of his breathing. He could detect no mind as such, no domain of the mental, only a vast experienced (or experienceable) world, with some of it amazingly close and fleeting—that is, events in his body—which is all he can pin down about his think*ing* or experienc*ing* of the experienc*ed*.

In the last pages of the abridgement of *The Principles* (1892) James declared that "the waters of metaphysical criticism leak into every joint" of his proposed natural scientific and dualistic framework for doing psychology. He must completely rethink what self, mind, knowing, and world are. Pursuing relentlessly (with his artist's eye) what actually shows itself in experience, James happened to look into the blue of the sky. What figured in his thinking and perceiving life—the blue—was just what was there in the world he found at large; and what was peculiarly himself was his body possessed in a certain way in these moments by what was seen. Something that approaches adequate description of his "mental state" might go like this: skyified-my-head-is-turned-upward-into-the-blue.

He ruminated on this breakthrough insight for twelve years and began to publish its implications in *Essays in Radical Empiricism*. His empiricism was radical in that he saw relations as equiprimordial with entities related, and the difference between mind, or minding, and body as only a matter of somewhat different relations between the same energic properties related. The very hardness of a stone, say, that characterizes its history in the world at large, also figures in the ongoing history of the knowers, ourselves; we call a stretch of this history our perceiving the stone. That is, the hardness is numerically identical in the two contexts. It is hardness "thought of in a thinking" only because it is not stubbornly located in the world after the immediate perceiving of it; that is, it might be remembered in conjunction with other energic properties, and because it might be entertained fancifully: I imagine pinching it into powder with my fingers. But regardless of these "powers of mind," we are not merely *in* the world, we are *of* it, that is, constituted of its very own properties or "specific natures."

He called these energic properties pure experiences. He referred to them sometimes as neutral. That is, they are neutral between mind and matter, between subject and object, between self and other. They are anterior to, and more basic than, these very distinctions. Falling into different historical careers or contexts, they constitute mind and matter, and self and other. Selves are not just subjects over against objects.

Already we can see how James's emerging thought opens out onto a world very different from European scientific and technological thinking, particularly from the seventeenth century to our day. His thinking is non-dualistic: there is no veil of mental "sense data" dividing us from the world. Since in knowing we directly encounter the things themselves known, are irradiated by their exfoliating envelopes of energy, then when knowing things taken to be paradigmatically regenerative—such as snakes or bears—we are irradiated with their regenerative powers. At least this is so if we do not close ourselves off and detach ourselves in contempt or panic—or insist that scientific objectification is the only way of knowing them. Already we gain a glimpse of how a shamanic cure might work, when it does so.

Let us say a bit more about this domain of immediate encounter and intimate communion with the rest of the world—times of immediate engulfment—occasions before we have had time to reflect and neatly contrast the context of pure experiences that is our perceiving and thinking selves with the context that is the rest of the world, the world at large. It is easy to skip out of the moment of immediate encounter or interfusion before we grasp it. To repeat, James said that pure experience is neutral between knower and known, that it antecedes and makes possible the very distinction between "subject" and "object." But almost inevitably we slip into dualistic and mentalistic and atomistic assumptions embedded in our grammar. We say, "I regard it"—and we think of ourselves as a subject over against an object. But thereby we miss the immediate experience of excited interfusion that a healer such as Black Elk must tap if the cure is to work.

Before James, Emerson had already seen much of this. For example, to ride into a forest is to feel that one has disturbed something that had been going on, and that one is being watched.[2] So it is misleading on this primal level to say, "I regard it," or even "It regards me," or "We regard each other." It is better if regard floats in the situation; there is interfusion of energies. The same with respect to motion. As James wrote, "When clouds float by the moon, it is as if both clouds and moon and we ourselves shared in the motion."[3] Or, when we sit in a train in a station, looking out a window we cannot tell if it is our train or the one next to it that moves. Motion simply happens. I am as much moved as mover—or rather, the distinction collapses. The dualism of agent/patient or active/passive, collapses, along with that of subject/object and mind/matter.

* * *

At age nine an Oglala Lakota, Black Elk, experienced what he called his Great Vision. Ill, lying for days in a kind of coma, he experienced the cosmos spread around him in the most personal way, though of course in his people's terms as well. With a sensuous vividness and meaning that, he said, defied words to tell completely, he experienced himself oriented, aligned, authorized, and empowered by the six cardinal directions as they appeared to him in the form of the Six Grandfathers: The Powers of north, east, south, west, and of the upper and lower worlds. At the center of the vision was the World Tree, pulling all the Powers within itself and emitting them again amplified in its blooms. (This is a universal image in shamanic experience. For example, Emerson appropriated *Yggdrasil* from the Norse legend of World Tree; *Ygg* = *Egg*).

Enclosing this vast scene, extending "as far as sunlight and starlight," was the Hoop of the World, with the Hoop of Black Elk's people enlaced in it. Within this nest Wakan Tanka had intended the Lakota to brood and to raise their children in integrity with the Whole. (*Wakan Tanka*, commonly rendered in English as *Great Spirit*, should probably be rendered as *Great Mystery*, for *spirit* carries dualistic overtones, suggesting something above and beyond "mere" matter.)

Of course Black Elk's own account should be read (it has been translated by Black Elk's son and recorded by John Neihardt and his stenographer daughter). Yet I must employ enough of the detail in this chapter to connect it to William James's theoretical account of pure or neutral experience—what James called "the mysterious sensorial life."[4] Without the concrete detail we slip out of the operant level—the primal and immediate level—of experience, and lose ourselves in airy abstractions such as Mind and Spirit (or the Great Spirit). Lost in Western dualisms, we miss the actual visceral and total involvement that constitutes shamanic healing experience.

For example, when Black Elk's words are translated as "the Other World behind this one," did he mean something like "non-natural" or "supernatural" in the typical Western sense? The whole context of his words indicates that he did not, that he meant an interlacing of the worlds much more intimate and sensuous than Europeans typically imagine. When he recounts how Crazy Horse got his name, he explains that in vision or trance his cousin was seeing "in a sacred manner," and in this mode of seeing, his horse shimmered "crazily." This does not mean that his horse was nonphysical. It rather suggests, following James, that the horse itself was being seen in a more dilated and revealing way— seen as the exfoliating node of energies that *is* the horse as it interacts or interfuses with us and the rest of the surroundings.

I must at least mention a few more of the concrete details if we are to have any chance to grasp what actually went on in Black Elk's first healing: the appearance of the Sacred Pipe in his vision, the smoking of which bonds participants with the Powers of the world; the appearance of Virgins in one or other of the Four Quarters, which connotes, I think, the power of new or fresh life in its very possibility; the need to finally enact (if that is a tolerable word) portions of his vision for the people to witness—an enactment necessary for the very reality of the vision and its efficacity, its consensual being or its "objectivity" (to use a very European-parochial word).[5]

When the nine-year-old Black Elk recovered from his coma-vision people realized that he was changed, but he was reluctant to disclose the reason (perhaps he felt unworthy or unbelievable). In fact, over fifty years later Black Elk told Neihardt that he was telling the whole story— "all that can be told"—for the first time. Given the desperate plight of his people following their Pyhrric victory over Custer in 1876, and ten years after the vision, Black Elk felt compelled to heal if he could.

After fasting and immersing himself in a sweat lodge for several days, followed by lamenting on the plains during a cold and stormy night, Black Elk experienced a kind of replay of the vision, or portions of it. The next day, in a more or less wakeful state and in the company of a trusted friend, he sought in the area items that had appeared to him in the replay of the vision. In his vision he had, for example, seen a four-rayed star herb on the side of a gully. So he and his companion went there "in the full light of day" and found it, dug it out, and preserved its roots by wrapping them in sage. For some reason that he did not know at the time, Black Elk told Neihardt, he knew he would have need of it. And lo, later that very day, his fellow Lakota, Cuts-to-Pieces, reported to him that his young son was very sick and asked Black Elk to minister to him.

Before we sketch Black Elk's first cure, let us ruminate on two matters. Given engrained ancestral dualisms, Europeans tend to think of visions or trance states (if they take them seriously at all) as experiences of a transcendent domain, something outside the merely natural or physical. This completely misleads us about the power and scope of shamanic trance and vision. Recall what I said above about the meaning of Crazy Horse's mount: He was seeing it more completely than in everyday vision. I think that these apparently strange modes of perceiving can keep us housed in what James called "the instant field of the present"—the state of immediate encounter and actual interfusion with things, before reflection and abstraction has had a chance to neatly divide self and other, subject and object, and we have had time to forget the interfusion, the exchange of energies between things themselves. Studies of shamanic healings can give new life to phenomenology, to Edmund Husserl's rallying cry, "*Zu den sachen selbst*," that is, to the things themselves.

The second matter is this: Shamans, it is said, have the power to heal only because they themselves have passed through a death or near-death experience, have themselves been reborn or regenerated. Clearly this was true of Black Elk. I imagine that it applies to some extent to William James. We know that he was incapacitated for about a year with some kind of nervous collapse after receiving a medical degree from Harvard; apparently he was institutionalized for some of this time (the hospital records are still sealed, a colleague informs me). Moreover, the limits into which he ran in developing his natural scientific psychology stymied and shocked him for several years. Then he suffered heart trouble in the last years of the last century, and wrote much of his monumental *Varieties of Religious Experience* (published in 1902) while in bed.

Yet for all of James's deep insights into shamanic experience, his ability to free the European mind to explore its cognitive and curative powers, it would probably be stretching things to call him a shaman. (Gary Snyder recounts that in India some are thought to be both philosophers and shamans, which *might* accommodate James.)[6] In the end he was, I think, too untrusting of his own abilities to achieve what he called "mystical experiences" and to channel them in therapeutic ways. And we need not limit these ruminations to his personal life. Gaps show up in his theoretical work.

For example, he simply wrote that "mental fires don't burn mental sticks."[7] James should have said, I think, that mental fires don't *necessarily* burn mental sticks; that is, one of our mental powers is to fancy that they don't. But in the actual perceiving, the immediate minding, of an actual fire burning actual sticks, we *must* perceive it as burning them. And in fact, in the original experience at close quarters, the perceiving is itself hot. Even remembering the fire—and remembering that perceiving is not reduced to a mere "mental image" in the traditional dualist sense but excites reflexes—quickens the pulse and leaves a residuum of this in the neural pathways of the body.

A second matter, at least equally important for understanding the limits of James's abilities for grasping shamanic healing, is this: His grasp of what might be called the mythic mode of experience never quite jelled, I believe. That is, we need not merely *fancy* that mental fires don't burn mental sticks. When Moses heard God's voice speaking from the burning bush—burning without being consumed—it was not a fancying, but an overwhelming experience that stretched beyond ordinary modes of awareness and touched without grasping a reality beyond everyday distinctions and limitations, something like the Eternal. The story goes like this: "And when Aaron and all the children of Israel saw Moses, behold, the skin of his face shone; and they were afraid to come nigh unto him."[8]

* * *

Now let us grasp as best we can Black Elk's first cure. Each concrete detail and the sequence of these details is significant, but I can recount only some of them. The sick boy lies in the northeast sector of the tepee. Black Elk proceeds into the space through the entrance, which faces south—the direction believed to be, lived as, the source of heat and life. Four virginal young women accompany him, as does a male colleague who carries the sacred pipe and the four-rayed herb. Black Elk first offers the pipe to the Six Powers, then passes it to all who accompany him to smoke. Someone beats a drum as another offering is made to Wakan Tanka ("its sound arouses the mind and makes men feel the mystery and power of things").

Black Elk carries a wooden cup full of water and a few flakes of red willow bark, and proceeds around the outer perimeter of the inner space until he faces west—where the sun sets each day and dies, as each of us must do some day. (In doing this he acknowledges his own mortal reality, and probably his own near-death experience at the age of nine.) He addresses the Grandfather of the West with the sacred pipe. He then proceeds to the north—"where the white hairs are," where the cleansing cold wind of the north teaches endurance—and there addresses the Grandfather. He participates ecstatically in this Power of the north.

At about this point the sick boy smiles at him, and immediately Black Elk, who had been somewhat unsure of himself, feels power come up through the Earth, the lower world, and through his body: "I could feel something queer all through my body, something that made me want to cry for all unhappy things, and there were tears on my face." (One can only think of James's idea of the will to believe. Why can it be a fault to believe before evidence comes in, as some Western intellectuals think, when with regard to certain crucial matters of living, the belief that one holds profoundly influences the evidence that comes in?)

Black Elk drinks from the cup with the flakes of red willow bark and instructs one of the virgins to give it to the boy for him to drink also. He proceeds to where the boy lies and stamps his foot four times. After some incantations in pulses of four, he put his mouth on the pit of the boy's stomach and sucks through his body the cleansing wind of the north— the wind that teaches endurance.

Black Elk arises and proceeds to the east—the source of light and understanding—and addresses the Grandfather there. He then instructs one of the virgins to go to the boy and to assist him in rising and walking. This the boy does, with great difficulty. Black Elk then exits to the south, where he had first entered, having completed the cycle through the Four Directions and the Six Powers, not waiting to monitor any further progress made by the boy.

The next day Cuts-to-Pieces tells Black Elk that his boy is much improved. The elderly Black Elk told Neihardt that the boy lived until the age of thirty.

* * *

At this point most persons of European ancestry will almost automatically speak of "the power of positive thinking"—if they give this idea any credence. An ostensibly more sophisticated response would be to invoke "the power of the symbolical." Perhaps an explanation of Black Elk's story would go something like this: "After all, the boy was dreadfully sick, his life cycle was about to abort. Black Elk's circulating around the floor of the tepee vividly symbolized a completed life cycle, and this inspired the boy to make great efforts to regain his threatened life cycle. The boy succeeded."

Such responses are well intentioned and not simply false. But such talk blocks any real understanding of the healing transaction, for what does "the power of positive thinking" mean concretely? The phrase is an airy abstraction. In giving the impression that an explanation is provided, it blocks further inquiry; it is worse than if nothing had been said. The same applies to the ostensibly more sophisticated talk. Symbols are typically understood dualistically as mental or spiritual, and we are left with the problem insurmountable by dualism: How can such mental or spiritual activity possibly influence the body?

Only James's antidualistic approach brings us to the threshold of what was actually happening. Despite the apparent celebration of mind in dualism, placing it isolated on a pedestal makes it grow increasingly pale and impotent in the face of hard science's ever-deeper exposure of the powers of the physical. Increasingly in ever-spreading North Atlantic civilization it is assumed that the real world is the "external" world, the world minus our full, minding selves. But we *are* our bodies, I believe, and our bodies include, of course, our massive functioning brains embedded electrochemically in the rest of the body and in the rest of the world beneath, around, and above us.

The idea of an external world is itself an abstraction, a partial account. As Black Elk lived ecstatically in the far reaches of the four cardinal directions and of the upper and lower worlds, he did not conceive of these Powers as "in the mind." In the moment's interfusion of energies he was *identical* with them. His career and theirs intersected and were one. And as the sick boy participated believingly, ecstatically, in Black Elk, the Powers become his ecstatically.

The "symbolic" approach is particularly inadequate to grasp any healing transaction, particularly the climactic moment in which Black Elk drew the North Wind through the boy's body by sucking it through his abdomen. We might say, "The sucking didn't really do this, but only symbolized it." But this again repeats the dualistic abstraction that the north wind is really only what it is minus our mindful participation in it. No, it is more plausible to say that Black Elk drew the North Wind through the boy's body. To say this is to understand the wind in its full amplitude as including how it figures in the human nervous system, what it means to us in the interfusing moment *and* over time. As the North Wind works on, in, and through directly perceiving and then memorializing humans, it leaves a potent residue in the body that communicates and radiates directly from body into body in the ritualized situation.[9]

Since the healing apparently worked, it is probably that the world's regenerative energies radically augmented the boy's immunological or regenerative powers. The engaged energies realigned him in what Emerson called Circular power returning into itself, the regenerative universe. James was less sweeping in his terminology, but he escorted us methodically to a commanding viewpoint for surveying the surprising ramifications of sticking close to pure experience, to what he called the immediate, naive, pragmatic.

THREE

Pragmatism and

Specific Issues in Bioethics

11 Mental Illness: Rights, Competence, and Communication

BETH J. SINGER

THE ISSUE of mental patients' right to refuse treatment with psychotropic medication is primarily a legal one, but it involves many philosophic issues. Whether this prima facie right should be honored or abrogated is a question that arises primarily in connection with patients who have been involuntarily hospitalized, but even these patients have been held by the courts to retain the right to refuse medication unless and until they have been demonstrated, in a formal legal proceeding, to be incompetent. The decision by the New York State Court of Appeals in *Rivers v. Katz* is now accepted as definitive. The court held, in overturning a trial court ruling, that the due process clause of the New York State Constitution grants a fundamental right to refuse unwanted treatment, and that this right may be overridden only in strictly limited circumstances.[1] Ellen Clayton summarizes the court's finding as follows:

> The court acknowledged that the state, in the exercise of its police power, may administer drugs to avoid danger to the patient or to others. . . . [It] . . . rejected the argument, however, that the police power extends to protecting the "[s]tate's interest in providing a therapeutic environment, in preserving the time and resources of the hospital staff, in increasing the process of deinstitutionalization and in maintaining the ethical integrity of the medical profession" at the expense of the patient.
>
> The court also significantly limited the power of the state as parens patriae to give unwanted treatment. First, the court held that this power extends at most only to incompetent patients and made clear that the fact of commitment is not a presumptive finding of incompetence. Rather, the determination of incompetence is a judicial conclusion made after an administrative review with counsel and in which the state bears the burden of providing clear and convincing evidence. Moreover, the matter does not end with a determination of incompetence. Instead, a court is to authorize treatment only if the unwanted therapy "is narrowly

tailored to give substantive effect to the patient's liberty interest, taking into consideration all relevant circumstances, including the patient's best interests, the benefits to be gained from treatment, the adverse side effects associated with the treatment, and any less intrusive alternate treatments."[2]

According to *Rivers*, the courts may override a patient's right to refuse medication in order to avoid danger to the patient or others. In what follows, I raise questions as to what this should be taken to mean and the scope of its applicability. I also discuss the meaning of competence (*competency* in some sources).

Posing a danger, whether to self or to others, is almost universally used to justify hospitalizing patients against their will.[3] In relation to the refusal of medication, the primary consideration is usually an evaluation of the patient's competence or capacity (with *competence* defined as a group of capacities). For instance, under the laws of the state of California, patients who are involuntarily confined are given a document informing them that they have the right to refuse treatment with antipsychotic medication. The document continues:

However, you may be treated with antipsychotic medication over your objection in the case of an emergency or upon a determination that you do not have the capacity to refuse treatment, in a capacity hearing held for this purpose. The capacity hearing will be conducted at the facility where you are receiving treatment by a hearing officer [a superior court judge, a court-appointed commissioner or referee, or a court-appointed hearing officer]. The hearing officer will determine whether you have the capacity to refuse medication as a form of treatment. You may apeal the determination of the capacity hearing to the superior court of the court of appeal.

You have the right to be represented at the capacity hearing by a patients' rights advocate or legal counsel. This person will assist you to prepare for the hearing and will answer questions you may have about the capacity hearing process.[4]

Incompetence makes impossible the kind of informed consent (and, by implication, informed refusal) that is required by the courts. As noted by Jessica Willen Berg, Paul S. Appelbaum, and Thomas Grisso, "The notion of competence in the medical context stems from the law of informed consent, which has evolved over the past three decades into a complex doctrine designed to promote patients' autonomous decisionmaking."[5] In a footnote the authors add, "Valid informed consent also requires an element of voluntariness, or absence of coercion, and a competent patient."

But autonomy in making decisions is more than voluntariness or the absence of coercion, and a bit later I discuss this concept, too. Competence itself and the criteria by which it is measured, widely discussed in the literature, have been described in many different ways. "What has not emerged from the standard accounts," according to the medical ethicist Baruch Brody, "is a proper account of the capacities that constitute the patient's competency to participate in health care decision making."[6] Summing up the capacities generally appealed to, Brody says:

They seem to be as follows. (1) *The ability to receive information from the surrounding.* (2) *The capacity to remember the information they have received.* (3) *The ability to make a decision and give a reason for it.* (4) *The ability to use the relevant information in making the decision.* (5) *The ability to appropriately assess the relevant information.*[7]

Brody is not writing specifically about mental patients, but these criteria seem applicable to them as to others. I think the list needs to be amplified, however. The right to refuse medication is a right to participate in decision making regarding treatment. It is therefore a right to discuss the treatment plan with the caregiver. For that reason, I believe the capacity to participate constructively in these discussions is a component of the sort of competence that is requisite for making decisions concerning the acceptance or rejection of treatment. But the right to do so should also entail a right to have one's views considered seriously. I expand upon this idea a bit later.

The capacity for discussion is complex. Ideally, as applied in the present context, it would include the ability to seriously consider what is being recommended, the reasons given for it, and the effects it can be expected to have; the ability to offer an equally serious and sincere appraisal of the recommendation and the factors that enter into it; and the ability to engage in respectful critique of all the opinions offered in the course of the dialogue, including the patient's own.

Inseparable from these capacities is the ability to engage in mutual questioning and answering. I refer to this complex of abilities as a capacity for dialogic reciprocity.[8] It is, of course, an ability or power that persons possess in varying degrees and that they do not always exercise as fully as they might. Moreover, the level of a patient's capacity would have to be assessed on the basis of his or her performance in a very stressful situation. It is therefore quite a demanding standard. Nevertheless, in relation to the treatment decision it is an important one, and in being difficult to measure precisely, the capacity for dialogic reciprocity does not differ sharply from other factors that are already taken into consideration. It could not be the sole criterion of competence, yet it cannot help but affect the other abilities that are employed as criteria.

In an article on competency to refuse psychotropic medication, despite her overall approval of what she takes to be the generally operative legal standard, Elyn R. Saks concludes that considering different competency standards is important not only because they could have practical consequences, but also because studying them may further theoretical understanding.[9] Neither the capacity for dialogic reciprocity nor the other criterion I suggest in this chapter is intended as an alternative to those generally in effect; both are recommended as supplementary, and the procedural context in which they would be assessed is designed not only to elicit them, but also, reflexively, to help the patient cultivate the capacity for communicative interchange.

I am aware that, as Saks notes, "giving psychiatrists more scope to find incompetency," which adding to the list of criteria might be thought to do, "[is] likely to result in more findings of incompetency."[10] But if I am correct, even though engaging patients in an extended dialogue concerning what is being prescribed for them could uncover the inability of some to participate in such a reciprocal exchange and could therefore be counted as a mark of incompetence, it might help to produce greater understanding and even enhance the communicative ability of such patients. If it did, it could result in a higher rather than a lower rate of patient compliance.

As summarized by Saks, the law's treatment competency standard is fundamentally a matter of cognitive understanding: "That standard, briefly stated, is that a person is competent to make a treatment decision if she comprehends the caregiver's explanation of her condition and the treatment, and forms no patently false beliefs—'delusions'—about her condition and the treatment."[11]

Noting that the protection of autonomy presupposes that patients "are the best judges of their own interests," Berg, Appelbaum, and Grisso stress that "[e]mbedded in [this] notion of autonomy are concrete requirements of capacity."[12] They continue: "To the extent that a patient's capacity is impaired with respect to abilities necessary to exercise autonomy, that person is less able to participate competently in the decision-making process." But, they contend, "Presently there is a lack of both an authoritative framework for thinking about legal competence and clear standards for it."[13] Concerning the requirement of understanding cited by Saks, Berg and associates ask, "[W]hat degree of incapacity suffices to establish incompetence under an 'understanding' standard? How much understanding is necessary and what does the patient need to be able to

understand?" In addition, "Do different situations warrant the application of different standards or the demonstration of different levels of ability?"[14]

In an earlier paper Saks had elaborated on the concept of understanding, identifying four categories: pure understanding, modified
understanding, understanding and belief (or "sophisticated understanding and belief"), and full reasoning.[15] Even though they acknowledge that
"Saks's categorizations are closely linked to language found in cases and
statutes," Berg and her coauthors contend that "they do not adequately
distinguish between different capacities."[16] In short, "[a]lthough the law
focuses on cognitive impairments, there are no uniform standards among
the jurisdictions to identify the relevant abilities that, when impaired,
constitute incompetence."[17]

Drawing on the work of two of them, Appelbaum and Grisso, Berg
and associates present four other "potential components of competence
standards" that also, they hold, reflect what is found in the law. These
are: "(i) ability to communicate a choice, (ii) ability to understand relevant information, (iii) ability to appreciate the nature of the situation and
its likely consequences, and (iv) ability to manipulate information rationally."[18]

These components were employed in an extensive review of American cases, "The MacArthur Treatment Competence Study," and the
resulting data seem to Berg and her coauthors to support the judgment
that taking into account both the third and fourth of these components
(the "appreciation" and "rational manipulation" components) leads to a
more adequate standard, since in the cases under review it identified persons as suffering from schizophrenia who were not otherwise identified,
and discriminated with a fair degree of accuracy between those patients
and others suffering from depression and angina. Yet, despite the greater
accuracy of the abilities identified in these components as predictors,
these abilities are not precisely measurable either, and at least for the present it would seem that whatever our standards, we must rely on the
judgment of trained, alert, and careful participant-observers to apply
them in appraising the competence of patients to decide for themselves
whether or not to accept medication.[19]

Even if we accept Appelbaum and Grisso's more careful formulation
of the legal standard of competence, the capacity for dialogic reciprocity
goes beyond them. It is more than purely cognitive, and it involves
greater communicative powers than the ability to communicate a choice.
The capacity for mutual responsiveness is central to all effective communication with others and thereby affects cognition and the way one uses

what one knows or seems to know (which is how I construe the "rational manipulation" of information).

As far as I know, despite legal provisions for hearings to determine competency, this capacity has not, as such, been identified or taken into account in any relevant medical or legal context. For instance, voluntary patients in California are told that they will be treated with antipsychotic medications only after they have "completed the *informed consent* process." Concerning this process they are given the following information:

Before you consent to any antipsychotic medication, your doctor must explain to you:
(1) the reasons for taking this medication and what benefits you can expect
(2) that you may withdraw your consent at any time
(3) the type and amount of medicine and how often it must be taken
(4) the common side effects from taking this medication and what effects you can most probably expect to experience
(5) alternative treatments that are available (if any)
(6) the potential long-term side effects of taking the medication[20]

Note that no explicit provision is cited here for discussion of the information that is presented or for any exchange of ideas concerning it. The patient is simply instructed, in a note on the back of the booklet describing these and other rights, "If you have any questions or complaints regarding your rights please contact [name, address, and telephone number of a patients' rights advocate]."

I believe that patients should have a right to mutually responsive communication about what is being prescribed for them, and that the capacity to participate in such communication should be a criterion used in evaluating their competence. I propose this not simply because the capacity in question is a crucial element in social interaction in general, but on the ground that the degree to which it is or is not operative in the communication between patient and caregiver is an important factor in the patient's response to what is prescribed and affects his or her decision to accept or reject it.

But there is more involved than this. As the word *reciprocity* implies, the capacity for dialogic reciprocity must be exercised by the caregivers even as they try to evaluate it in—and to foster its exerise by—their patients. The process in which any treatment plan is presented should be carefully designed not simply to maximize communication between caregiver and patient, but also to make clear to the patient that he or she is being given a voice in this process. What is called for is genuine dialogue, joint consideration of every statement made by either party. I would also argue for a similar, mutually responsive method to be employed subsequently in appraising the efficacy of treatment and determining whether the prescribed medication should continue to be used.

As I said earlier, employing this method might even help to enhance the patient's capacity. However, despite the important role I assign to dialogue, I am not talking about its use in treatment as such—that is, about psychoanalysis or other forms of psychotherapy. What I am concerned with is the importance of communicative ability as a standard of patient competence and the centrality of the communicative process in any deliberations regarding the prescription of medication. In addition to being demanding on the part of staff as well as patients, discussions of the sort that the attempt at reciprocity would require are time consuming and, as many writers have noted with regard to other careful or elaborate procedures, would be expensive. Still, if they resulted in greater acceptance of medication and therefore in fewer rehospitalizations, patient care would, in the end, cost less.

In its fullest sense, dialogic reciprocity involves even more than what I have suggested thus far. This chapter is at least partly about rights. But I am concerned not merely with the right of hospitalized patients to refuse treatment or their right to receive it.[21] The rights to receive and to refuse treatment have been codified and become legal rights that must be judicially enforced, but when I speak of rights, including patients' rights and in particular the rights involved in dialogic reciprocity, I mean what philosophers call moral rights. The principle of dialogic reciprocity itself involves respect for certain basic moral rights.

The idea underlying the principle of dialogic reciprocity is derived from George Herbert Mead's analysis of communication.[22] Mead took communication to presuppose the ability on the part of each of the parties involved to take the attitude of the other[s]—that is, to see the object of communication as the others do. This means that to understand another's gestures (by which Mead meant primarily, but not exclusively, vocal gestures), we must implicitly respond as they do to that to which they refer (we must have this response within ourselves), even if we do not do so overtly. By implication, to understand gestures that are made in response to one's own, we must be able, as we say in the vernacular, "to see ourselves as others see us." Absent this shared understanding, communication is impossible. Dialogic reciprocity includes this, but goes beyond it. It is not necessarily presupposed by the kind of mutual understanding Mead intended, but facilitates it.

The reciprocity I am talking about involves mutual respect for the autonomy and authority of all the participants in a discussion, a respect that I argue should be accorded to them as a matter of right. What is common to this concept and that of Mead is a shared attitude, in that each participant must have (and express) the same attitude of respect for his or her own authority and autonomy as for those of the others. The concept of authority as I am using it here differs sharply from the usual notion of authority as the power to impose one's judgments on others. What I mean by it is closer to a presumed authoritativeness, or, in a slightly weaker sense, legitimacy: acceptability as a contributor on a par with all the other participants in the dialogue.

Respecting a person's authority in this sense can be thought of as a type of empowerment: empowerment to have one's contribution to the discussion taken seriously, even if it may be subsequently rejected or overridden. *Autonomy* is one of the terms we find used in connection with informed consent and patient competence, but although in connection with action I understand it, as others do, to connote self-determination, in relation to communication I give it a somewhat broader sense, namely that of judging for oneself. This usage also differs from the ways in which it has been used and defined by philosophers.[23]

To exercise autonomy is not to maintain a closed mind. In order to exercise dialogic reciprocity, one must remain open to the possibility of modifying or revising one's judgments.[24] A key feature of mutually responsive communicative interchange is that when we engage in it we are also reflecting, engaging in communication with ourselves, which Justus Buchler terms "reflexive communication."[25]

Mead describes this in terms of a dialogue between the "I" and the "me," a dialogue in which we alternately speak (or, in the language I prefer, judge) as the self we have become in the course of previous social communication and interaction ("me") and as a self who is responding to that self ("I"). Not being bound by the "me," the "I" can respond critically and in new ways, so that the attitudes or judgments the self has acquired or come to accept can be either changed or reinforced. That is, reflexive communication can be a process of learning and development. In the exercise of dialogic reciprocity we reflect autonomously and critically on our own judgments as well as those of the others with whom we are in dialogue. Therefore, we are open to change, even though the dialogue may result in strengthening our original position.

As I noted earlier, the essence of dialogic reciprocity is respect on the part of each participant for the autonomy and authority of all. Not only must each display this respect for the others; each must expect the same respect in turn. On grounds that I can only briefly summarize here, I have argued that respect for personal authority and autonomy, in the specified senses, should be accorded to all members of every community as a matter of right.[26] My argument is basically that only if they respect one another as autonomous and authoritative will those who are associated with one another come to accept a common set of social norms.

The hospital community would not be an exception to this principle. Admittedly, the behavior of those who are severely mentally ill can often be such as to sharply limit the extent to which these rights can be observed or even to make it impossible to observe them. But patients are no less worthy of respect than anyone else, and treatment communities (which I take mental hospitals to be), like all others, require normative regulation. Not only is it morally and legally unacceptable, it is not possible to govern any group of people completely by fiat or by force, and the understanding and acceptance of the respective roles of patients and staff and the powers and responsibilities of the various staff members is dependent on the social norms that govern all of them.

Therefore, my general argument for the rights cited is applicable here. Although patients may not understand these rights intellectually—many rights are respected in practice without being conceptualized, a fact that has been overlooked—patients as well as staff members should, as far as possible, be both accorded these rights and expected to respect them.[27] Nevertheless, my main concern is not the hospital community as such, but the narrower context in which treatment decisions are arrived at, and there the rights of autonomy and authority should play a special part.

My primary contention has been that the capacity for dialogic reciprocity is a necessary condition of cognitive competence. There is no mechanical measure of this capacity, but the extent to which a person exercises it, exhibiting the ability to listen to others, to consider what they are saying, to raise questions, and to respond thoughtfully with the expectation of being similarly listened to, is observable and can be evaluated, even if not as precisely as we would wish. Moreover, employing the method of dialogic reciprocity enables and requires caregivers to review their evaluations as discussions with their patients proceed.

The exercise of this capacity does not entail accepting what others say uncritically: Mutual criticism is a feature of the sort of dialogue I intend, as is self-criticism. But in that treatment must be discussed and the patient has a presumptive right of refusal, demonstration of at least some ability to participate constructively and responsively in this discussion

is required. (Some would say rationally, but on the grounds of vagueness this term has been subject to so much criticism that I prefer not to
employ it.)

This means that an evaluation of the patient's capacity for reciprocal
communication should be employed in determining whether or not the
patient should, in the end, be granted the legal right to refuse the proffered treatment. At the same time, an increased capacity for this kind of
communication can be viewed as one of the goals of psychiatric treatment, and, as such, would be a measure of its success or failure. All of this
implies that the communication process must be studied and that more
precise standards of communicative competence need to be established.

The *Rivers* decision referred to at the beginning of this chapter permits
the state to employ the motive of avoiding danger either to the patient or
to others, which is routinely applied by the courts to justify involuntary
confinement and to justify the administration of drugs. This seems to
imply that posing such a danger may be employed by caregivers as a criterion in connection with the right to refuse treatment. But posing a danger or threat of danger, whether to oneself or to others, seems almost
universally to be defined in terms of physical harm, and posing a danger
to oneself seems to be construed as either attempting or threatening suicide. For instance, Carroll, Schneider, and Wesly quote a decision handed
down by a state court: "Although attempts to predict future conduct are
always difficult, and confinement based upon such a prediction must
always be viewed with suspicion, we believe civil confinement can be
justified in some cases if the proper burden of proof is satisfied and dan-
gerousness is based upon a finding of a recent overt act, attempt or threat
to do substantial harm to oneself or another."[28]

The authors go on to say, "In most jurisdictions, and as noted by the
Lessard court, . . . a person may be committed not only on the basis of posing a *physical* threat to others but also on the basis of posing a threat to
oneself, *either by attempting or threatening suicide*" (italics mine).[29] In a note
they quote another source that elaborates the criteria for commitment in
such cases, as follows: "(1) the person in question must be proven, on the
basis of convincing scientific evidence given at a fair hearing with appropriate due process guarantees, to lack capacities of rational choice and
deliberation; and (2) these incapacities must be *shown* to be highly likely
to lead to danger to the person's life and limb or to the life and limb of
others."[30]

In discussing the issue of paternalism in connection with involuntary
commitment, the authors similarly construe harm to self in terms of suicide. Regarding the necessary and sufficient conditions for paternalistic

interference, they argue for taking the capacity for rational decision making into consideration as well as for "the consequences of an act [being] in some way irreversibly harmful to oneself." And they continue, "[I]t would be unjustified to commit a person involuntarily for an indefinite period of time *only on the basis that the person is suicidal*" (italics mine).[31]

I believe a question must be raised as to whether, to pose a serious threat, either to oneself or to others, actual or predictable behavior need literally be a threat to "life and limb." Can the danger include anything short of attempting or threatening to put an end to that life? Should it be defined so as to include behavior that can be shown, on the basis of the patient's past history or of credible scientific evidence presented in a fair hearing in which due process is observed, to be highly likely to worsen the patient's condition? Even if it would be ruled out by the courts as justification for involuntary hospitalization, should the motive of avoiding this kind of harm nevertheless be employed to justify abridging the right to refuse treatment?

No one can be forced to swallow pills. But we can make clear the danger entailed by the failure to do so. The ability to appreciate and evaluate what is known about the expected consequences (positive and negative) of the proposed treatment and of following it or failing to do so is already taken into account in evaluating competence. When psychotropic medication can be shown with a high degree of certainty to be beneficial and failure to utilize it to have negative consequences that outweigh potentially undesirable side effects, the issue of danger to self enters in. (By implication, since the behavior that results from the acceptance or refusal of the medication will affect those close to the patient, there is also a secondary question concerning the potential for harm to others.)

Provided the patient had had the opportunity to discuss the issue in a dialogue governed by the principle of reciprocity, a dialogue in which his or her rights of autonomy and authority as well as those of the caregivers were respected, I would argue for including "danger to self," in the broadened sense I have suggested, as one of the criteria to be employed in determining whether or not an individual's right to refuse psychotropic medication should be honored.

12 Genetics and Pragmatism

HERMAN J. SAATKAMP, JR.

GENETIC and pragmatic explanations seem to march not only to different drums, but in opposite directions. Looking to the past, genetic explanations rely on an analysis of one's heritable nature to account for current traits and behavior, whereas pragmatic explanations look to the future, relying on the consequential radiations of actions to determine their significance. Combining such explanations produces a Janus face looking in two directions.

If there also are two pairs of feet struggling toward opposing destinations, there is little likelihood of making progress by bringing together genetic and pragmatic explanations. On the one hand, one might argue that such a combined approach will not succeed in theory or practice because of internal conflicts. On the other hand, if pragmatism is seen as a future-oriented, consequentialist position from which one determines the value and significance of genetic explanations, then the two perspectives are compatible, and bringing them together may be viewed as an outcome of the bipolar nature of human life that naturally unites one's heritage and one's future.

I argue for this latter perspective. Specifically, I maintain that certain characteristics of pragmatism provide (1) the basis for evaluating and understanding genetic explanations of human traits and behavior, (2) a guideline for parents making decisions about the future lives of their children, and (3) a thoughtful assessment of social policies that may be fostered by the new genetics. Finally, I also maintain that the pragmatic position has serious limitations that require consideration.

The New Genetics

The success of the well-publicized Human Genome Project is a basis for concern and hope in the area of human reproduction. If one supposes, as I do, that genetics is the foundation of all animal action, and that, when coupled with environmental assessments, genetic explanations also may provide an adequate account of animal behavior, then the promise and threat of the new genetics become clear. Against the backdrop of repeated difficulties and failures in social policies and social research, the new human genetics may provide practical and specific guidelines for parents and societies that wish to choose characteristics and behavioral patterns for future generations.

To a limited extent, this is already true. Through genetic testing parents can screen out certain possible futures for their children (for example, Tay-Sachs disease, Huntington's disease, Down's syndrome, and thalassemia) by first detecting a genetic marker for the trait and then either not implanting the embryo (if in vitro fertilization is being used) or aborting the fetus. Negative eugenics of this sort will become more readily available as better techniques are found for determining these characteristics in the early embryo stages and as the Human Genome Project completes its mapping and sequencing tasks.

Among the currently available techniques, amniocentesis provides parents with choices they did not have before its development, not only in terms of ruling out certain genetic maladies, but also, more controversially, in determining the sex of their children. But amniocentesis has serious limitations. Amniotic fluid samples are taken through a needle introduced into the uterus between the tenth and sixteenth weeks of pregnancy. There is approximately 0.5 percent risk of miscarriage, and it normally takes a few weeks before the parents have the results of the test. Hence, any parental decisions based on amniocentesis must come in the second trimester, at the earliest.

Other alternatives offer quicker information, within days, and earlier testing possibilities, but carry a higher risk of miscarriage. For example, CVS (chorionic villus sampling) is a sampling of the outer layer of the placenta, the chorion, and has approximately 5.5 percent chance of miscarriage. Currently several researchers are developing tests for fetal cells that circulate in maternal blood. If successfully developed, this technique will remove or significantly reduce the risk to the fetus, and parents will have an alternative for gathering considerable information about the developing embryo in the early stages of pregnancy.

So far, the tests available are used primarily to rule out horrific and brief futures for children, and there is little, although some, disagreement over the importance of gathering this information for parental use. Who wishes to see a child born who will live a brief and painful life? But obviously the issues become more complex if one focuses on lives that are full but limited (for instance, by Down's syndrome and Huntington's disease).

As difficult as the present issues are, the difficulties will be raised to new levels as parents become able not only to screen out certain characteristics, but also to include traits in their children they consider positive. Such traits include not only socially privileged ones, such as body build, but perhaps traits of sociability, aggression, intelligence, sexual orientation, and more. Practically, one may argue that if individual citizens have more positive traits, the prospects for a civil society to flourish will be higher.

Of course the great concern raised by this possibility is the specter of eugenics and the haunting and ghastly features of Nazi eugenics, a disciplined tragedy that chose the parents who could have children and systematically eliminated humans who should not. The new eugenics is changing the focus to choosing future children, not the parents of those children; rather than killing adult humans, the focus is on reducing or eliminating the prospects for negative genetic traits to be carried to the next generation as well as fostering positive genetic traits for future generations. Various approaches eliminate developing embryos in the early stages of development either through in vitro fertilization, in which embryos free of harmful traits are selected over other embryos to be implanted, or by abortion. The status of the embryos not chosen for implantation is already an issue in many in vitro fertilization clinics, and eventually is likely to lead to more precise medical and governmental guidelines.

In focusing on choosing children rather than parents, are we making our prospects better than previous eugenic tragedies? Given the history of our successes and failures in shaping the world to human purposes, there is no clear answer to this question, but pragmatism offers more hope than do ideological perspectives now being used to address the promise and problems of the new genetics.

Some may think this speculation is fortune-telling. Little progress in explaining complex human behavior has been accomplished through the new genetics. But the new genetics is new, and the most recent advances offer a chance of detecting and altering traits and behavior (such as aggression and bipolarity) that to date have eluded other types of research and social policies. As evidence and technology become available for choosing the characteristics of children, responsible parents (with the means of doing so) will not ignore these alternatives any more than they knowingly ignore proper nourishment and care. In this sense we are entering a new era of eugenics that, as Philip Kitcher and Glenn McGee argue, seems inevitable for parents who have the best interest of their children at heart.[1]

How are we to assess the new genetics, and what guidelines may help us in fostering personal choices and social policies? Therein lies the place of pragmatism. In the last few years there have been many advances in understanding genotypes and their resulting phenotypes, particularly in the area of genetic abnormalities. Within a decade these major advances are likely to be viewed as small steps toward a much grander understanding of human actions. Pragmatism offers one approach to evaluate the significance of these advances and to provide a basis for making individual and social decisions.

Pragmatism and Genetic Explanations

Pragmatism, like any large intellectual area, is not easy to describe. If one searches for defining characteristics, there are few if any that go unchallenged.[2] But there are several earmarks that appear essential to pragmatism and provide a foundation for assessing the new genetics. Two of the most general characteristics of pragmatism are its general view of philosophy and its nonideological tenor. Pragmatic philosophy focuses on problems of human finitude, placing human action in the context of its cultural and natural environment; it is a philosophy not bound by disciplinary lines, and it aims at ameliorating the human condition. Because of the contingency of human knowledge and experience, pragmatism does not ascribe to a formal ideology, but rather claims that it represents common sense and a common good within the pluralism of human experience.

The basic nonideological but moral tone of pragmatic thought can be more accurately described as maintaining the priority of the good over truth and as strongly favoring some form of individualism. To clarify the meaning of truth, Peirce says, "Consider what effects, which might conceivably have practical bearings, we conceive the object of our conception to have. Then, our conception of these effects is the whole of our conception of the object."[3] James adds that one knows whether one's conception is true if the practical consequences are. Pragmatism removes truth from traditional correspondence and coherence theories and places it squarely in the radiating consequences of beliefs and actions. In so doing, pragmatic truth does not conform to the ordinary notion that truthful statements reflect the reality in the world, but rather pragmatically true statements become true if the expected consequences occur.

These consequences may be good, bad, or neutral, and in this sense pragmatic truth is distinguishable from considerations of the good, and Peirce's more rigorous and limited application of pragmatism appears not to give the good a place of priority over truth. However, pragmatism, particularly in James and Dewey, is deeply interested in structuring personal and social life for the best consequences. This is one of the reasons Santayana believed that James's and Dewey's philosophies were rooted in moralism rather than a thorough naturalism, since more traditional naturalists give little priority to individual experience let alone a central priority to individual human experience.

Although it is a controversial claim, a cardinal trait of pragmatism—and one that makes it a strong candidate for assessing the new genetics—is its placement of the good as having priority over the ordinary sense of truth.[4] What difference does it make if I know the way the world really is, but such knowledge does not lead to a better way of living for me and for my culture or species?

By focusing on whether the radiations of knowledge and actions are good or not, the pragmatist also raises the difficult question of the role of the individual in making such determinations. Due to the advances in genetics and the neurosciences, understanding how individuals can choose or determine particular actions is more complex than anyone imagined even a decade ago. Here again, it appears that pragmatism and the new genetics march to different orders.

Genetics looks for common traits among individuals. Each human has a similar chromosomal structure, and abnormalities are distinguishable from this common structure. Individual traits appear to be lost, and, if genetic explanations extend beyond mere background information to causal dependency (as is presently claimed for Huntington's disease and Tay-Sachs disease), individual decisions and environmental influences are eliminated as determinable characteristics in explanations of animal behavior. But pragmatism moves in quite a different direction. Individual experience, rooted in James's radical empiricism, is at the forefront. The pragmatist recognizes many of the commonalities of human and animal experience, but there is an unshakeable belief that individual experience is fundamental and that it is best to allow individuals to make their own decisions. Dewey's commitment to democracy and education was based on this belief. Rather than force a social policy with good consequences on society, Dewey worked to foster an educated public that individually would make informed decisions about their lives and their participation in a democratic culture.

The priority of the good over truth coupled with the centrality of individual decisions leads the pragmatist to strongly favor allowing individuals to make decisions about their own futures without coercive social factors. In light of popular accounts of the new genetics, pragmatism's reliance on individual actions and decisions may seem both old fashioned and out of step with the new science. By placing the weight of the future on heritable traits, genetics appears to eliminate the pragmatic approach. Such reasoning, although popular, is in error, and, if it prospers, could lead to a future as ghastly as the disciplined and ordered horrors of the Nazi eugenics. An examination of the genetic explanations of complex human behaviors can be helpful here.

The popular but largely false model of genetic explanation is a simple one: genotype causes phenotype. Within this model current traits and behavior are explained by the presence of a specific, identifiable genotype inherited from one's parents. All heritable traits, including characteristics and actions, are thought to be causally determined by one's genotype, with little, if any, influence from the environment or culture. Single-trait phenotypes are models for this form of explanation. Dimples, the color of one's eyes, earlobe attachment, widow's peak hairline, hitchhiker's thumb, and other traits are determined by a single gene whose presence determines whether these traits are exhibited (provided the environment fosters the life of the individual long enough for the heritable traits to appear).

Single-gene explanations are easy to understand, because the complexity of environment and culture appears to be excluded from them, and one can model simple cause-and-effect accounts that are intuitively clear: If a specific gene is carried on a chromosome, either somatic or germ line, then a particular trait will inevitably characterize the individual carrying that heritable gene. As we shall see, multifactorial traits are not as intuitively clear nor as easily couched in simple cause-and-effect language.

If the new genetics can characterize complex human behaviors (aggression, sexual orientation, intelligence, sociability, and so on) by reference to single genes, then the popular genotype-phenotype explanation will be the simplest key to understanding, predicting, and controlling these behaviors. And certain phenotypes appear to follow this formula, particularly Huntington's disease (Tay-Sachs disease and trisomy 18 are other candidates).[5]

An overlong CAG repeat near the tip of chromosome 4 will inevitably lead to Huntington's disease, an autosomal dominant neurodegenerative disorder with symptoms of worsening gait, uncontrollable movement, cognitive decline, and personality changes leading to insanity. It usually occurs between thirty and fifty years of age, and an individual with the disease normally dies within ten to fifteen years after its onset. If an individual has the CAG codon repeats, then regardless of the person's environment, family, or culture, that individual appears destined to a very difficult ending of life. No doubt this accounts for the high rate of suicide among people with Huntington's disease.

If this were the full story and if it served as the model for other complex human behaviors, the role of genetic explanation would be one of causal determinancy with little or no role for environmental influences or individual choices. But it is not the full story. At present, the march of Huntington's disease in an individual's life cannot be altered. Everyone with the genotype will have the phenotype. The onset of the disease and its length vary, and for a while some thought these characteristics might be environmentally influenced, but recent research suggests that the number of CAG repeats may be an indicator of these factors.

A few years ago PKU (phenylketonuria) was viewed in much the same way. This is a genetic disease that impedes children's ability to metabolize the amino acid phenylalanine and leads to severe retardation. Today, as a result of special diets, children with PKU develop normally. By altering the children's dietary environment, the oversupply of phenylalanine and the lack of tyrosine can be prevented, and the tragic alteration of the children's cognitive capacities can be avoided. One can hope the same will be true of Huntington's disease and other devastating maladies that now appear inevitable.

The lesson here is that a simple model of causal determinacy between genotype and phenotype is easy to understand and may appear to be the best we can do given our current knowledge. But there is always the possibility that by separating the genetic anomaly from its phenotype we can discover environmental influences that will alter the onset, length, and severity of the malady. From a pragmatic perspective, there may be far better consequences if we continue to look for environmental influences that shape a phenotype even if we have found a single genetic characteristic that sets it in motion. However, the likelihood of finding single genetic traits that determine most complex human behaviors appears unlikely. Even for multifactorial characteristics such as physical height, it appears that there is both a multifaceted genetic base and complex environmental influences. Therefore, the pragmatic insight into the complexity and contingency of human life warns against looking for any overly simplistic or single-chain type of determinism.

The pragmatic insight also calls attention to the human tragedies that have resulted from simplistic reasoning, or, as Dewey might have put it, from not acting intelligently. Santayana's oft-repeated epigram merits one more echo: "Those who cannot remember the past are condemned to repeat it."[6] Surely many of the historic tragedies of eugenics occurred because of a simplistic view that if we control the makeup of parents, we will control the production of children with positive attributes.

The new eugenics, far more scientifically based than Nazi eugenics, tempts one to believe one can control the complex characteristics of future generations by simply controlling genotypes. This cause-and-effect approach not only is misleading, but also, based on current evidence, is wrong. Even if the current evidence did not fully support the conclusion, the pragmatist might well argue that better consequences will come if we continue to pursue not only the Human Genome Project, but also the environmentally and culturally important features of human life. A fuller, more humane, and more creative approach to understanding human behavior is more likely to result than if we make individual and social decisions based on a simplistic model that assumes the phenotype is rigidly determined by the genotype.

One may wonder what is gained by this pragmatic insight other than the recognition of the complexity of scientific explanations (not an unimportant point). After all, the multifactorial accounts of climatology provide reliable bases for making weather predictions, but no one supposes that the weather is determined by anything other than natural causes; it is not free or indeterminate merely because our predictions are based on probabilities. Winds or clouds have no choice in the matter. Are humans any different?

Even if we knew all the genetic and environmental factors in human behavior, we still might be able to predict only with a certain probability what the resulting phenotypes would be, but that would not provide credence for the claim that social policies should be based on individual decisions. Indeed, it might call for structuring individual decisions to match social goals, much as in the form imagined by Plato in his *Republic* or in a more rigidly and scientifically organized way than envisioned by early eugenics movements in the United States, England, and Europe. In such structures individual decisions would not be the determinants of social policies, but the reverse would hold, and some may argue that the new eugenics supports such an ordering.

Why should one hold to the pragmatic principle that individual human experience should be the principal basis for choices and social policies? This is no simple question, and it cannot be answered adequately in a short chapter. However, the outlines of a pragmatic response are clear. First, one may recall James's arguments that it is better to believe in free will than not, even if one cannot prove it. I will not recount his argument, but will simply note that the belief in freedom of the will is more likely to result in persons taking responsibility for their actions. If the evidence for and against free choice is not decisive, believing in free will is the better option leading to better results.

Second, the new genetics brings a twist to the question of individual freedom that needs to be sorted out and also promises considerable advances in understanding human action. It is a double twist that places greater weight on human responsibility than on human freedom and highlights the question of how responsible human beings are fostered by society. Earlier these issues had a different form. Responsibility was viewed as resulting from free will, a will not determined by antecedent conditions. But, as we learn more about the causes of complex human actions, there appear to be few alternatives but to consider all actions as natural results of forces within us, our environment, and our culture.

Previously many of the questions concerning the individual and society were approached from the metaphysical certainty that individuals formed societies, and the principal problem was to explain why they did so. Within the new genetics and the evolutionary studies of human behavior, individuals with heritable traits are seen as being generated within a society and an environment, and the difficult question is why only some individuals are responsible persons in their environment and their culture. That is, previously the fundamental question seemed to be why individuals created societies, and now the fundamental question is how individuals are created within societies.

Each of these issues has a long intellectual history. In terms of freedom, many scholars have noted that the question is not whether individual actions are caused, but what is their cause. Surely persons are causal forces in the world, and the extent to which one's own nature causes actions will play a significant role in determining whether an action is considered free or not.

However, in an odd sort of way, even if the notion of freedom is reconsidered or some notion of it abandoned as no longer tenable, this will not remove our responsibility for actions. If I know that rearing children in a hostile and harsh environment is likely to have detrimental effects, that knowledge makes me more responsible for raising children in a certain way than if I did not have the knowledge. If I know that many complex human actions are shaped by our genotypes in concert with the environment, that knowledge places a serious weight of responsibility on my shoulders for shaping genotype, environment, and culture so that humans flourish.

This is a responsibility that other generations did not have, at least not in the sense that we do, because we now have strong evidence for this belief. Hence, if a notion of freedom that relied heavily on some mysterious, nonnatural cause is eventually abandoned, that may only increase our responsibility for our actions, particularly if individuals are viewed as causal forces bringing about changes within our environment and our culture. And we may be helped in this matter by other advances in understanding human development in the areas of biochemistry, evolutionary studies, and the social sciences.

Ironically and dramatically, the genetic focus on human commonality highlights the issue of how responsible individuals are cultivated. There is no question that individuals come from societies, coming into the world with heritable traits waiting to shape their lives and environment, and also waiting to be shaped by the environment. The biological and societal commonality of humans—of all living cells, for that matter—is the given. But why do some individuals become responsible and productive persons, whereas others do not? That may prove to be the driving question for the next level of understanding human development, and the pragmatic principle of common sense and the common good may well be our best guide.

In summary, pragmatism advises us (1) to not overlook the complexity of the interplay between genotype, environment, and culture, (2) to pursue not only the genetic base for complex human actions, but also the environmental and cultural forces, (3) to focus on the responsibility of ameliorating the human condition by intelligently utilizing scientific and cultural knowledge, and (4) to redirect current research to understanding the development of responsible individuals within the biological and social commonalities.

Pragmatism and Parents

Perhaps the most difficult issues raised by the new genetics are those facing parents. If our knowledge of genotypes linked to heritable traits is increasing significantly, how should parents use that information? The selective process of finding a compatible mate previously seemed to be a social function largely bound by one's economic and social status, loosely described in external characteristics: personality, beauty and charm, apparent initiative and intelligence, and so on.

But the slightest piece of cellular material or bodily fluid can provide a far more detailed account of heritable traits and some assessment of possible futures for one's children as well as oneself. In the near future, mail-in tests or shopping-mall stores named Genes R Us will not have to exist for people with the economic means to gain far more information about their own genotype than any previous generation had. That information is likely to come with new technologies that will help shape the future lives of children—and the future lives of each succeeding generation.

Is this "playing God"? Yes, perhaps, but primarily it is taking the role of parenting seriously. If the means for determining many aspects of the future lives of one's children are available, do parents not have the obligation, within reason, to use those means and the results wisely? If I know I have a particular heritable trait that may dramatically harm or enhance the lives of my children, that knowledge carries a responsibility. But what am I to do with the responsibility?

Rather than enunciating a specific set of parental principles, the pragmatist normally resorts to accounts of the complexity and contingency of human knowledge, of the interplay between nature, culture, and environment that make it difficult, even impossible, to draw rigid guidelines or principles for parents to follow. Hence, on the pragmatic account one should minimize overreaching social policies that force parents and medical institutions into ironclad approaches, thereby leaving the door open for individual decisions and creative alternatives. If doing so leads to some results that are less than desirable, that is to be expected, but the overall results should be better. In order for parents to make the best decisions, they need information and an understanding of that information.

The pragmatist places great importance on the free flow of information, on education that equips individuals for intelligent action, and on the general belief that all individuals will seek the good of their children. For the pragmatist rationality is rooted in the desire to avoid harm, particularly harm to those closest and dearest to one. A significant corollary to this form of rationality is that it is embodied. It is not an abstract mental construction, but it is a rationality embodied in the physiology of the individual and in the relations of that individual with the environment, society, and culture.

Pragmatists realize that even if we have the proper information and understanding, the immense difficulties of making these decisions will not be lessened. Ironically, they will be greater. Certain traits will no longer result from random occurrences or be the products of uncaring fate; in the new genetics more and more characteristics will be subject to parental choices and parental care.

Genetic counselors know the difficult decisions parents make, particularly when their decisions are based on partial knowledge of their own heritable traits and on partial understanding of the probabilities that these traits will be passed to future generations. Guilt, concern, and control are all issues, but fragmentary scientific knowledge coupled with the difficulty of understanding and acting on complex mathematical probabilities weakens the foundation of all such decisions. In the past we have been surprised when "good" parents have sometimes had "bad" children or when a genetic malady suddenly appeared in a family with no known historical pedigree for it. Now parents may have more responsibility for knowing their own heritable traits and for doing what they can not to harm their children's futures and, if possible, to enhance them.

Obviously there will be many difficulties with parents' having these responsibilities—and not merely the difficulties of having to make such important decisions. Think of the expectations that will be placed on a child if the parents have taken all precautions to raise a bright, personable, productive individual. But what if the child does not meet these expectations? Already parents sometimes have very high expectations of their children based on what may soon appear to be surface evidence. Sending children to the best schools with expectations of high achievement does not always work out, and parents and children experience not only disappointment because of these pressures, but also serious harm that can last a lifetime.

One can assume that the potential for harm will increase as we take more responsibility for the traits and behavior patterns of our children. If children's personalities and behavioral traits could truly be engineered, imagine what remarkable expectations we would have of our future generations. However, one must also consider the alternative of ignoring the opportunities and responsibilities of the new genetics. If we do so, are the results likely to be better or less problematic? The answer is no.

In summation, pragmatism suggests that parents (1) should not be bound by ideological approaches to parenting or to moral decisions, (2) should get genetic information and wisely use it in shaping their lives and that of their children, and (3) should accept responsibility not only for wisely using the new genetics, but also for shaping our society and environment so that future generations may flourish.

Rigid ideological approaches to human reproduction and the development of responsible individuals are not likely to match the difficulty or complexity of the actual circumstances of human life. Embodied within each of us are habits and a heritage that have been tested since the arrival of the human species. Each newborn child is the leading edge of generations of ancestors, possessing some heritable traits from his or her lineage and some newly recombined chromosomal formations. Each child develops, grows, and dies, leaving his or her own legacy, usually including the transmission of genotypes to future generations. Narrow and doctrinaire approaches to child rearing and morality are unlikely to match the complexity and creativity of this long-standing natural process.

Choices concerning the new genetics are unlikely to be altogether clear cut, and some parents will be more adventurous, while others will take a more cautious path. The likelihood that either approach will be entirely correct is small. Hence, pragmatism suggests that parents learn as much as they can about the influences on themselves and on their children and make the best decision possible in the context of that complexity.

Gathering information will not be enough; one also needs to be able to understand the information, interpret it, and use it. Education will play the most obvious role by enabling individuals to make wise decisions based on the evidence available. Even if much of the evidence is incomplete, based on mathematical probabilities, and difficult to decipher because of medical and scientific jargon, parental responsibility will not be lessened, but rather will be increased simply because greater knowledge carries greater responsibility. Coupled with the responsibility to understanding the important implications of the new genetics will be the obligation to shape and structure society and the environment so that future generations can flourish. Genetic information may be of basic help in this endeavor, but an appreciation of the way human life is structured by social, cultural, and environmental influences will be equally important.

Pragmatism and Social Policy

Just as no specific principles for parents are entailed by the pragmatist approach, it provides no ironclad guidelines for social policy. Although the pragmatist focus is on educating individuals for intelligent action, that clearly is not enough. Socially we raise our children in a caring, trusting environment, even teaching them myths such as that of a white-bearded jolly gentleman who brings presents to good children at the winter solstice. But part of becoming an adult is to understand that the world is not entirely populated by people who have a loving interest in children's well-being.

There are people who have little capacity for caring and who, worse yet, enjoy bringing pain to others, even their own children. Some of these individuals are locked up, and some are not. Furthermore, there are individuals whose cognitive capacities lessen their responsibilities. There are also groups of people—hate groups, cults, and sects—with such narrow interests that the good of those beyond their interests is not to be calculated. Fanaticism of all kinds narrows the perspective of caring to a small, mean domain. In addition, not all family structures are caring and supportive of children. Today the myth of the nuclear family is widespread, particularly in the United States, but there is substantial evidence that many families are quite harmful to the future lives of their children.

Hence, social limits must be placed on individual decisions, because not all individual decisions are equal. But what those limits should be is not easy to determine, particularly regarding the new genetics. The United States continues to set severe limits and prohibitions on embryo and fetal research. Should those limitations be expanded and applied to genetic research? Should parents have the right to full knowledge of their own genotype and that of their children? Should there be limits on the actions parents can take based on such knowledge? Must medical institutions provide not only genetic information, but also the services requested by parents?

One does not have to recall the difficulties of the abortion issue to imagine the difficulties likely to develop with the new technologies and information that will be available following the completion of the Human Genome Project.[7] The patenting of DNA products already is raising remarkably difficult social issues concerning business interest in agricultural life, and one can imagine what may lie ahead regarding human life.

Pragmatism has no ready solutions to these issues and counsels against following anyone who does. Education, care in fostering the development of our children, and securing a safe environment and a nurturing society are all goals of pragmatism. A principal pragmatic tenet is that social decisions should be made by those who will be most affected by such decisions; that is, individuals should decide for themselves, and parents should be permitted the greatest latitude possible to make important decisions about the future lives of their children while still maintaining a stable society and healthy environment.[8]

The Limitations of Pragmatism

Briefly and without the benefit of a lengthy treatise, I have argued that pragmatism provides some of the best criteria for understanding genetic explanations of human traits and behavior, for aiding parents in making decisions about the future lives of their children, and for guiding social policies. However, although pragmatism may be our best hope, it has serious limitations. One obvious limitation is the lack of specificity of its recommendations; this is a genuine weakness if one is looking for absolutes or guidelines not subject to wear and tear.

Normally the pragmatist will argue that specificity will be supplied by the circumstances. Besides, in this case we are anticipating new circumstances and therefore cannot provide the particulars as yet. Genetic counselors, researchers on the Human Genome Project, hospital ethics committees, and parents are presently making specific decisions regarding particular issues, and as these become larger societal issues, we are likely to find governmental, educational, medical, and other societal institutions developing specific guidelines, much as was done at the beginning of the genome project. Although the lack of specificity may be a weakness of the pragmatist's approach to the new issues that are arising, the pragmatist also sees it as a strength that will permit adaptability and creativity.

But there is another limitation that may be more serious. Pragmatism may be entirely wrong. By emphasizing the priority of the good over truth, pragmatism opens the door to fictions that bring good results until confronted by the reality of the natural world, a world that has no central focus or concern for human experience. One is reminded of the account—by Nietzsche, I believe—of the contented cows that spend their lives placidly in a pasture; each day food and shelter are provided as needed, until the day comes when the cows are taken to the slaughterhouse. The cows did not know of the undercurrents in the social and economic structures that shaped their lives.

For several millennia we humans were in the same boat, realizing only recently that the most basic threats to human existence are not social structures and wars, but microorganisms that undermine the very basis of human life through disease and death. Now we are learning more about the genetic base of our lives, but this is a small piece of knowledge in an ocean of living beings. Human experience seems a slight matter in the remarkable natural history of the development of the living universe and of the process that structures genetic development. Perhaps, like the cows, we know little of an impending, uncaring, natural evolution or doom that awaits us. We may be in complete error if we assume we have control over our fate in any fundamental way, and particularly if we assume that human intelligence is equal to any dilemma, natural or social, that may confront our species.

Even so, the pragmatist argues that since such events are beyond our control and current experience, we need not be concerned. If we are doomed to a microorganic cataclysm, it would be better to live as if we were not, as if our actions and choices mattered, as if the future were in our hands. This is certainly correct. But one may hope that if one enlarges the pragmatic perspective by playing down the centrality of human experience and individualism, both humility and joy will be the resulting human trait. And these two traits, which are not common characteristics of pragmatism, could serve as a corrective to the task-oriented and sometimes joyless pragmatic accounts of the human condition.

The do-good and constant-improvement orientation of pragmatism seem to portray one unending task after another as the human dilemma, leaving little room for play, enjoyment, and delight in the moment, art, or pleasure. The philosophy of Santayana, more than any of the classical American thinkers, seems the best corrective to a pragmatism that was shaped by the task-oriented capitalism of the past two centuries. He thought that there are many tasks at hand, and some things are genuinely in our control, but one principal goal of life is not an endless succession of activities and moral tasks; it is to celebrate living and to enjoy our children.

All our hopes of shaping the future may be an illusion, but the aesthetic delight of being alive is real. It is one of the most humbling and joyful experiences of our species, whether we understand it or not. In fact, in terms of the quality of life, experiencing the joy of life is more important than understanding it (to paraphrase Santayana's thoughts on the nature of beauty). One hopes the new genetics provides us with a better understanding of aesthetic delight in our lives and that of future generations. If it does not, so much the worse for the new genetics and for pragmatism.

13 Genetic Enhancement of Families

GLENN MCGEE

LATELY IT SEEMS a whole commercial culture and social conversation have grown up around "enhancements." Some are quite controversial: Prozac and other antidepressants have been increasingly reported to be performance enhancers, and, as Peter Kramer points out, are even prescribed for that purpose.[1] Lawrence Difler's recent essay highlights an increase in enhancement-based rationale for use of the stimulant Ritalin, originally prescribed to combat attention deficit disorder.[2] Some enhancements only barely raise our collective ire, such as the now well-established use of cosmetic surgery to modify appearance, the selection of offspring gender, or the sale of "genius" gametes by one California sperm bank. Still others seem uncontroversial or seem not to count as enhancements at all, such as the use of private schools, vaccinations, and vitamin supplements.

Bioethicists have attempted to draw distinctions between enhancements and the conventional development of genetically determined potential, and to differentiate enhancement from restoration or therapy. In the former case, struggling for a rationale as to why cosmetic surgery is fundamentally different from and more objectionable than a new haircut, Kathy Davis argues that through cosmetic surgery patients attempt to change the kind of persons that they are.[3] In the latter case, Norman Daniels and others attempt to distinguish enhancement from therapy or restoration, developing an idea they term species-typical functioning. In an era of limited resources, species-typical functioning is the attempt to divine from aggregate medical data and data "in society a theoretical account of the design of the organism" that describes "the natural functional organization of a typical member of the species."[4] Bringing an organism to within species-typical parameters is therapy or restoration, whereas improving on those norms is enhancement.

Elsewhere I argue at length that attempts to distinguish between conventional development of potential and artificial enhancement rely on an outmoded account of human nature and of genetic causality, and that species-typical functioning misses the point that health and illness are experienced and defined in terms of their meaning in human social experience.[5] Parents and others engage in a variety of attempts to enhance human life, and the important differences between these enhancements seem tied to their social context. In this present chapter I focus on the ethical implications of genetic enhancement in parenting.

The reason for this focus is partially technological: Many current and proposed genetic services will be useful primarily, or first, in a reproductive context or for children. For example, most genetic tests have immediate implications for would-be parents. As tests, technologies, and gene therapies begin to move into the less conventional realm of improvement, parents will be the first to make choices about the best means and most appropriate ends of enhancement.

My reasoning is also personal. Parenthood can feel like a laboratory in enhancement. All of us with children experience the pressure to develop the life of an infant, a young person, a young adult. Children present themselves to us as so many interwoven needs: needs for support, for care, for attention. The struggle to parent feels like a perilous and wonderful dance as we balance the need to transmit and inculcate values and culture with the need to give children the freedom to define their own character. As we make choices about our children, we pick up some cultural lessons that work not only for mundane parental decision making, but also for the radical possibility of making, perhaps sooner than we think, some systematic choices about the enhancement of our children through genetic technologies.

It may turn out, in this quest for some social improvement, that genes are among the least effective tools for advancing personal, familial, and social goals. Technical failings in all previously initiated trials of gene therapy suggest that our powers to induce genetic modification have perhaps been exaggerated. Is it likely that even an effective genetic therapy would revamp the human species? Not especially. Nor is it likely, conversely, that altered genes will destroy our human nature. Conventional social institutions, such as schools and churches, have a much more immediate effect on who we become, and we "conventional" parents can botch up child making quite well without gene therapy.

There is plenty to be frightened about, though, when conversation turns to eugenics. The fear is not of genetic control, but of socially prescribed blueprints of perfection, enforced by intolerant scientists cum bureaucrats. We have seen the results in our own century, and can at least glean from the misadventures chronicled by Daniel Kevles and others that a scientifically styled "perfect society" stratified by genes makes little sense in a world in which genetic variability turns out to be a virtue—and in which specialization and rigidity spell extinction.[6] There are also plenty of practical examples of the danger of replacing parental responsibility with overarching social control.[7]

How, then, can we put history's lessons to work in making responsible use of our social aim of improvement? First, we have to separate the dreams of eugenics from the hopes of families. The quest to improve humanity is not mere aberration, the deluded dream of social engineers. The *Newsweek* description of perfection (tall, blonde, powerful, smart children, made to order) is shocking, in part, because it is lifted directly from fashion magazines and television. Our culture pursues notions of perfection in everything from eye color to weight to "swagger." We invest billions of dollars in the attempt to make people more intelligent and less aggressive.

We call this attempt public education. As with eugenics, the goal of education for children is to design and inculcate skills and norms in the behaviors of offspring, from sexual mores through beliefs about history to respect for the law. Athletic activity and school lunches are designed so that children will grow up to be stronger, more capable, and smarter. Those who do not perform well in school are "failed" and miss out on college, better-paying work, or social success. That families and the social order should abandon the aim of improving children is unthinkable. Libraries, nutritional and environmental regulations, and the matrix of social and political institutions we have crafted testify to the importance of this goal.

Because we make big social blunders, our programs, visionary plans, and political ambitions often do not provide the "new world order" that is promised. Great plans for our children's futures can also be doomed by shortsightedness, avarice, and cowardice, or merely turn out to be unworkable or inapplicable to environmental and cultural conditions. Nonetheless, the hope for continuing improvement, "making the world better for our children," remains central to human progress and is present in the rhetoric of markets, politics, religion, and even medicine. We learn from our mistakes and work for a better future. Therefore, the deadly and not-so-deadly sins[8] we need to avoid along the road to enhancement are not all related to genes, test tubes, or the Nazis. The five I explore here are instead sins we learn to avoid as parents and social stewards: the sins of calculativeness, overbearingness, shortsightedness, hasty judgment, and pessimism.

The Sin of Calculativeness

Consider, for a moment, your memories of childhood. Parents (or guardians) send children thousands of messages about appropriate behavior, communicating their hopes and fears. Some give an inordinate amount of advice and counseling.[9] Some even set up elaborate systems of rules and procedures to instill certain habits and values. You might have been awarded two dollars for mowing the lawn, cleaning your room, and washing the dishes. You might have lost your driving or entertaining privileges for misbehaving. These thoughtful, organized systems provide a network of beliefs and structure a child's developmental environment. But they are not the whole experience of being a child.

In fact, you may have learned much more from the character, rules, and goals of your parents by watching what they in fact did than by obeying or disobeying the rules that they set for you. Or the most vital and formative experiences of your childhood may not have had anything at all to do with the detailed plans that your parents agonized over. A brief, unpredictable outburst from a parent may outweigh years of regimented education. The sudden death of a grandparent or parent may change the entire family ethos. We commit the sin of calculativeness when we overemphasize the importance of planning and systematic choices in parenthood.

Like most sins, calculativeness is as much impractical as it is immoral. It is extraordinarily difficult to know what actions and words will register in the minds of our children. How will the whole package fit together: the way we treat them, the food we feed them, the genes we give them, and the rules we set for them? The most complex and sophisticated plans for a child's future can turn out to be the least effective, and we may send messages that are much more mixed than we know.

At times we cannot even be sure what we want for (and from) our children. Children can be instruments in our own efforts to work out our childhood insecurities, ambitions, and fears. Our own frustrated efforts to get to Harvard may become our children's yoke. The abuse of a father becomes a son's abuse of his own child. The approval of friends and neighbors can influence the way that we dress and teach our children. Parents can effortlessly create tortuous paradigms that children are expected to live up to.

Our beliefs about the "perfection" of our expected children may be much simpler or grander than we can articulate. The hopeful, infertile couple who expresses the fervent wish for any biological child, saying,

"All we want is a healthy baby," may not be fully conscious of the reasons why they seek not only health, but also biological relation. A father who spends weeks teaching baseball to his son might actually prefer (at some deeper and more inarticulate level) that he and his son be able to have a nice conversation or share a common goal. Because parenting is subtle, sophisticated, and enormously complicated, it is not at all surprising that parents should be unaware of our own motivations—or even that we should act in ways contrary to our deeply held desires. Parenting habits are as complex as any human patterns of behavior, and they can be malleable or rigid, conscientious or the thoughtless repetition of our own parents' behaviors.

Though genetic tests and therapies may not have the capacity to advance the intelligence and attractiveness of our children, faith in the efficacy of genetic technologies could lead parents to deemphasize important parts of parental responsibility. In addition, a faith in genetic modification of offspring could encourage the emphasis by parents of narrow, artificially defined traits. Parents could have hopes of transmitting, in a simple and systematic way, all of the currently fashionable traits to their children, relying on the common images of "perfection" in the public. These images of perfection are not taken from the dreams of dictators or from science fiction novels. They are present in advertisements, polls, television programs, and movies.[10] Based on the images in *Cosmopolitan* or *Men's Health,* the "perfect" male baby would grow to be six feet tall, 185 pounds, and disease free. His IQ would be 150, and he would have special aptitudes in biomedical science. He would have blonde hair and blue eyes. He would be aggressive and could play NFL football, NHL hockey, and NBA basketball, but would also enjoy poetry and fine wine.

The parent who might opts for such systematic control over the creation of a child puts faith in the ability of "genetic parenthood" to create a child that has particular traits. The more ordinary ways of parenting offer no such systematic options. The hereditary possibilities available with "conventional" parenthood revolve around a mixture of similarities (traits already in our family) over which we have little control. We may ask, "Will our baby have my ears or hers? Our toes?" We do not know, and we have little control over the answer. By contrast, genetic parenthood seems to offer a different kind of control. Using this option parents could utterly abandon similarities, replacing them with choices that were reasoned in advance. If we thought that we could systematically impart to a child an IQ of 150 instead of whatever mental traits we carry, we might opt to change our hereditary gift.

The "sin" of making these calculated choices would not be rooted in the idea that they might actually work, giving our children IQs of 150 or the appearance of gods. That much is unlikely to emerge from the polymerase chain reaction, gene splicing, and vector technology of 1998, and it may be conceptually impossible for reasons we described above. The sin would be in understanding a child to be the result of systematic choices, and thus allowing genetic choices to define the child's telos. The faith that genetic enhancements can alter character (removing homosexuality or increasing thoughtfulness, for instance) could lend itself to a parenthood of oppressive control. Parents who choose traits as calculative consumers might come to devalue the essential connections of relatedness and sameness in the family relationship.

Though it may not be articulated in the fashion of our day, parents also want their children to be like themselves. This is evidenced by the celebration of every child as a "perfect" child, beautiful and appropriate exactly because it represents the particular union of two particular people.[11] We share names and houses and values with our children, as well as important biological and cultural habits. The essential fact of this sharing is not its biological element. Adoptive parents also appreciate similarities in their children, and secure it through familial patterns of values transmission. The sharing of similarities among members of a family could be diluted by genetic choices. A parent who is expecting a "brilliant child" could value that child only for his or her accomplishments rather than for the child's struggles and growth.

One of the problems of our calculativeness has to do with efficacy: Whatever our social goals, the likelihood of achieving them through genetic interventions would—or should—include calculations about how best to spend our money. The propensity to use genetic interventions should then be measured against other means of achieving our social goals. In the case of intelligence, it is amazing that we are willing to spend millions of dollars on the search for genes that code for calculative efficiency, whereas Head Start programs go unfunded, teachers are underpaid and overworked, and even smart children graduate ill prepared for the job market and uninspired by democracy.

The Sin of Being Overbearing

Hans Jonas and Joel Feinberg refer to a child's right to be open to as much freedom of identity as possible. They fear that genetic engineering, by stylizing children along the lines of rigid parental expectations, could steal this right. Children would be born into a world in which their ultimate choices had been made by parents before their birth. Although Jonas's fear hinges, in part, on the power of genetics to accomplish this feat, his insistence on children's continuing need for freedom is important. Genetic expectations, as noted earlier, could carry tremendous weight, as parents might hope that children would become the sort of persons they had engineered. Already parents who have used in vitro fertilization technologies to implant embryos with the sperm of especially intelligent, artistic, or athletic donors have expressed expectations of greatness from such children, insisting on constant study, endless piano lessons, or daily tennis practice.

How can we distinguish between responsible hopes and overbearing ambitions in reproductive enhancement? A pragmatic answer begins with the recognition of the essential continuity between hopes connected to genetic engineering and everyday hopes. The parent who wants a daughter who is a beautiful ballerina will want one whether or not genetic technologies are in the picture. Likewise, parents whose guiding motivation is that their children find and pursue some kind of flourishing will be reluctant to use genetic improvements or conventional means of overdetermining identity through reproduction.

The decisions of parenthood are not always explicit, and they are made in a social context, so that parents are constantly exposed to suggestions from all quarters about the kinds of babies that are "good." Fortunately, there are also extensive pressures in society for the maintenance of randomness and the celebration of hereditary difference. The sentiment that each baby is perfect conveys this pressure, as does the choice many parents make to refuse unnecessary ultrasound exams, waiting to know a baby's gender until birth.

We have to emphasize the responsibility that comes with new information before we spill it onto the table and write it into the chart. Parents must ask themselves regarding each new test and procedure, "Why do I want to know about X?" Honest answers may turn up more than parental curiosity. If tests for gender, intelligence, and other traits cultivate a parental mentality in which traits take center stage, it will pay to consider the danger of such planning and expectations. However, as J. S. Mill, William James, and Derek Parfit have made so plain, there must be tolerance of different ways of approaching human natures. Whenever tests and procedures will not compromise a child, plural approaches to genetic modification must be allowed. No single simple solution will work. It makes no sense—and is generally counterproductive—to issue wholesale policy restrictions of any genetic research that is positive or enhancing in character.

Experiments in biological engineering must be tempered by respect for diversity and for each individual child. Overbearing parents can reduce a child to an instrument of their own ambitions or insecurities. This is no more appropriate when exercised through genetic technologies than when implemented by a parent who insists that a child accompany him to Klan meetings or refuse appropriate medical treatment in the name of religious beliefs a child cannot endorse. Children must be allowed to imagine and grow, and the balance to be struck is between instilling the values that parents hold and allowing the growth that could pull children away from those values. The desire for sameness can be a crippling expression of parental ego, just as the desire for a fashionably beautiful child can express self-loathing in the parent. The key is to avoid extreme measures through biological or any other means, and to temper decisions made before birth with the recognition that every child has a right to make some decisions about his or her own identity.

The Sin of Shortsightedness

As much as we plan for and anticipate the future, we cannot be sure what our children should or will become. We simply cannot anticipate the world of tomorrow. Within the past decade an empire has been destroyed, Europe has formed an economic alliance, genetic testing has been developed, and computer speed has increased ten thousand–fold. Economic and political prophets failed to predict a major market crash, the United States went to war with a third-world country, and a U.S. physician began an assisted suicide service. Fashions have changed, as have language, science, philosophy, psychology, and secondary education. Our heroes have also changed: Alan Alda was in, but now he is out; George Bush moved from an 80 percent to 34 percent approval rating in less than a year. What will the next decade—a mere ten years in the life of a child—hold in store? If anyone thinks he or she knows, odds are that person has a shortsightedness problem. This is fine unless it becomes the basis for designing that person's descendants.

One advantage of the conventional uncertainties in parenting is that just about all of our rules and practices can be changed to fit the exigencies of a changing world. For example, business schools grew to their apex during the early 1980s, then began to shrink as fewer employers recruited business majors. Savvy students quickly transferred from "entrepreneurship" fields into the humanities and environmental sciences. Parents with a stubborn, outmoded desire for a business school education for their children ended up with unemployed progeny or children on Prozac.

Younger children are even more malleable than college students, and infants will accept the most conditioning of all. A child is receptive to language, math, rules, values, and abstract ideas. If conditions change, a child adapts. One danger of genetic engineering for positive traits, then, is the sin of shortsightedness: How can we know which traits to lock in through genetics in a world where fashions fade quickly and rigidity is a disadvantage?

An intelligent approach will militate against hasty and acontextual decisions. Just as it is difficult to plan the inculcation of values and character in children, hard to know what action or word will register, so too is it difficult to single out characteristics that will make a child's life better. In the first edition of Mueller's *Out of the Night*, one of the most important treatises on eugenics, the geneticist favored breeding children who embodied the traits of Lenin and Marx. In his later lectures, he dropped Lenin for Descartes, Marx for Lincoln. Political currency plays a role in our notions of perfection.

When we examine the plans of contemporary genetic optimists for a gradual but total revision of human nature, what is most striking is their confidence that we already have the wisdom to select the best traits. Like Plato, writers such as Leroy Hood and Brian Stableford assume that human nature is immutable and determined prior to birth, so that genetic engineers have merely to figure out how to manipulate stable biological materials in order to accomplish wondrous things.[12] A human with scales and gills would help us to live in the sea, Stableford writes, where we would be able to exploit its unending resources. But to which oceans does Stableford refer? We have turned much of the sea into a colossal dump for industrial and commercial waste. How much would we have to give up to live in this deep, dark ocean? Why would we want to live there?

The description of genetic engineering as a one-stop shop for human improvement sometimes depends on wildly unrealistic political and scientific plans. Such grand schemes are not only difficult from a genetic standpoint; they can simply be icons of poorly thought-through political visions for human growth.

A parent who desires a smart child might actually be able at some point to increase the calculative speed of that child's brain. At present, scientists often compare the power of our minds to the power of computers. Computers are better when they are faster, so much of this research has focused on creating a faster brain. In ten years, though, we may learn that calculative speed is a hindrance to thoughtfulness, imagination, and vision. A child could thus be robbed of the ability to adapt, stuck with a trait that would hinder his or her ability to work with flexibility in the changing world—all the while trying to live up to parental expectations of brilliance.

Moreover, it is not always wise to assume that more of a good thing is better. Genetic diversity has tremendous value, because it provides the opportunity for those of many hereditary backgrounds to employ differing approaches toward maximization of the potential of a given environment. If dozens of children were created from the genes of an Einstein, would the world be a better place? Einstein was the product of a particular set of parents, experiences, and inspirations. In suburban Dallas as child of an oil baron, a cloned Einstein might as easily end up driving a truck or selling horizontal drilling rigs as becoming a brilliant physicist. He might live alone and homeless. Even with an optimal environment, young Clonestein might find that his progenitor's approach had been all but replaced by a different mode of analysis, as differing approaches to problems rendered his style of physics less capable of explanation and control in physics.

Just as it is important for parents to allow children to develop in individual ways, there is reason for parental plans to allow for a changing world. Highly directed parental ambitions for children, such as ambitions for success in a particular sport or with a particular musical instrument, can result in crushed hopes for parent and child. There are only so many slots on college and professional basketball teams, and not many will go to men who are five feet seven inches tall. Only one in a million musicians attends Julliard. It would be no advantage to choose male offspring, which most Americans report that they would, if suddenly 60 percent of live births were male.[13]

Children need support—not pressure—in pursuing their own dreams within the context of family and culture. Diffuse parental hopes are more appropriate than are focused ones. Children need to learn courage and self-esteem, and they need to be critical and functionally literate. They should have the support of their parents as they learn and grow.

The Sin of Hasty Judgment

In College Station, Texas, there are acres and acres of "test fields." In these fields the "Aggies" of Texas A&M University see to it that there are more hybridized and genetically engineered crops than in any other region on earth. It is here that the supertomato was first grown. Cantaloupes are genetically crossed with watermelons, and cows have been cloned and genetically modified in literally thousands of ways. College Station is also home to amazing new strains of disease, which began to thrive on these same new crops. Genetic engineering in agriculture has been a proving ground for the possibilities of modification of humans. The results are somewhat revealing: Genetically engineered fruits and vegetables are frequently much more vulnerable to diseases and parasites than are their "conventional" cousins, and they rarely taste as good as nonhybridized, nonengineered strains.[14] Engineering of plants and animals can also result in the transmission of dangerous materials into the human and animal food supply.

The perfect baby, like perfect soybeans and perfect corn, could turn out to be markedly imperfect. How difficult would it be to live an engineered life? Hans Jonas cautions us regarding the danger of freakish accidents in genetic engineering, of the kind discussed in Cambridge, Massachusetts, and at Asilomar.[15] Ironically, the more important accidents may be more likely to occur after the birth of an apparently healthy, improved baby. Although medical technologies could make alterations in the physical characteristics of a newborn, we can hardly hope for the viability of those traits in our complex world.

For example, wild strawberries have a much better chance of surviving against infection and parasites than engineered strawberries. The reason is that although genetic engineers controlled for particular traits, they could not control for the dozens of conditions that face a strawberry. Wild strawberries pack a variety of genetic habits, including resistances. These resistances help them to have stable interactions with a range of circumstances. A genetically engineered strawberry, on the other hand, is a hit-or-miss proposition, with engineering emphasis placed only on particular traits.

A child who was engineered to possess positive traits might end up suffering unexpected and disastrous ills. It is extremely dangerous to move too quickly in the direction of changing human traits lest we forget to control—or forget that we can not control—for the vast variety of human environmental conditions. Just as the gene that presumably causes sickle-cell anemia codes for resistance to malaria, the gene for sonar hearing might interfere with the genetic pattern that codes for opposable thumbs or sex organs. In a strawberry the sin of hasty judgment can lead to new diseases and bad-tasting fruit; in a human child this sin could have more complex results that would be catastrophic for the family.

There is also a more general point to be gleaned from our recent experience with agricultural engineering. The genetically enhanced tomato was delicious and tender when raised in lab conditions, but tasted rubbery in "real-life" conditions. Seedless watermelons also suffer from diminished flavor when removed from the laboratory. By analogy, imagine the beautiful, intelligent, even-tempered girl who might be developed by genetic engineering. Could she survive in an imperfect world with bad water and fatty foods? Would others hate or envy her? On paper, genetic engineering looks enticing. In practice, what makes one person more attractive or intelligent than other people is more random and depends on their quirks as well as their assets. A perfect child would find the world of imperfection, disease, disasters, and emotions deadly or unsatisfying.

A pragmatic approach urges more cautious progress toward improving humans. Just as parents should promote malleability in their parenting, there must be room for imperfections and developmental choices. The child who is genetically crafted to resemble 1997's models of perfection may find the world of 2014 intolerable. Instead, parents should aim to continue to update their style of parenting to match the demands of natural and social conditions.

This means that some modifications may indeed become advisable, but only on condition of reversibility. However, we would want to insist on the reversibility of the modification and to carefully examine its side effects prior to clinical trials.

The Sin of Pessimism

In his essay "The Moral Equivalent of War," William James argued that although war is to be avoided at all costs, humans seem to need to exercise aggression and domination during their lives.[16] He termed the channeling of these powerful impulses into other activities "the moral equivalent of war." The notion of moral equivalency is useful here. Reproductive genetic enhancement may present new choices, but these choices are suffused with the "moral equivalence" of activities already present in the context of parenthood. The moral dominion of parenthood creates the context for reproductive genetic interventions. Therefore, while exercising caution is intelligent, we need not treat genetics as a radically different endeavor, a slippery slope to biological castles and Frankenstein.

The categorical opponents of genetic enhancement, Paul Ramsey and Jeremy Rifkin being the most notable, have developed rigid rules to enforce the sanctity of human genetic coding.[17] Such an ethic does little to guide our actions; it is simply naive in the light of other social pressures to apply scientific results, obtain improvements in life, and have healthy children. Ethics cannot ignore science: The problem with putting the values that are present in our culture to use in our culture is that those values can sometimes be, as John Dewey said, "undermined by the conclusions of modern science."[18]

We also would do well to consider Dewey's charge that "if intelligent method is lacking, prejudice, the pressure of immediate circumstance, self-interest and class interest, traditional customs, institutions of accidental historical origin, are not lacking, and they tend to take the place of intelligence."[19] For example, the few fetal diagnoses available now are so expensive that only the wealthy use them. As a consequence, a disproportionate number of children with Down's syndrome are "almost certainly born to the less affluent."[20]

Our claim that some eugenic selection is already present in social engineering intimates another danger, then, of uncritical genetic research: It may be engineering that benefits only the powerful and wealthy. If society chooses not to concern itself with reproductive enhancement, we make a choice: to leave science to the scientists and its application to political pressure and happenstance. Consider the application of genetic research in its political and economic context: Where there are therapies, there will always be pressures on a physician to offer them. The day that a gene for homosexuality is announced, it will be too late for bioethics to put a "spin" on whether or not that gene is useful. Bioethicists need to join the conversation about appropriate research before it becomes technology.

If pessimism is sinful, though, abject optimism is not its antidote. Even assuming that certain isolable ailments could be dealt with by genetic engineering, the approach to avoiding the not-so-deadly sins must be intelligent and cautious; we must work toward developing protocols and therapies experimentally and gradually. This approach takes seriously the caution implicit in the hands-off attitude of those who would leave genetics to nature without surrendering the hope to make our condition and our nature better a little at a time.

Social conversation concerning the enhancement of children is possible, and technological advancement is desirable in pediatrics. First, though, bloethicists' conversation about expensive and sophisticated genetic technologies must be connected to public conversations about parenthood. This requires us to abandon the search for an exotic ethics of enhancement and get our hands dirty in the mundane world of the ordinary parents who will make decisions about genetic interventions and the meaning of growth and flourishing in the family and the community.

14 Pragmatism and the Determination of Death

MARTIN BENJAMIN

The individual has a stock of old opinions already, but he meets a new experience that puts them to a strain. . . . The result is an inward trouble to which his mind till then had been a stranger, and from which he seeks to escape by modifying his previous mass of opinions. He saves as much of it as he can, for in this matter of belief we are all extreme conservatives.
William James[1]

What serious men not engaged in the professional business of philosophy most want to know is what modifications and abandonments of intellectual inheritance are required by the newer industrial, political, and scientific movements. They want to know what these newer movements mean when translated into general ideas. Unless professional philosophy can mobilize itself sufficiently to assist in this clarification and redirection of men's thoughts, it is likely to get more and more sidetracked from the main currents of contemporary life.
John Dewey[2]

RECENT DEBATES over the determination of death illustrate these observations by James and Dewey. From about 1850 to the 1960s there was general agreement about the determination of death. An individual was pronounced dead when breathing and heartbeat had permanently ceased. In the mid-1960s, however, advances in medical knowledge and technology were enabling physicians to maintain respiration and circulation in patients with total loss of brain function. This new experience, in James's words, together with the development of organ transplantation, was placing considerable strain on our old opinions about the determination of death. The result was an inward trouble of mind from which physicians sought to escape by modifying our previous mass of opinions. This modification—declaring patients with heartbeat and respiration but total loss of brain function dead—saved as much of the previous mass of opinions as possible, confirming James's observation that "in this matter of belief we are all extreme conservatives."

Yet the change has not remained stable. Debate over the so-called definition of death continues to this day. An explanation is suggested by the passage from Dewey. Adopting new criteria for death required certain modifications and abandonments of intellectual inheritance that were not at the time adequately considered. Those in the forefront of change gave insufficient attention to the philosophical question of what these modifications and abandonments meant when translated into general ideas. This question ranged beyond the more-or-less immediate practical concerns of physicians. Therefore, to adapt Dewey's words, *until* serious men (and women) not engaged in the professional business of philosophy attend fully to the philosophical dimensions of the determination of death—and *until* professional philosophers adequately assist in this clarification and redirection of their thoughts—the debate is likely to continue.

In what follows, I develop this suggestion. I begin by explaining the controversy over the determination of death. Then I identify the general ideas—the possible modifications and abandonments of intellectual inheritance—at stake in the debate. I conclude by proposing a clarification and redirection of our understanding of the determination of death and defend it on pragmatic grounds.

Background

In the not-so-distant past, respiration and circulation were considered the principal signs of human life, and their cessation was considered the mark of death. Individuals were pronounced dead when they had permanently stopped breathing or their hearts had stopped beating. In the mid-1960s, however, developments in mechanical respiration (together with related supportive measures) gave physicians the capacity to maintain respiration and circulation in patients who had undergone total and permanent loss of brain function. Such patients—patients who were totally and permanently unconscious—were, according to the prevailing criteria, living human beings.

In 1968 a landmark article published by an ad hoc committee of the Harvard Medical School identified reliable clinical criteria for identifying respirator-dependent patients who have lost *all* brain functions, including primitive brain stem reflexes.[3] Patients satisfying these criteria, the committee said, were in "irreversible coma." The committee then proposed that patients in irreversible coma be declared dead and removed from the respirator. The publication of this article gave currency to the misleading term *brain death*.

Brain death, in the first and most literal sense, means the death of an organ, the brain. But death of an organ is one thing, and death of the organism of which it is a part quite another. Yet the term soon came to be used to refer to the latter as well. That is, a patient pronounced dead by use of the so-called Harvard criteria for irreversible coma was often said to be brain dead. The result was a misleading impression that there were now two kinds of death—ordinary (heart-lung) death and brain death.

The confusion may be avoided by scrupulously restricting the expression *brain death* to the death of the brain and using the term *brain criteria* to refer to the criteria for pronouncing a respirator-dependent patient with absolutely no brain function dead. Such a patient should be considered dead in the same way—and for the same reasons—as a patient whose heartbeat and respiration have permanently ceased. This important clarification, however, required taking account of certain philosophical considerations that in the late 1960s were given insufficient attention.

The motivation for the Harvard ad hoc committee's recommendation that irreversible coma (or the death of the brain) be accepted as a criterion for determining the death of the patient was clinical, not philosophical. First, the increasing number of respirator-dependent patients who met the Harvard criteria was becoming a burden on limited medical, technological, and financial resources. This seemed wasteful insofar as physicians believed such patients could no longer benefit from treatment. Second, the development of organ transplantation was increasing the demand for kidneys, hearts, and other organs. Transplant surgeons wanted permission to remove healthy organs from irreversibly comatose respirator-dependent patients without being accused of murder. And third, waiting to pronounce such patients dead according to traditional heart-lung criteria prolonged the limbolike status—and related emotional costs—of friends and family members awaiting the inevitable.

After publication of the Harvard criteria, states began reconsidering their statutes on death. By 1980 twenty-four states had incorporated brain criteria. Then in 1981 a presidential commission undertook a comprehensive review of the "medical, legal, and ethical issues in the determination of death." The commission eventually endorsed brain criteria and, together with the American Medical Association and the American Bar Association, recommended adoption by all states of a model statute, the Uniform Determination of Death Act (UDDA):

An individual who has sustained either (1) irreversible cessation of circulatory and respiratory functions or (2) irreversible cessation of all functions of the entire brain, including the brain stem, is dead. A determination of death must be made in accordance with accepted medical standards.[4]

Brain criteria for the determination of death have now been incorporated into the law of most states. Health professionals, lawyers, legislators, and the public generally agree that a patient who has lost all brain function is, despite respirator-assisted breathing and heartbeat, dead.

Continuing Controversy

Yet the debate has not ended. As specified by the UDDA, the new criteria require "irreversible cessation of *all* functions of the *entire* brain, *including the brain stem*" (my emphasis). But beginning with the case of Karen Ann Quinlan in 1976, the condition now dubbed a persistent vegetative state (PVS) has become both more prevalent and widely known. Patients in a vegetative state are unconscious because the parts of the brain necessary for thought and consciousness are no longer functioning. The state becomes permanent when it becomes irreversible.[5]

Such patients are totally and permanently unconscious. Yet they do not satisfy the current criteria for death; they have not lost *all* brain function. Because their brain stems continue to function and because the brain stem can regulate respiration, blood pressure, and a number of other vegetative functions, in the absence of cerebral function patients in a persistent vegetative state are often able to breathe and maintain their heartbeat without the assistance of a respirator.

Are such patients living or dead? According to the law, they are alive. The general criteria for death proposed by the Harvard ad hoc committee, endorsed by the president's commission, and adopted by the states explicitly require the permanent loss of *all* function of the brain, *including the brain stem*—and patients in a permanent vegetative state have functioning brain stems. But a number of bioethicists have recommended that such patients be pronounced dead[6]. Total and permanent loss of consciousness—and not total and permanent loss of *all* brain function, these bioethicists maintain—is what marks the line between human life and death.

The controversy is usually characterized as a debate over the definition of death. Defenders of the status quo are said to accept a "whole-brain" definition of death, while their opponents propose we adopt a "higher-brain" definition. This characterization is, however, misleading.

The disagreement does not center on definition, but rather on what Dewey described as the "general ideas" underlying the "modifications and abandonments of intellectual inheritance" required by a "new scientific movement." The new scientific movement is, in this instance, the capacity to diagnose total and permanent loss of consciousness in patients for whom respiration and heartbeat may be medically maintained (in some cases, for over thirty years). The underlying general idea is whether being alive is, for the likes of you and me, solely a matter of biology or whether it also involves consciousness (or the potential for consciousness). This is a philosophical question, not simply a matter of definition.

The Main Question

We have no trouble understanding what people mean when they speak or write of the death of a human embryo, a lawn, a dog, a language, or an entire culture. In each case the entity to which the word *dead* (or one of its cognates) is applied has ceased to exist as a thing *of that kind*. The conditions of existence and death of any entity—be it a human embryo, a lawn, a dog, a language, or a culture—are determined by the kind of thing that it is. "Death" is the cessation of life, a ceasing to be. When we are puzzled over what it means to say, "Karen Anne Quinlan is dead," the problem centers not on the meaning of *dead*, but rather on the entity to which we refer; exactly what *kind* of entity is it, and what are the conditions of its existence? Are we referring only to a human biological organism, or are we referring to something else, something whose conditions of existence include consciousness or at least the potential for consciousness?

The so-called definition-of-death debate, then, is really a debate over how we should conceive the individual subject to which the words *is dead* are applied. Exactly what is it that ceases to exist when we say someone like you or me is dead? This is the difficult, unavoidable philosophical question generated by the capacity of modern medicine to sustain respiration and heartbeat in patients who are totally and permanently unconscious.

We owe the misplaced emphasis on definition, I suspect, to the fact that the terms of the problem were set by those who first encountered and addressed it—members of the medical community. Clinicians are understandably more comfortable talking about definitions than they are about opposing philosophical conceptions of the human individual. But the philosophical questions are now unavoidable. What exactly is it that has lost life or ceased to be when we say that someone like you or me is dead? What is so important about whatever has been lost when we pronounce death to justify the enormous difference between our treatment of the living and the dead? These are not, on reflection, easy questions. And there may be no single answer to them that ought, at this time, to be embraced by all of us, insofar as we are informed and rational. Still, we will not reach closure on the determination of death until we can satisfactorily address them.

Death of the Organism as a Whole

Though the Harvard ad hoc committee did not address these questions, eleven years later the president's commission did. Essential to human life, the commission argued, is the integrated functioning of the circulatory system, the respiratory system, and the central nervous system:

Three organs—the heart, lungs, and brain—assume special significance . . . because their interrelationship is very close and the irreversible cessation of any one very quickly stops the other two and consequently halts the integrated functioning of the organism as a whole. Because they were easily measured, circulation and respiration were traditionally the basic "vital signs." But breathing and heartbeat are not life itself. They are simply used as signs—as one window for viewing a deeper and more complex reality: a triangle of interrelated systems with the brain at its apex.[7]

The subject of life and death is, then, the organism as a whole. The organism as a whole is alive when there is the integrated functioning of the circulatory, respiratory, and central nervous systems. The organism dies when the integrated functioning of these three systems is permanently disrupted. Permanent loss of any corner of the "triangle" soon leads to permanent loss of the other two.

According to the president's commission, then, adoption of brain criteria does not require a change in philosophical understanding. The subject of life and death has always been the organism as a whole, conceived as the integrating functioning of the circulatory, respiratory, and central nervous systems. Each set of criteria—heart-lung and brain—represents a different "window" for viewing the same state, death of the organism as a whole. "On this view," the commission wrote, "death is that moment at which the body's physiological system ceases to constitute an integrated whole. Even if life continues in individual cells or organs, life of the organism as a whole requires complex integration and without the latter, a person cannot properly be regarded as alive." The commission considered and explicitly rejected "higher-brain" criteria because, among other things, even if it could be shown that "higher" brain function is necessary for consciousness, the cessation of higher brain function "often cannot be assessed with the certainty that would be required in applying a statutory definition [of death]."[8]

Finally, the commission acknowledged with some pride that its proposal was "deliberately conservative." The UDDA incorporates legal recognition of a new way to diagnose death, but it does not put forth a new philosophical conception of death. Brain criteria identify the very same thing heart-lung criteria have traditionally identified—death of the organism as a whole. Therefore, in modifying our "old opinions" to accommodate a "new experience that put them to a strain," the commission sought to save as much of our "previous mass of opinions" as it could. "For in this matter of belief," as James put it, "we are all extreme conservatives."

Death of the Person

But, proponents of higher-brain criteria contend, the capacity to sustain biological life long after an individual becomes totally and permanently unconscious requires more extensive revision of our previous mass of opinions than the president's commission was willing to acknowledge. A "person"—where the word *person* designates the kind of being whose continued existence is generally of the utmost importance to us—may be dead even though the organism as a whole is alive.[9] What really matters to us, when we consider our own lives and the lives of others, is continued existence as persons, not continued existence as personless organisms.

Consider, for example, the following situation. In one part of a large urban hospital, infant Andrew is born with anencephaly. Anencephaly is a rare congenital condition marked by absence of a major portion of the brain, skull, and scalp. Anencephalic infants have functioning brain stems, but because they lack functioning cerebral hemispheres, they do not and never will experience any degree of consciousness. Andrew, though "alive" by current criteria, is totally and permanently unconscious. Without highly aggressive care, Andrew is likely to satisfy the UDDA's criteria for death within a few days, if not hours. Even with aggressive care, he is unlikely to live for more than a week or two.

In a nearby hospital lies infant Helen. Helen has hypoplastic left heart syndrome, a congenital malformation very likely to lead to an early death. Apart from her seriously defective heart, Helen is healthy. Though his brain is seriously defective, Andrew has a healthy heart. Suppose, as may in reality be the case, it is surgically possible to replace Helen's defective heart with Andrew's healthy one. Such an operation is likely to significantly extend Helen's life. The surgeon cannot, however, wait until Andrew is pronounced dead. By the time Andrew satisfies the current criteria for death, his heart will have seriously deteriorated. So the question is whether, if both Helen's and Andrew's parents give their informed consent, it would be wrong for a surgeon to remove Andrew's heart and transplant it to Helen.

If by "wrong" we mean illegal, the answer is clear. Under current law, removing Andrew's heart would be an act of murder. Andrew is a living human being, and the cause of death would be the surgeon's cutting into his chest and removing his heart. But is removing Andrew's heart to save Helen's life a significant moral wrong? Indeed, might it not be wrong not to do the operation—wrong not only for Helen and her parents, but also for Andrew's parents? How, if Andrew is totally and permanently unconscious, would he be wronged by removing his heart? Removing his heart will not cause him pain or suffering, nor will it deprive him of a valuable future. As far as pain or prospects for future experience go, Andrew is no different than any cadaver organ donor. Why, then, should it be okay to save a life by transplanting the heart of a patient who satisfies whole-brain criteria for death, but wrong to save a life by transplanting Andrew's heart?

The Council on Ethical and Judicial Affairs of the American Medical Association reports: "In a survey of leading medical experts in ethics, two thirds of those surveyed stated that they consider the use of organs from anencephalic infants 'intrinsically moral,' and more than half stated their support for a change in the law to permit such use."[10] I am inclined to agree; and when I ask why the law should be changed, the answer that springs to mind is that there is an important sense in which Andrew is already dead. Though Andrew is certainly a living human organism, something central to my understanding of the wrongness of killing is missing in this and similar cases.

Exactly what this is comes into sharper focus when we shift our consideration from an infant with anencephaly to a patient in a permanent vegetative state. Both anencephalic infants and patients in a permanent vegetative state are totally and permanently unconscious. The main difference is that total and permanent unconsciousness is congenital in the former and acquired in the latter. Therefore, if anencephalic infants are to be pronounced dead because they are totally and permanently unconscious, we shall have to do the same with patients in a permanent vegetative state. Is there good reason to consider these patients dead?

Imagine you have just been diagnosed with a terrible disease that will soon ravage your body and end your life. A surgeon then comes along who offers the possibility of a dramatic new operation guaranteed to stop the disease in its tracks. There is, however, one very serious side effect. The operation is very long and the anesthetic very powerful. One of the consequences is that, although the disease will be cured, you will emerge from the operation in a permanent vegetative state. But, the surgeon cheerfully emphasizes, at least you will be alive! The operation will cure the disease, and your life will be saved. Finally, let us suppose, the operation is very expensive. To cover its costs you will have to use up your entire life savings and sell all your possessions. The question, now, is, will you agree to undergo the operation?

When I put this question to myself, the answer is clear. Whether or not I have the operation, it seems to me that *I* will be dead. That is, *I*—the being whose motivation for having the operation is to live to meet my grandchildren, watch them grow, finish the book I am working on, enjoy conversation and travel with my wife, and see the Chicago Cubs win the World Series—will not survive in either case. Whether I have the operation or forego it, I—whatever exactly *I* refers to here—will be dead. Though my body will survive the operation, I—the person whose body it is—will not. The only difference from my perspective is whether the doctors will get my money or it will go to my family. And there is no question that I want it to go to my family.

The same general point can be made from a third-person perspective. Suppose someone develops a "permanent vegetative state drug"— a tasteless chemical compound that makes anyone who imbibes it totally and permanently unconscious. Then someone deliberately places this drug in the drink of one of your dearest friends or relatives. Soon after drinking it, your friend or relative becomes totally and permanently unconscious. The heinous perpetrator is then caught. How should he or she be charged? Should the charge be murder? If you (not unreasonably) answer yes, is it not because you believe that your friend or relative (the person you loved, whose well-being and future you valued, and whose company you cherished) is now dead? How persuaded would you be by a defense attorney arguing for a lesser charge by pointing out that your friend or family member still enjoys integrated functioning of the circulatory, respiratory, and central nervous systems and, on no less authority than that of a presidential commission, is alive?

As these examples suggest, there may be an important difference between a living human biological organism and whatever it is we regard as the subject of life and death when we say of ourselves or some other human being, X, "X is alive" or "X is dead." What, then, is the subject of the predicates *alive* and *dead* when applied to beings like you and me? Is it a biological organism (the class of which includes you and me, together with anencephalic infants and permanently vegetative patients) or, as my examples suggest, is it what I am calling a person? And can, in a small number of cases, the organism as a whole survive the death of the person? There will be no closure on the determination of death until there is closure on these fundamental questions.

Before considering a philosophically pragmatic response, we must consider an important objection to the personhood conception. Whether a person is in a permanent vegetative state, the objection correctly maintains, cannot be assessed by all physicians with the same degree of certainty as the death of the organism as a whole. But ease of application and a very high degree of certainty are necessary for criteria for death to be incorporated into the law. Therefore, the personhood conception must be rejected.[11]

The objection is, however, overstated. In the vast majority of cases, defenders of the personhood conception can point out, it is as easy to diagnose death under the personhood conception as it is under the biological conception because the two conceptions employ the same criteria for death. A person is dead if he or she sustains either: (1) irreversible cessation of circulatory and respiratory functions or (2) irreversible cessation of all functions of the entire brain, including the brain stem. Either the first criterion or the second is sufficient for total and permanent loss of consciousness. Indeed, it is the death of the person that provides the most plausible rationale for use of these criteria.

At the same time, the personhood conception explains why these conditions, although sufficient for pronouncing death, may not be necessary. Individuals in a permanent vegetative state are also totally and permanently unconscious (even though they have not undergone either irreversible cessation of respiration and circulation or total and irreversible cessation of all brain functions). If the most plausible rationale for the use of heart-lung and "whole-brain" criteria is that they give us a way to identify total and permanent loss of consciousness, anencephalic infants and others in a permanent vegetative state must also be regarded as dead, for they too are totally and permanently unconscious.

Therefore, even if we have doubts about our capacity to clearly and definitively diagnose a permanent vegetative state, the personhood conception may provide a more plausible rationale for our current criteria for death than does the "death of the organism as a whole" conception. Second, if we are willing to defer to neurologists, we will, after various periods of testing and observation, be able to identify with a high degree of certainty many cases of permanent vegetative state. Third, it is quite possible that more specific and reliable criteria for diagnosing a permanent vegetative state will emerge from further studies of large patient populations or the development of more refined technology (such as positron-emission tomographic [PET] scanners, which can detect decreases in cerebral cortical metabolism consistent with unconsciousness and deep anesthesia).[12]

Pragmatism and the Subject of Life and Death

How, then, should we conceive the subject of human life and death? Is it a biological organism, or is it a person? Whatever the answer to this question, pragmatists would say, it will not be discovered in a fixed, external reality, independent of and prior to our efforts to live and make sense of our lives in a complex, dynamic, social and natural world. "The trail of the human serpent," as James once put it, "is over everything."[13] Our conception of human death turns on our conception of the conditions of existence for beings like ourselves; and our conception of these conditions turns in part on a wide variety of factors, including human biology, our scientific and technological capacities, our beliefs about the world, and our reasonable aspirations, given our full set of values and principles. None of these elements is fixed or independent of the others. Significant changes in one will often occasion revisions in the others. There is, moreover, no way for us to show that any particular stage in this evolving web of reflective action and active belief is the last or final stage.

Which conception of the human individual—and its related conditions for existence—best coheres with the complex network of actions and beliefs giving shape and meaning to our lives? Is it principally a biological conception, centering on the integrated functioning of the organism as a whole? Or is it a social-psychological conception, centering on consciousness?

To fix this question pragmatically—to bring it "down to earth," as it were—we must ask ourselves such questions as, What really matters to us with respect to questions of life and death? Are we, when push comes to shove, deeply concerned with the continued existence of the integrated functioning of the circulatory, respiratory, and central nervous systems, independent of its contribution to consciousness? How willing are we to sacrifice other important values and principles—not to mention economic and social resources—to sustain the integrated functioning of a human organism as a whole? What conception of the subject of life and death provides the most practical and unified approach to the largest number of bioethical issues? And, most generally, what conception best coheres with the largest number of things that we are, on reflection, strongly inclined to do and believe? Though detailed and complete answers to these and related questions are beyond the scope of this chapter, my hunch is that conceiving the subject of life and death in terms of personhood will provide a more satisfactory answer to this family of questions than conceiving it in terms of biology alone.

First, when we ask what really matters to us with regard to human life and death—why, for example, we believe murder is so very wrong (and a physician's prima facie obligation to save life so very right)—the most plausible answer, it seems to me, turns on what Donald Marquis identifies as the "loss of a valuable future": "The loss of one's life is one of the greatest losses one can suffer. The loss of one's life deprives one of all the experience, activities, projects, and enjoyments that would otherwise have constituted one's future. Therefore, killing someone is wrong, primarily because the killing inflicts (one of) the greatest possible losses on the victim."[14]

But neither anencephalic infants nor those in a permanent vegetative state can be deprived of all of the experience, activities, projects, and enjoyments that would otherwise have constituted their future because they are, due to the absence or permanent loss of cerebral functioning, incapable of experiencing, doing, planning, or enjoying anything. If the loss of all possible experience, action, projects, or enjoyment is what makes killing prima facie wrong and the prospect of such experience, action, projects, or enjoyment what makes saving life prima facie right, both murder victims and patients are best conceived as biological persons, not simply as biological organisms.

Second, acceptance of the UDDA has not entirely eliminated the "inward trouble" of mind to which the Harvard criteria and the UDDA were a response. Many of us are, for example, troubled by the prohibition against transplanting hearts from anencephalic infants like Andrew in order to save the lives of infants with hypoplastic left heart syndrome like Helen. Moreover, we question spending over a billion dollars per year for an increasing number of permanently vegetative patients while millions of Americans are denied access to health care because of an inability to pay.

We are also disturbed by the fact that each year hundreds of persons in need of new hearts or livers die on waiting lists while the hearts and livers of patients in permanent vegetative states keep on going until they satisfy the UDDA, at which time their organs are no longer biologically suitable for transplantation. To what extent should we be willing to trade off the lives of infants like Helen, the resources used to maintain permanently vegetative patients, and the life-saving potential of their organs for the sake of the integrated functioning of various sets of circulatory, respiratory, and central nervous systems?

Finally, a shift from a mainly biological conception of human life and death to a more social-psychological conception may lead to plausible and coherent resolutions to a wide range of bioethical issues—from abortion and embryo research on the one hand to euthanasia and assisted suicide on the other. Exploring the ramifications of such a change—its overall human and economic costs, benefits, implications, and so on—may also lead to a better overall understanding of ourselves and of the value of our lives.

Whatever the results of such an inquiry (and I do not expect that it will soon be completed), it addresses one of the most basic, far-reaching philosophical questions of our time. Unless "professional philosophy can mobilize itself sufficiently to assist" in clarifying and redirecting our thoughts about these and related issues, it runs the risk, as foreseen by Dewey, of becoming "more and more sidetracked from the main currents of contemporary life."

15 Dying Old as a Social Problem

JOHN LACHS

WE LIVE in times of unprecedented change. Improvements in nutrition, in public sanitation, and in the treatment of disease have enhanced the quality of life and extended its length beyond all but the wildest expectations. We live longer and, in material terms, better by far than any previous generation.

Methuselah was supposed to have lived more than three times three hundred years, but believers who read about him in the twelfth century were glad to make it to thirty. Yet for us average life expectancy at birth rose from 47.3 years in 1900 to 68.2 in 1950. It has continued to rise since then, topping 75.8 years in 1995, with no indication that a peak has been reached. Optimistic estimates suggest that the human life span can and will, before too long, be extended to 150 or even 200 years.

The elderly population in industrialized nations is increasing far more rapidly than the population as a whole. From 1900 to 1994 the population of the United States tripled, but the number of those over 65 years of age grew elevenfold, to 33 million. The number of the oldest old increased even more impressively, growing to 3.5 million persons in 1994, which is 28 times greater than the number of people 85 and over who lived in 1900. Conservative estimates indicate that by 2030 more than 20 percent of the U.S. population will be over 65.[1]

Such advances come at a price. Many of the elderly need personal assistance even with everyday activities. On some occasions, life can be extended only at a great loss of its satisfactions. On others, the lives saved are such in name only and families and institutions end up caring for biological organisms whose human potential has been wrecked. Though longer life offers vast benefits, it also protracts the debility of old age and creates a population of elderly people plagued by chronic diseases. Loss of autonomy, successive organ failures, and intractable pain suggest that rather than living long, many of these individuals are just slow to die.

The seamy downside of our success in extending life is that a small but significant number of the very sick and the very old want to die, but cannot. Many more people are likely to suffer from a surfeit of life in the coming years. The number of people over 65 in the United States is projected to increase to over 80 million in the next fifty years, and the number of those over 85 possibly to 10 million. No matter how fast and how far medical technology will have progressed by then, this will leave hundreds of thousands of people who are tired of battling for life or at least sincerely believe that existence no longer benefits them.

Arguing that one has a right to one's life and can therefore terminate it at will misses the personal dynamics and the social complexities of the situation. This renders attacks on the right to die largely beside the point.[2] Asserting a right may be useful against an intrusive government or as protection from aggressive neighbors, but it has no place in a community structured by the ideal of uniting the values of individuals with the common good. Maintaining, from the other side, that the state has a preeminent interest in the lives of its citizens misses the point no less. The government must be devoted to the good of citizens first, and to their lives only to the extent that they deem them to be conditions or ingredients of that good.

How, then, should we think about people who no longer wish to live? Clearly we *must* think about their plight, because the problem will not go away. But we must not approach complex issues in a simplistic way. Satisfying as it is to take the moral high ground by announcing the that all life is sacred, such gestures will not take us very far. No one actually believes this—or, at least, no one believes it, acts on it, and lives long enough to explore all of its merits. Even people who refuse to eat meat kill and dine on broccoli without a moral qualm. Since we cannot survive on stones and mud, it is ineffectual or insincere to pretend that we respect life of every sort.

A look at our practices reveals that we do not even treat human life as sacred. We wash living cells off the face, allow ova to die unfertilized, and spread thousands of trillions of sperms around the world without maximizing their chances to grow into new organisms. We remove diseased organs without mercy and kill both healthy and cancerous cells. Would health massage, cosmetology, and the tonsorial art—never mind medicine, dentistry, and surgery—be possible if we thought all products of the human genome must remain inviolate?

But this, some will insist, is a wilful distortion of what earnest people mean: They maintain that only the entire human body need be respected, not its parts. This defense exposes the fundamental and lamentable error to which sanctity-of-life arguments lead. The operation of the entire body is no more an end in itself than is the integrity of its organs; their value derives from the support they provide for a human life. Confusing a human life with the life of a human body is a pernicious mistake, and it remains a baffling irony that religious people who believe in the transcendent destiny of the soul should be the ones most apt to make it.

There must have been a terrible inversion of values in the last fifty or one hundred years to focus the attention of deeply believing Christians on the body in its vegetative function. Insisting on the inviolability of intact individuals and protecting the weak, the underprivileged, and the disabled are in the best tradition of religious caring. But these are defenses of the body only incidentally; their primary purpose is to honor the wishes, the needs, and the ontological status of persons. There is, accordingly, nothing to justify the move from meeting the needs of persons to protecting the presumed rights of the bodies connected to them. Bodies have no rights and, when their sole function is biological, no persons own or inhabit them to give them standing.

Adulation of the body is, moreover, a singularly pagan practice. It shows itself in the heartrending activity of safeguarding the bodies of persons killed by years of coma. Worse, when even biological function ceases, we embalm the body, enhance its look with makeup, and put it on display, claiming identity with the departed soul. "Doesn't he look good!" mourners can then exclaim as they walk past the open coffin, feasting their eyes on the simulacrum of a human being, on what is no more than a clump of matter soon to rest underground.

Few seem to reflect on what such practices reveal about our beliefs, and, as a result, our judgments remain unchallenged and incoherent. We confuse biological activity with human life and assign the value of the person to the body. In this way we blind ourselves to the sensible and natural line between an intelligently operating organism and that creature reduced to its minimal functions or, in the end, to a gravitating heap.

The principle of the sanctity of all life remains, therefore, an empty slogan unless those who wish to rely on it as a guide to policy or to morality provide a clear account of what sort of life they have in mind and what manner of beings are to enjoy it at what cost. A more promising approach is to avoid reference to absolute principles altogether, examining each class of cases on its own to see how far it advances or hinders human well-being. Although there may be other values that rightly command our allegiance, we cannot go far wrong in stressing the importance of human flourishing.

The long experience of the race and our personal experiments afford us ample information about the range of human goods. The first and perhaps most remarkable fact that commends itself to our attention is the central, privileged role people play in defining or at least in discovering their good.

Like flowers, humans are scattered to grow in directly self-governing, operationally independent organisms. Although tied to their fellows by bonds of need and love, adult individuals constitute systems that are in some respects complete. They are able to act on their own and, experiencing the outcomes, to make suitable adjustments in their behavior. Though by no means insular, they nevertheless occupy integrated small worlds with an element of privacy unique to each. This is what we normally mean when we say that people live their own lives and die their own deaths, fill out their worlds and close them down, with others grieving or cheering them on, but only distantly involved.

This ineluctable element of subjectivity makes individuals specially situated, even if by no means invariably accurate, judges of their own good. Under normal circumstances they are in a better position than anyone else to know what they wish to accomplish, what pleases them, and what they are prepared to give up to obtain such satisfactions. People find their own private and idiosyncratic value structures familiar and intuitively right; others, by contrast, may not be able to understand how anyone can enjoy or treasure such odd things.

Only under special conditions can others offer us valid insight or useful advice: In times of great stress or passion, for example, we can discount or overlook what caring others plainly perceive. Even psychologists, working from a general knowledge of the range of human goods, have nothing to match the detailed and specific information individuals possess about what is of significance to them. And the best among those who dare to offer advice quickly learn to say only what in the depths of our souls we already know.

The principle that, other things being equal, people are the best judges of what they want out of life provides a sound and sensible basis for dealing with them. If we must remember this principle when our friends seek a better life, we should not forget it when they face death. We should be satisfied to let them chart their own courses, convinced that probably no one knows better what they want than they and that, in any case, they will be first in line when it comes to suffering the consequences of their decisions.

Such decisions are momentous and irreversible, so no one should have to make them without the caring support of the community. But loving concern is one thing, meddling obstruction of the process quite another. Legislation that wrests the decisions from individuals situated in their communities is a blunt and objectionable instrument for the expression of caring.

The vast literature directed against suicide suffers from a very poor argument, repeated and judged conclusive even by such sensitive defenders of liberty as John Stuart Mill.[3] Since killing oneself is irreversible, these philosophers maintain, it cannot fall within the autonomous decision-making power of individuals. Consistent thinkers, including Mill, decline extending freedom to any act whose consequences make its reversal impossible, such as selling oneself into slavery and killing not only oneself, but anyone. Such consistency is commendable, but it quickly reduces the argument to absurdity. For it is astonishing that murder and slavery are the only irreversible acts these philosophers can find, when we are surrounded by them on all sides.

Actually, since time itself cannot be undone or turned around, all human acts have a sort of finality. Lies and infidelities can be only forgiven, never erased. We can never recapture the squandered opportunities of youth, nor can we atone for occasions on which the time came to act but our hearts froze. Choosing the wrong place to live, the wrong mate, or the wrong profession may seem easy to fix by going back to square one and starting again. But though the start may feel fresh, it does not undo the damage of the past; the third spouse may at last be right, but the sadness and pain of the first two always remain.

Something dies in us with every passing day and, though the loss is not of everything at once, as it is with death, it is of almost everything cumulatively over time, leaving little for the final act to take. Being no longer able to do some things is a natural consequence of aging, and it differs only in degree from the inability to do anything consequent upon death. And when death comes at the end of lengthy illness, it stops fewer activities than did the onset of disease. So irreversible loss attends nearly everything we do, and if we don't trust people to make sensible decisions about death, we should not trust their other choices either.

This argument against suicide cuts, therefore, equally against all significant freedom. If the irreversibility of death disqualifies people from choosing it, the irreparable loss that comes of marrying the wrong person renders choice of mate impermissible. If people should not be allowed to choose the time and manner of their exit, they must not be permitted to decide about attending college, buying a house, and having children either. Tyrants can in this way enlist the fundamental structure of reality to justify their rule.

Mill, I suspect, was in the end less bothered about the irreversibility than about the momentousness of the consequences of what we do. This concern is particularly legitimate and understandable in the case of death. Unfortunately, however, assessments of the damage death inflicts tend to be one dimensional.

Thinkers typically focus on events that are heartrendingly sad instead of examining a broad range of cases. But the value of terminating life, as the value of anything, must be examined in context: Each death must be judged individually, by reference to the life it ends. Those who take the untimely departure of loved ones or teen-age suicide as their model are sure to be misled. The vast loss these represent is a poor guide to assessing the appropriateness of painlessly slipping away at the sick end of a long life. Condemnation of suicide loses its plausibility the moment we consider the daily life and prospects of at least some of the people who seek it.

The fact that individuals are particularly well situated to know what is of value to them does not imply that caring others are always ignorant. Detailed observation of their choices reveals a great deal about what people prize. In the case of healthy teenagers, moreover, it is obvious that the bulk of their life is ahead of them, and the flimsiest knowledge of psychology suffices to convince us that their depressions will lift after a while. Even if *Weltschmerz* or disappointed love distorts their vision by darkening their days, their otherwise bright prospects justify us in not standing idly by when they propose to take their lives in ill-considered haste.

Similarly, we can have significant knowledge of the condition of old people suffering from a painful terminal disease. Even if we lack what may be, in their case, exquisitely certain knowledge of what they want, we can understand their situation and assess their prospects. Romanticizing affirmations of the beauty of life are revoltingly out of place here. Their present may consist of drugged stupor and their future of a few more weeks of suffering. Their condition has almost nothing in common with the situation of young people temporarily distressed: It is not subjectively dark, but objectively bleak.

Our proper inability to honor the desire of the young for release from life must not blind us to what may well be a sound and sensible wish on the part of people who are both sick and old. Multiple organ failure leaves individuals—like derelict ships at sea—without rudder and destination, marking the days until the final storm floods all compartments. Whoever sees the world from their perspective understands that continued life can do them little good and that the harm quick death would bring is less by far than that caused by life to an unwanted child.

It strikes me as unseemly to try to delegitimate the desire for death by claiming that its source must be depression. Reasonings built on such conveniently loose psychological concepts do little more than confirm one's preexisting judgments. But even if we disregard this obvious point, the argument can be compelling only if depression constitutes an invariably inappropriate response and if it always clouds the faculty of judgment. Both of these conditions, however, are open to doubt.

Depression may well be perverse when its cause is easily removed. If reasonable effort promises to eliminate the external circumstance or personal failure that stands in the way of getting what we want, depression is an irrational response. But when one's condition is genuinely hopeless, it would be strange not to get depressed. Painful and inevitable death *is* depressing, and the mad response to it is cheerful acceptance, not a crushing sense of impotence. The feeling of being cornered is, moreover, under the circumstances a deeply insightful assessment of one's situation. So, quite apart from the general arguments of such pessimists as Schopenhauer for the view that only the dejected perceive the world the way it truly is, when the prospects for life are dim, depressed people, seeing doom and gloom, render strikingly accurate accounts of their reality.

I conclude that if we honor the ordinary, sensible wishes of people we care for or love, under the right circumstances we must honor their choice of death as well. We must be careful that this choice is not unduly influenced by the desires of others, and particularly that it does not originate in what is increasingly talked about as the duty to die.[4] We can understand that the wish not to be a burden to those we love can play a powerful role in the decision to die at an early stage of a debilitating or terminal disease. But it is well worth remembering that we live in a world of relative plenty, so economic considerations should not be allowed primacy in such decisions. And, on the psychological side, those who love us may never be satisfied that they have shown their caring unless they have an opportunity to see us through a large portion of our decline.

People who bemoan the tendency of terminally ill people to seek early release from their suffering, attributing it to erroneous beliefs or personal weakness, need to spend more time trying to understand its social causes. In a world busy with work, caring for the sick falls to paid specialists. There is no room in the house for debilitated older people and no time to tend to their wishes. They are shipped to the hospital, to the hospice, or, at best, to isolated facilities providing "assisted living"; the place of the nurturing home is taken by the nursing home. Familiar surroundings and routines are replaced by antiseptic rooms that permit no privacy and few activities beyond those needed for physical existence. Tended by indifferent strangers, the old and the sick grow sick at heart and find it pointless to live through days that lack hope and meaning.

In different circumstances, natural, even slow, death could be seen as a wonderful affirmation of the enduring values of family and love. The continuity of life, visibly displayed as responsibility and strength pass from the old to the young, provides a peace words cannot describe. Seeing the energy of children and grandchildren gives hope that all is not lost, that one's life survives in the successes of others. Under such conditions, there is point to living on: A bit of joy and a ray of hope suffice to brighten the day. We see that few of those dying in the midst of their families and feeling their love seek early death or assisted suicide. The nurturing community provides reasons for living and removes the horror of a lonely death.

Our highly mediated society has made different arrangements for taking care of the old, and the problems we face with end-of-life decisions constitute a portion of the price we pay for them.[5] Concentrating the old in special housing developments, isolating the seriously ill from family and friends, and orchestrating the dying process under the supervision of professionals distance vulnerable people from their roots. Many of them cease to want to live even when they are relatively healthy; why live on if the people who matter are beyond reach and the sights and sounds and activities that filled the days with small satisfactions have long disappeared?

No radical change in these social arrangements is likely to occur in the foreseeable future. We shall have to settle, instead, for modest improvements in how we tend the old and the ill. Those interested in reducing the pressure for legalizing euthanasia and the incidence of suicide among the sick would find greater success by working to make the lives of terminal patients more meaningful than by trying to pass legislation. Remarkably, retirement home operators have so far shown less than full understanding of the social and spiritual needs of the persons entrusted to their care. Only recently have a few facilities started to invite groups of children to visit and to provide cats and dogs for their residents to love. Such humanizing touches bring the old closer to the sweet energy of life and give them small but potent reasons to get up in the morning. Active people who have shouldered responsibility all their lives cannot be expected to convert themselves into the human equivalents of the potted plants that sit in their still rooms. No one wants to live long without purpose, without some pride in self-reliance, and without the sense of being needed.

There are similar signs of promise in how the "management" of death is beginning to change. Economic reasons have led hospitals to discharge the very ill to die, if at all possible, in their own homes. Seeing life and death in the same well-loved or at least familiar surroundings provides comfort and consolation. The ritual of friends coming to visit or to say good-bye confers a sense of touching completion on life. Excruciating pain is easier to bear than abandonment; in any case, so long as one is in the loving care of those one loves, the pain can always be stilled.

Our first concern in dealing with a rapidly aging population must therefore be to provide the support of community to all who face old age and painful death. This support must be more than the anonymous readiness to pay taxes for the treatment of those lacking means. It has to take the form of personal caring, the sort of human relationships that make living worthwhile. Dying people need to feel what we seek throughout our lives: appreciation of the significance of what we have done and who we are. This standing in the eyes of the community, this importance of our passing individuality, is the ultimate recognition we want from our friends and from those who hold jobs in the institutions of the world. Sadly, few ever feel such acknowledgement even at the height of their power. Lacking it near the moment of death kills the soul before the body is ready to go.

To provide this standing in the generous way suffering friends deserve, we must learn to honor the momentousness of dying. Infernal busyness protects us from feeling the nodes of life; we go through the world without savoring the great occasions that make for the pathos and the deep mystery of existence. Religion called these moments sacred, but its decline left us unable to apply such vital concepts. One of the weaknesses of secular society is that it has nothing to offer in their place. As a result, life loses some of its depth and nearly all its articulation: everything happens on a single plane, without the exaltation and the celebration grand events deserve.

At the very least, we must recapture the experience of death for ordinary life. We cannot celebrate the event if it remains hidden from sight in the cancer wards and operating rooms of hospitals. It needs to be a public part of reality, socially fought, bravely faced, and openly discussed. It must become a part of the school curriculum, as well, so young people can feel its weight and not fear its secrets. If we can appropriate it as a natural event in every person's history, we can rally with sympathy to the sides of those whose time has come. Just as knowing the pain of hunger creates solidarity with those in need of food, expectation of our own death brings us into a special community with those whose expectations are about to be fulfilled.

The second task in dealing with the growing number of old and sick people in our midst is to respect the choices they make about their lives and deaths. They have a special competence to know what they want and an inescapable responsibility for the consequences of their decisions. Accepting their word cannot, of course, mean leaving them alone to sort things out as best they can in the privacy of their souls. What they want affects us, as well, and in deciding they need to know that their continued existence and the quality of their daily lives are of vital significance to others. Caring prevents suicide and the need for euthanasia.

We cannot underestimate the human capacity for following the crowd. At times in the history of humankind, suicide was contagiously easy. One lesson of the recent Dutch experience may well be that euthanasia can come to be viewed as a quick solution to multiple problems. We must not let the human tendency for imitation foreshorten the lives of our loved ones. Caring for them conveys the notion that they are wanted, but nothing deters the desire for death more than the thought that one's work is not yet complete. The greatest argument against early death is how much those suffering, in spite of their pain, can still contribute to our lives and how much we can do to enrich theirs. Soon enough, we will no longer be able to walk hand in hand, but it matters deeply that we treasure the companionship while we can.

In the teeth of the best efforts of the community, however, sometimes the pain, the bewilderment, and the degradation of disease become too much to bear. Alzheimer's patients whose moments of lucidity grow further and further apart, cancer sufferers whose pain can be stilled only by sinking their minds in a pool of haze, those afflicted with ALS who watch in horror as the paralysis of their bodies approaches the lungs and heart may well judge that it is pointless to hope and struggle on. Respect for them requires that we permit the last word to be theirs.

At such an advanced stage of debility, this is neither abandonment nor lack of caring. We must understand it, rather, as an expression of love. Love wants the other's good as the other defines it. There is no doubt that some people at the distant edge of life decide or recognize that it is better not to be. In condemning their wish to die or failing to give them aid, we allow our own energy and hatred of death to speak. That is the voice we must still, partly to help those we love today and partly to prepare for the time when our own predicaments may reveal the rightness of their stance.

16 Community, Autonomy, and Managed Care

JACQUELYN ANN K. KEGLEY

IN HIS ESSAY "The War Is Won, but the Peace Is Not," Albert Einstein wrote, "Everything has changed but our ways of thinking, and if these do not change, we drift toward unparalleled catastrophe." These words capture well the way things are in the health care delivery system in the United States today. Profound environmental shifts in health care have occurred under the umbrella of the notion of "managed care." These shifts, I believe, must be critically and proactively analyzed so that this new environment can be shaped to be more reflective of ethical medical practice and moral care, as well as more hospitable to the realization of the principles of autonomy, beneficence, and justice.

However, this will not be the case if there is not a paradigm shift in the way we think about the issues confronting us in health care today. These issues include the tension between serving patients' needs and making money, the conflict between cost containment and just allocation of scarce health care resources, the division of loyalties faced by physician-employees, the blurring of distinctions between health needs and desires, the schizophrenia faced by persons as patient-consumers, and the troublesome interaction of medical versus economic and public versus individual conceptions of appropriate and/or necessary health care.

I contend that what is needed to sufficiently address these and other pressing concerns in the new health care delivery system is a new paradigm, a new way of thinking and analysis, which challenges the operative framework of economic self-interested individualism. Indeed, the trends in health care delivery are not at all surprising given this view, which features the individual person as *homo economicus*, the individual rational decision maker who weighs and balances issues in terms of cost-benefit analysis and self-interest and which stresses free market mechanisms and contractual relationships as appropriate notions for all domains of human endeavor.

In contrast to this framework of self-interested individualism, I suggest a paradigm shift from a highly individualized notion of the person and personal decision making and of community and communal decision making to an understanding of the person as a decision maker always within social contexts and social roles, whose autonomy and individuality are hindered or fostered by social context and whose choices impact more than just self. Genuine individuals are fostered by supportive and vibrant communities which, in turn, are the result of the actions and choices of authentic and autonomous individuals.

Good decision making is a subtle balancing of the individual's good and communal good, of the good of a particular group and the broader public good. Communities are not mere collections of individuals and of individual self-interests, but rather the result of individual and communal interaction and dialogue. Communities share some common goals and values and interests across time and generations, and genuine communities are concerned for both individual and community growth and fulfillment. Community building through communal dialogue and decision making should be at the center of the new health care delivery system, and both individual health and health care and public health and health care should be of concern.

Further, the roles of both health care providers and patients need to be reconceptualized in terms of such concepts as mutual interpretation, mediation, loyalty, and a set of professional and personal virtues. Medicine as an institution also needs reconceptualization from a critical care, individualized, hospital focus to a holistic functionality, public health-community health focus and to a notion of a flexible continuum of care across stages of life.

In what follows I briefly characterize the present health care environment and the framework of economic self-interested individualism, giving attention to some of the inadequacies and difficult issues. The remainder of the chapter is devoted to sketching the new paradigm shift and some of its implications for the new system of health care delivery.

Managed Care, Managed Competition, and Managed Costs

It has been said that the business of the United States is business. It is not surprising, therefore, that another area of American life has become captive to the march of aggressive business entrepreneurship. This change occurred somewhat rapidly as escalating health costs demanded a more efficient delivery of medical services, which led to the "managed care" movement. *Managed care* as a term refers to various organizational arrangements that bring together four groups: the health care provider, the patient (known as the consumer, the insurer, the reimburser for costs of care, and the purchaser of care, an entity that buys care and is usually a large employer organization or a government agency, such as a county.

Capitation is a key concept of managed care. It involves the negotiation of a fixed dollar amount for health services for a specified number of patients regardless of the care delivered, and the financial risk for actual cost of care is shared by the provider and the insurer.[1] About 85 percent of the health care delivered in the United States is now delivered under a managed care system.

However, changes have continued as health care delivery has become "corporatized," namely as large medi-giants have integrated health care facilities, medical services, and insurance.[2] This shift has brought about other kinds of changes. For example, health care decision making has shifted from individual physicians to third-party bureaucrats, resulting in what some have called the "deprofessionalization" of medicine[3] as well as a confusion of loyalties for physicians who traditionally were advocates for their patients, but who now face over-ruling of their medical decisions and even financial disincentives and loss of position.

Additionally, medical services have become rationalized, quantified, and routinized. "Diagnostic-related groups" (DRGs) were the first step in this regard. These involve the notion that complex medical processes can be strictly categorized and quantified for the purposes of determining reimbursement for care and days of hospital care. Therefore, every pneumonia case was assumed to be the same in terms of types of care required and days needed for recovery, regardless of individual patients' circumstances.

At the forefront of this move toward standardization and routinization today is HealthSouth Corporation, led by Richard Scrushy, which has a chain of rehabilitation and surgery centers, mostly outpatient, that offer a wide variety of "cost-effective" and "consistent" health care procedures. Mr. Scrushy uses sports figures and razzle-dazzle advertisement to create what he envisions as the Holiday Inns or MacDonalds of health care, with "readily accessible standardized care across the country."[4] Managed care has metamorphosed into big business.

Yet the corporate model does not always easily fit health care. While HealthSouth Corporation gears up for a market capitalization of $6.6 billion and Mr. Scrushy earns a salary and bonuses of nearly $7 million, other entrepreneurial health care firms have seen their market values and earnings plummet. Some observers of this conclude that health care, which has long been primarily a nonprofit enterprise, is simply harder to manage and control than other businesses. For example, Rick Wade of the American Hospital Association says, "One thing that amazes people is the health-care field doesn't always obey the laws of markets and commodities."[5] Perhaps a stronger judgment is in order—namely, that the corporate model is inappropriate for health care.

However the judgment is made, the developments in health care delivery are causing alarm in various sectors of American society. For instance, in August 1997 Congress rushed through a bill prohibiting managed care companies from imposing "drive-through deliveries" on new mothers. Federal law now guarantees maternity patients at least forty-eight hours in the hospital. At least one member of Congress, Rose DeLaurio of Connecticut, has introduced a bill requiring health plans to allow at least forty-eight hours of inpatient care following a mastectomy. Such federal piecemeal tinkering with the abuses of managed care is, of course, not practical, and it seems to foster third-party medical decision-making as well as standardized, categorized care. Yet, citizen concern about abuses may spur further such moves by the federal government.

Legal issues also have become somewhat confused in the new health care environment. Although medical decision making is increasingly in the hands of nonmedical bureaucrats, physicians—rather than health maintenance organizations (HMOs) and chief executive officers (CEOs) or other executives—are liable for medical malpractice. The HMOs argue that they are not practicing medicine, but merely making decisions about insurance coverage. This troublesome fiction and dilution of responsibility, I believe, leads to further breakdown of provider-patient relationships and of trust and loyalty within the health care system. Rather than the traditional long-term commitments of physicians and patients to health care plans for a lifetime, there is now provider-employee turnover and patient-consumer shopping. Accountability and measures of health care outcomes will be very difficult under these conditions.

Another troublesome fiction in today's health care delivery environment in the United States is the notion of quality assurance. One aspect of this idea is the need for objective measures by which health plans can be compared. A second and closely related notion is that of measures of quality of care or medical outcomes. This whole area is problematic. First, the two major agencies—namely, the Joint Commission on Accreditation of Healthcare Organizations and the National Committee for Quality Assurance—that oversee quality assurance are private agencies controlled by the industries they regulate.

Further, "quality" is difficult to measure, and there is disagreement on its meaning. For example, a traditional notion of quality care involved process and structure; that is, the emphasis was placed on the provision of care by a competent practitioner with certain qualifications and training in an appropriate setting, generally a hospital situation, using commonly accepted procedures in accordance with accepted medical practice. Therefore, the medical profession was the primary overseer of this kind of quality care.

The new stress, however, is on outcomes, with attention focused on the effects of care on the patients' health and satisfaction. Again, there is disagreement about definitions of *health* and *outcomes*, and "objective" data on such is notoriously hard to compile, much less to convey in a meaningful way to patient-consumers.

Further, "quality assurance" involves a sleight of hand that Robert Kettner of the *Washington Post* identifies as a confusion of "cost-savings" with "quality improvement." He writes: "The essence of managed care today is to confuse cost-savings with quality improvement, as if they were the same thing. But sometimes 'quality' medicine requires the plan to pay, while cost-savings may come at the expense of needed treatment."[6] Quality care is not necessarily cost effective. We will discuss this issue further as we talk about justice in health care and rationing.

Another troublesome confusion fostered by the drive for quality assurance is the confusion between the notions of quality of care and getting more for our money, so that quality assurance becomes a kind of consumer's guide to health care. This notion of health care as a product and patients as consumers has a number of troublesome implications. For example, it increases the difficulty of distinguishing between health care needs and health care desires and wants.

Seeing health care as a supermarket of individualized health care products does not seem to promote the idea of cost containment, and it leads to a disregard for the health care needs of those who are poor and cannot buy health care products. It could lead to notions of cheap health care goods versus quality health care goods, with the complementary division between those who can afford quality health care and those who cannot. Commodification of health care goods and the objectification of persons has already occurred with surrogate motherhood, which many argue views surrogate mothers and babies as goods to be used and bought, respectively.

All of these concerns about the new developments in health care delivery in the United States might well lead one to the conclusion that the term *managed care* is an oxymoron. A similar conclusion has been reached by some with regard to the term *business ethics*. Indeed, another danger of the present situation is the possibility that the ethics of managed care might be reduced to issues of business ethics—namely, concerns such as truth in advertising, trade secrets, workers' rights, loyalty, and whistle-blowing.

Such issues probably have a place in the new hybrid "managed care," but ethical issues in health care delivery need to be much broader in scope and focused on different questions. Health care, after all, is of fundamental moral importance.[7] It is a primary social good, for health care is essential both to the functioning of society and its members and to individuals and their abilities to pursue goals in life and to fulfill their life plans. Health and its protection and health information are important conditions for the actualization of individual autonomy, and health, defined partly as social functionality, is crucial to a society's development and fulfillment. Further, as a primary social good, the fair distribution of health care resources is key to promoting justice for all in a democratic society or any other.

The principle of beneficence is another important consideration, because health care is about reducing pain and suffering and preventing premature loss of life. Further, the principle of loyalty and concepts of personal responsibility and professional integrity, all key to the traditional fiduciary physician-patient relationship, cannot be ignored in seeking to provide true caring in our health care delivery system.

In this sketch of the new paradigm for health care I hope to deal, though somewhat briefly, with each of these issues. Before turning to this task, however, I first need to outline the contours of the operative philosophical framework of economic self-interested individualism—a framework, I believe, that is inadequate to deal with the new health care delivery environment and fosters a number of its deleterious aspects.

The Economic Self and Market Justice

The assumed framework for much social, ethical, and public policy discussion in the United States is that of self-interested individualism. Central to this view is the belief that the individual is the authoritative judge and jury of his or her own life; the individual is seen as rational, autonomous *homo economicus*, who makes solitary decisions after cost-benefit analysis in terms of self-interest. Autonomy is primarily seen as "negative liberty"—that is, as protection from coercion or interference—and the rights of the individual are often conceptualized as implementation of this negative liberty; that is, they are to guarantee certain freedoms, and they imply a duty of others to honor these rights.

Closely connected to the concept of "individual liberty" is the belief in *laissez-faire*. namely, non-interference with individual choices, behaviors and actions by government and others except when others' rights and liberties are threatened. In economics, *lassiez faire* translates into trusting to the mechanisms of the free market to drive forth the economy. Applied in social policy and in health care this translates to the conviction that markets and market behavior are the fairest and most efficient means of distributing social goods. This might be called "market justice."

In the area of relationships, including moral relationships, the contract becomes the model. Moral behavior means "honoring a contract which is fairly negotiated and agreed to by autonomous, consenting parties."[8] This model now governs surrogate motherhood relationships, as indicated earlier. As for communities, these are viewed as collections of individuals, and community interest is seen as the sum of the individual interests of its members.[9]

Although this characterization is overstated and simplified, it does aid us in pointing to some of the difficulties such a framework poses for the serious issues in our system of health care delivery today. First, in dealing with autonomy in health care decisions the emphasis has been rightfully on informed consent; but, framed in the individualistic context, stress has been placed on individual patient decision making, on individual competence, on noncoercion, and on the procedural process. These stresses fail to deal adequately with persons as social beings who usually make decisions in a context of interdependence and social roles, responsibilities, and values, whether a familial, occupational, ethnic, or religious context or some broader social context.

Not enough attention has been paid to fostering the conditions for adequate informed consent. For example, power inequalities in our society and in health care have a substantially negative impact on the ability of a number of Americans to make effective, informed choices about health care and life plans. This is true for black Americans and other ethnic minorities, for the poor and less educated, and for many women and children. Barriers to good informed consent, such as education, language facility, self-image, and paternalistic and prejudicial attitudes, all have an impact on the ability of these individuals to engage in informed consent. Indeed, the inadequate attention given to health education in the United States health care delivery system renders many individuals ineffectual in making informed health care choices, and therefore the conditions for true informed consent are lacking.

As for "rights," they depend on facilitative social and institutional conditions and on social and communal assent and willingness to implement the duties correlative with the right. Beth Singer, for example, argues that rights should be viewed as "operative social institutions."[10] Rights have to be successfully negotiated to become operative in a communal context. In a complex and pluralistic society like that in the United States, the failure to do this can result in disaster and the nonrecognition of rights. Two good examples are abortion rights and children's rights. Further, as the abortion issue also illustrates, an individualistic interpretation of "rights" leads too often to a clash of rights, an adversarial conflict of autonomous choices, an obscuring of the real issues and of the need for difficult and mutual communal decision making.

An individualistic economically oriented framework also ironically leads to a glossing over of two key features of our U.S. health care delivery system that have a heavy impact on escalating costs. One of these features is that we allow health care institutions to operate competitively when cooperative and collective action could reduce costs. A second feature of our medical system that contributes to cost escalation is the fact that we do not force anyone to take social and institutional responsibility for choosing and encouraging the use of high technology in the provision of care. Indeed, social and institutional responsibility is a difficult notion in a context in which social groups are conceived as mere collections of individuals.

Therefore, the blame for using costly technology is placed on individual physicians and patients, and the social mechanisms that foster and enforce the provision of high-technology care are generally ignored. This view fails to take regard of the fact that individuals' needs for and expectations about health care resources are shaped to a fundamental degree by societal conditions and forces. The following quotation from Marian Gray Secundy concerning the views of the minority elderly about aging and death makes the point very well: "It may well be that within the cultural practices and beliefs of some minority citizens our society could find a more positive model of the graceful acceptance of aging, an appreciation of what the elderly contribute to the community, and an acceptance of the inevitability of death. These conceptions in turn could guide resource allocations in more rational directions—for example, tilting spending for the elderly toward humane long-term care and toward medical interventions that enhance function in daily care units for patients who have no hope of regaining independent function."[11]

The notion of radical individualism focuses on individual health behavior and ignores the social preconditions of that behavior. Therefore, lung cancer becomes an individual responsibility, as do eating dysfunctions such as anorexia and bulimia, when in fact more attention should be given to the social forces—such as attitudes about behavior, the media, advertising, movies, literature, and folklore—that have made smoking and thin female bodies seem beautiful. Structural and collective change is minimized through victim blaming—for instance, seeing health problems as caused by behavioral problems or deficiencies of the victims. This kind of victim blaming may cause serious concerns in relation to genetic diseases. As more genetic screening becomes available, persons may face job discrimination because of genetic predispositions or conditions; the individual will bear the blame rather than society or the workplace, whereas social change could help solve at least part of the problem.[12]

Returning to Dr. Secundy's observation, we see that discussions of rationing health care for the elderly and of futility often focus on individual fault—that is, the fault of the patient or the physician for wanting to extend life and thus escalating the costs of care. Little attention is given to the way a market orientation has dramatized the role of the solitary physician-technician-scientist as our first and primary line of defense against the threat of death. Again, the behavioral deficiencies of individuals—for example, the elderly in their lonely struggle against death—are highlighted rather than the social factors that have made death into the feared grim reaper against which an individual must take heroic and technological action. There is no extended discussion of the social conditions that need to be provided for individuals to more adequately conceptualize death or the roles of the elderly and the young in a society in which productivity is the criterion of value and these two groups are seen as unproductive.

A new view of individuals as social beings, of health as an individual and communal concern, and of communal support and responsibility is needed if the real issues of health care delivery in the United States are to be adequately addressed. It is to this new paradigm that I now turn. This paradigm is based on my critical reflection on and reaction to the philosophy of Josiah Royce. I have developed this paradigm in detail as well as in specific reference to medicine in my book *Genuine Individuals and Genuine Communities*.[13] The implications of the paradigm for managed care are a further development of the work undertaken in the book.

Informed Consent: Individual and Communal

As indicated earlier, an individualistic notion of informed consent fails to take into account the need to provide facilitative conditions for the exercise of this very important right. Various barriers including power inequities, language facility, cultural differences, a feeling of powerlessness, paternalistic and prejudicial attitudes, and lack of education all hinder the exercise of adequate informed consent. Persons are social beings, and their decisions are always made in and out of a social context. Autonomy is something that is developed or hindered through various social conditions, and it grows and is enabled through continual facilitative and supportive acts of others.

To understand this one only need contemplate the difficulties abused women or abused children have in exercising their autonomy and making informed judgments about their situations. Poor self-images, self-blame, fear, and possible social censure all play roles in inhibiting these individuals from exercising their autonomous informed consent. Another interesting piece of evidence confirming the importance of social conditions to autonomy and consent in health care is the demonstrated fact that the use of and satisfaction with health care services among ethnic minorities increases with the presence of ethnically and linguistically trained health care staff.[14]

A more social understanding of informed consent would encourage training of health providers and HMO personnel in ways that would better equip them to deal with and respect their diverse patient population. This issue will be developed further as I discuss the roles of provider and patient as mutual interpreters and the need for professional and personal virtues.

Another obvious issue is the need for health education to help all individuals better understand the essentials of health care as well as the problems of limited resources. Also crucial are dialogue and community building concerning clinical diagnosis and care, beginning at the level of patient and physician and moving to the level of the family and other small social units such as employee groups, Medicaid patients, health plan members, and ethnic and cultural groups. The discussions should concern the meaning of health, priorities for health care, and common values and goals. Patients subscribing to a health plan or HMO should have a role in the management of the plan similar to the role of good PTA groups in the management of neighborhood schools.

Dialogue is already being tried and is demonstrating success. For instance, in Orange County, California, there is a Medicaid Managed Care Initiative that is engaged in facilitating dialogue between the Medicare population, public officials, and health care plan representatives on values and issues that are central in devising an adequate health coverage system for the county. To incorporate community values into the plan and its determination of coverage, focus groups were initiated that included ethnic representation from the African-American, Latino, Asian-American, and Caucasian communities, the Medicaid population, and a cross section of the general community. The values identified by the Medicaid population were dignity, respect, and fairness; those identified by the cross-sectional group were affordability and personal responsibility; and both groups identified quality and accountability as important priorities. Community input was sought in determining the values and goals of the plan in CEO recruitment, in marketing guidelines, in provider contracting structures, and in continuous quality improvement processes.[15]

A similar effort is that of the Rocky Mountain Centre for Health Care Ethics, which has facilitated dialogue among employers, patients, purchasers, and providers to forge a code of ethics for the managed care plan to be adopted in their community. This effort has involved various focus groups dealing with four sets of issues: economics and resources, relationships and responsibilities, information and education, and allocation of resources. In addition to developing a general code of ethics, the project has determined that an extensive community education program will be needed to best implement the plan that is finally devised.[16]

These efforts represent the building of communal consent and of community and are good examples of what I call enlightened provincialism—that is, the development of supportive communities with common goals and extension of these goals through time through dialogue and mutual interpretation. This involves a subtle blending of individual good and communal good and an extension of both individuals and communities beyond their own self-interests. The operative moral principle is the Roycean one of "loyalty to loyalty"—that is, the commitment to continual broadening of community through dialogue, mediation, and mutual interpretation.[17] This means that decisions made about autonomy, justice, health care, and so on, should be judged by their ability to broaden the conditions of autonomy and justice for other individuals and groups and to broaden the concern in health care for the basic functioning of the individual to a range of individuals.

I have spelled out the philosophical foundations of enlightened provincialism in my book *Genuine Individuals and Genuine Communities*, but here I sketch a few elements of what this communal-individual framework means for ethics in health care. First, there is an assumption of the inherent worth of individuals and their chosen life plans. It is these life plans and the stories embedded in them that constitute an individual's uniqueness and identification as a moral person.

Second and equally compelling is the fact of human interdependence. Individuals and communities need each other, and it is the community that must foster genuine individuality and the ability to realize individual life plans and goals. This means that there is a strong joint individual and communal responsibility for honoring human dignity and fostering the realization of the personal and social goals of individuals.[18] Common communal goods and a basic level of individual physiological, psychological, and social functionality are agreed upon in a mutual decision-making process and defined as "health." I discuss this more in the next section.

Third, if the resources of a family, social group, or society are such that limiting or rationing health care resources is necessary, the need for such must be clearly demonstrated in terms of achieving a communal goal while respecting individual human dignity in a process of open and participatory discussion and decision making. Rationing should be a shared common hardship, and applicable to all. Monitoring of rationing should be required, but mechanisms for such should allow continual, open, participatory discussion and evaluation of the results of the rationing measures.[19] The notion of solidarity—that is, the notion that all persons are equally responsible for sharing the burdens as well as the benefits of protection against death and disability—should be promoted. This notion is one apparently acceptable in European insurance circles and in their discussions of health care issues.

It should be clear at this point that I agree with the analysis of those who conclude (1) that rationing is already a part of our health care system, but it is implicit and not so identified, (2) that there are limited health care resources, (3) that these limits will not be overcome by elimination of various kinds of waste, and (4) that rationing decisions about health care are therefore inevitable.[20] Further, in the context of what has already been said, I agree with Leonard Fleck when he proposes that "rationing decisions do need to be made communally, if they are to be made fairly" and that every rationing decision, a decision that will have an impact on a specific individual's health and life, "should be endorsed at some level by the individual who will bear the burden of that decision."[21] Fleck has also identified two central characteristics of "unjust" rationing decisions: they are not self-imposed, and specific rationing decisions are made in arbitrary, subjective, and idiosyncratic ways.[22]

Community building and dialogue, then, become essential to justice in our health care delivery system and in dealing with rationing. First, such communal dialogue makes rationing decisions explicit and public.

The words of Uwe Reinhardt make my point: "The whole idea of managed competition is to delegate these painful decisions (about resource allocation for expensive, marginally beneficial, life-prolonging medical care) into the dark corners of the HMO. . . . This is a smart way of delegating painful decisions from the government to the private sector."[23]

Second, communal and public dialogue about rationing helps avoid fictions about the process. For example, rationing cannot be narrowly defined as denying an *"identified individual* significant health care for *economic reasons."*[24] Rather, it must be seen more broadly in terms of general health planning or utilization decisions, such as who will be admitted to or discharged early from an ICU. This is why individual and communal consent is an important part of utilization and general plan decision making. In this regard, the community must be broad to include all affected parties—lay, professional, and expert. The new type of thinking needed to deal with these issues is *not,* as David Eddy suggests, a "shift in medical thinking from quality to quantify."[25] Empirical evidence about outcomes is important in making treatment, rationing, and outcome decisions, but it is and should be only one important part of the communal dialogue about priorities.

A second key part of community building and dialogue with regard to the rationing question is that aspect of community called time-extension. David Eddy makes the point that "good" rationing decisions—those to which most reasonable people would agree—are those which are long-term decisions. Therefore, in switching from overused low-value practices to underused high-value practices and to determine various priorities for funding and treatment, the assumption is that the person making the decision is choosing for his or her future self and in making this choice does not have knowledge of his or her future health status. The person is self-imposing a limit on health care resources that may or may not have an impact on him or her in the future, but if it does this decision was an autonomous one and further, this person has most likely benefited from other decisions made in the past that freed up health resources.

The difficulty with the present health care system is that individuals do not necessarily have a long-term commitment to a health plan, and therefore the decisions they make now will not necessarily impact them in the future because by then they will have moved to another plan with different priorities. Yet they have made these decision for others in the original community.

Genuine community involves loyalty and commitment to common goals; abandonment of the community is betrayal. The paradigm being developed here assumes that loyalty is an important component of one's personal and professional ethical life. Loyalty, of course, is never blind, but rather is based on autonomy and on one's own life plan and chosen center. I will say more about this shortly, but briefly, mechanisms need to be developed to increase loyal commitment among patients and providers. I believe communal dialogue and participation in the shaping of health plans, priorities, and basic health care decisions will do much to foster loyalty.

Because I have briefly discussed rationing, I also need to briefly talk about justice. In the framework of enlightened provincialism, justice should be seen as the application of practical and prudential wisdom achieved through consensus building in a democratic, participatory, open-ended process. In distributing social goods the principles of autonomy and beneficence should be weighed and balanced in a way that honors the human dignity of the individuals involved while seeking to balance individual and social good in the context of the social circumstances of the specific individual and others also affected by decisions.

However, decisions need to be guided by the principle of loyalty to loyalty—that is, the commitment to create and foster conditions that broaden the possibility that others will have access to the good(s) in question. Individual and collective stewardship should be encouraged. Health care resources are a common social good that must be prudentially used by society and by individuals. There should be no open-ended individual right to health care in the sense of access to everything that is available. A balance needs to be sought in families, social units, and general society between preventive care, rescue medicine, and long-term care. Further, investments must be made by individuals and society in education about health care and health care choices in order to facilitate the making of informed choices and to protect stewardship.

Finally, enlightened provincialism promotes the value of caring. Human beings are necessarily interdependent, and caring should be viewed as a basic human need—a necessary condition, in fact—for adequate human development and for the development of self-worth as an individual. Justice as prudential wisdom requires that we support, encourage, and seek to broadly distribute this valuable and common good. Technological care is not ultimately the most valuable health care resource; the most valuable such resource is humane care and caring. And, contrary to the paradigmatic individualistic framework, we are not and need not be alone and solitary in our encounters with illness and death. These events are eminently individual, but also social and communal.

Disease and Illness: A Continuum of Whole-Person Functioning

Another part of our paradigm shift, and an aspect especially appropriate for discussions of managed care, is a shift in our understanding of health and treatment with an accompanying shift in ethical and professional attitude. More specifically, there needs to be (1) a shift in our understanding of health and illness from a model based purely on disease and critical care to the notion of illness and suffering as impacting the whole person, including the person's social setting; (2) a broadening of our view of care to include various forms of functionality as defined by the various parties involved, including the patient; (3) a new conception of treatment that fits a notion of a continuum of care and a reverse of the traditional attitude of fitting the patient to the treatment to a new attitude of fitting the treatment to the patient; and (4) a new notion of the role of health care providers that sees them as mediators, interpreters, and community enhancers.

Before turning to the explication of a paradigm shift in the understanding of ethical practice in health care, we seek to reconceptualize the notions of illness, health, treatment, care, and health care practice. Ethics, after all, is always practiced in a context, and one ethical duty we have is to mold an environment that we consider valid and facilitative of moral behavior.

Disease or illness, in the traditional health care model, known as the medical model, is primarily conceived as physically based in some organic dysfunction. This is even true of mental illnesses, in which the organic dysfunction is usually sought in brain mechanisms. The medical model implies nonresponsibility on the part of the patient due to the physical, external causation of the disease or illness, and the assumption is that the patient cannot get well on his or her own, but must seek expert help and knowledge based on scientific investigation and validation.[26] Accompanying this medical model is the notion of the "sick role," which connects illness with "abnormal social behavior or dysfunction."[27] The sick role implies temporary exemption from social responsibility with an obligation to get well as soon as possible by seeking technical/expert help because one cannot pull oneself together.

Therefore, *illness* or *disease* is usually defined in terms of a deficit in the physical form or psychological functioning of the individual. The individual's functioning is seen in a twofold manner: in terms of what society wants or expects from the individual and in terms of what the individual wants or expects from him- or herself. In health care practice generally the emphasis, as least explicitly, has presumably been on the individual, with the stress on autonomy and informed consent.

If we are honest, however, we admit that the notion of informed consent is still relatively new to the health care scene and that, as a matter of fact, paternalism has more often been present. This is the reason for the strong stress on autonomy and individual rights and the hesitancy to switch the emphasis to the community or others. Again, in my paradigm I wish to put equal emphasis on the individual and the community, and I would not discount in any way the need for attention to autonomy, informed consent, or rights. The need is for a reconceptualization of all three concepts in terms of the person as both individual and social. Being honest in a further sense, we recognize that the emphasis in health care has more often been on functionality in societal terms and less on functionality as defined by the patient.

How, then, might we redefine *disease* and *illness*? A good beginning, I believe, is to see them as a loss of autonomy and functionality in four realms of human endeavor.[28] First is the realm of "embodied meaning." Illness may cause loss of bodily and mental functionality that limits one's access to the world or distorts access so that the self is not completely functional in the world of other persons and things. Second is the realm of intersubjective life. Illness may inhibit one's fulfillment of his or her roles in the social world, including one's family and other personal relations.

Third is the realm of the will and life planning. Illness can prohibit the setting and achievement of personally chosen and significant goals, such as being a world-class athlete, or cause one to reassess one's goals and plans. Fourth is the realm of universal harmony. Illness can cause loss of connection with some ultimate meaning or being and thus feelings of emptiness, betrayal, loss of one's soul, and/or spiritual crisis.

From this scheme it becomes clear that restoration of health could have a profound effect in any or all of these different realms and in varying degrees and that, to a great extent, restoration needs to be in accordance with what illness and loss of functionality mean to the individual. Dialogue about what illness means to the individual is important, and a "values history and plan" should be incorporated into the person's medical record.[29] There is also an assumption that significant others, whether family or other persons, might be involved in helping to determine what restoration of health might mean to the individual.

Another implication of the receonceptualization of illness and health is that a new view of care and treatment needs to be developed to fit this more expansive view of health restoration, and to be more sensitive to individual and communal needs. Actually, therapeutic intervention in the era of managed care is changing, and the following characteristics seem to be emerging: (1) short-term care—that is, the use of crisis intervention to resolve desperate situations; (2) focused treatment—that is, identification and treatment of the target symptoms of the chief complaint; (3) goal-oriented intervention—that is, adequate resolution of the chief complaint if possible; (4) treatment designed only for the chief complaint; (5) episodic care—that is, resolution of acuteness and return for brief short-term treatments if needed; (6) emphasis on resolving "daily living" dysfunction; and (7) focus on stabilization.

Clinicians who wish to be engaged in ethical practice that benefits patients must deal with this framework in a collaborative and yet reasoned dialogue with patients and HMO officials. They also need to advocate for clear practice guidelines that, ideally, are worked out with participation by all involved in implementing the plans. These guidelines should take into account empirical data about outcomes, but also should involve reflective prudential wisdom about clear short-term and long-term gains or liabilities of the treatments and practices in terms of the four realms of meaning enumerated earlier as well as acceptable everyday functioning for the patient in terms of his or her values and roles, but not without consideration of the needs of others for treatment and resources. Dialogue with the patient and significant others is essential as well as joint dialogue, if possible, with HMO officials and others.

Clinicians and patients must be imaginative and innovative in seeking treatment practices that will deal adequately with patients' problems and will promote change for the better. Assumptions that traditional treatment practices are always best should be avoided. Treatment plans must be tighter, practical and specifically goal oriented, but all involved must be committed to reasonable access, quality of outcomes, and justice in distribution of health care resources. Vulnerable populations need to be protected, but protection and care must be critically and reflectively thought out; for instance, "intensive service" must be creatively separated and distinguished from shorter-term treatment, and various modalities of outpatient, community, and home treatment must be developed—again, if possible, in communal dialogue.

Further, health care providers need to work as teams, recognizing each others' talents, values, and resources. The same should be true for patients and their communal support groups. Again, human resources and caring can be as valuable or more valuable than technical care and resources, and each should play the proper role in treatment.

Justice in distribution of scarce health resources must be a continual consideration. The focus should be on establishing high-value treatments, even if underused, and decisions must be made about use of treatments that have lower value and yet may be costly in terms of distribution of the common health care resource. Discussion and practice should center on the establishment of a continuum of treatment and care based on a balancing of stewardship of resources with clinical and patient judgments about access to and quality of care. The goal should be to provide treatment and care in the least restrictive settings and to foster the timely flow of patients through various appropriate levels of care. Education should be a continual concern so that issues of value and appropriateness can be addressed, criticized, and understood and so that various perspectives—cultural, ethnic, professional, and personal—can be part of the overall decision-making process.

An important aspect of this kind of understanding of illness and its treatment is the notion of an interpreter, a role that should be played by various kinds of health care providers, but is equally appropriate for patients, significant others, and HMO personnel. An interpreter is one who takes on the task of building bridges of meaning and value between perspectives, people, and ideas. This is a complex and yet eminently ethical task, for it involves respect for persons and the honoring of autonomy and, if done well, it requires various virtues, primarily those of humility, compassion, patience, hope, prudence and courage.

In order to properly build bridges, an interpreter must have respect and regard for each person, each set of values, and each set of beliefs and ideas held by the parties among whom he or she seeks to build a "community" of meaning and value. For example, it should be assumed that the patient's experiences and perspectives are valid contributions to understanding the nature of his or her illness, its impact, and its meaning. Likewise, the patient's priorities, views of health, and life plan should be important components of treatment and care plans. It should be equally assumed that the views and values of managed care personnel are not just misguided and unethical. The interpreter's views also have validity.

The interpreter must have critical tolerance for all parties. That is, he or she must show respect for each person and idea and should give each person's ideas a fair hearing in the open forum of communal discussion even though these might not ultimately be implemented or only partially implemented. The goal of interpretation is to reach a consensus view that all can agree with in some way and that all feel comfortable implementing. In engaging in interpretation, the interpreter needs to be particularly sensitive to those who are vulnerable and whose voices may be silent or unrepresented, such as children or persons who are mentally impaired.

The role of the interpreter is not an easy one. It involves a set of virtues. A virtue is generally understood to be a "dispositional trait of character considered praiseworthy. I consider virtues crucial to ethical behavior and practice, because habits drive behavior in a crucial way and ethical habits can only foster better ethical practice, especially as virtues are the result of reflective and continuous practice. They involve attitudes brought to a situation and, as indicated in my earlier discussion of conditions for informed consent, attitudes can both hinder and facilitate good practice.

Virtues also imply consistency of practice and behavior, a trait important to ethical behavior and reasonableness. Further, as Aristotle made so clear, virtues are not blind habits, but rather are based on prudential wisdom, on assessment of the appropriate fit of a virtue to a given situation. Virtues involve balance and exercise of the "mean" in situations, not excess or deficit. For instance, in exercising courage—that is, action in the face of danger, such as might be taken by a whistle-blower—one acts neither rashly, with foolhardiness, nor without courage, as in cowardliness. In my view virtues, principles, and context all play key roles in ethical deliberation and practice.

The set of virtues needed by an interpreter are (1) *humility* to recognize that one's own and others' perspectives and meanings are only partial and are not the whole story; (2) *hope* that some consensus or harmony of views may be possible and that a fuller, more adequate understanding of the situation will be achieved; (3) *courage* to reach out to others and to risk having one's own values and ideas tested against those of others and to face possible failure if consensus cannot be reached; (4) *compassion* to try to understand, experience, and even sympathize with what is significant to the others involved; (5) *tolerance* to be able to confront, understand, and seek some common ground with values and views perhaps very foreign to one's own; (6) *patience* to persist in seeking to overcome resistance and confrontation for collaboration and mutual effort; and (7) *loyalty* to the concept of broader community, to the effort to harmonize conflicting loyalties and values so that a broader truth and value may be realized.

Interpretation, then, is clearly an ethical activity and one that is crucially important to ethical practice and moral care in the new health care environment. I will say more about virtues and ethics, but first I must make it clear that others besides the clinician could and should serve as interpreter. However, I believe that a person with expertise and some social power, such as the physician or another health care provider, has a fiduciary obligation to take on the role of interpreter.

Stewardship within the Context of Autonomy, Virtues, and Principles

Given the ethical nature of the interpreter's role, it seems appropriate to discuss a shift in our views of ethical practice to complement the shift in our conception of illness, treatment, and the role of health care providers. Traditional discussions of ethical issues in health care have, in the past, rightfully focused on principles of autonomy, beneficence, and justice. These principles are still crucial, yet I believe they need to be refocused for the new health care environment. Perhaps it is merely that these principles have not always been clearly understood and, of course, they are not so easily applied in concrete situations. Indeed, a major lesson of any discussion in ethics is that the world is complex, ambiguous, and uncertain; ethical situations are opaque, and therefore ethical practice requires practical wisdom and open, democratic discussion with representatives of all interests involved, if possible. This is why interpretation and its virtues are so crucial in the health care arena.

There is no doubt that the principle of autonomy ought to have priority in any discussion of ethics in health care. *Autonomy* is best defined as the right to make one's own choices. This, however, needs to be refined and expanded as follows: The right to make choices must be seen as circumstantial freedom; therefore, we can say that autonomy is the ability, under favorable circumstances, to act as one wishes for one's own good as one sees it. This makes clear the notion of a right as an "operative social institution" and the need for autonomy to be facilitated both by the environment and by others.[30]

Technology, for example, can play a key role in providing circumstantial freedom or in hindering it. Thus, the automobile and computer have permitted many more choices and ways to realize our freedom; however, their existence can inhibit our freedom either if we lack access to them or if someone deliberately uses them to rob us of our freedom. Drug technology has helped many mentally ill patients to become functional in certain senses, but drugs also rob us of freedom by bypassing our conscious will. This notion of autonomy as circumstantial freedom also returns us to the concept of health as functionality in various modes and to the need to work creatively to make persons as functional in as many ways as required by society and others—and above all, as expected and needed by the persons themselves.

It ought to be clear that respect for autonomy demands that we not interfere with the choice of another unless it seems justified. However, the justification must be solid and agreed to by others, including the person. This imperative for noninterference, nevertheless, must not be seen as a call to give in to a person's every demand. There must be distinctions between need and desire and persuasion; that is, the attempt to provide reasons for a different choice or point of view is always permissible and may, in certain situations, be morally demanded. The various levels of functionality and meaning I have described in my discussion of health and the notion of health care as a common social good and resource may be helpful in making a distinction between need and want. This context certainly is more promising than that which views health care as a product to be bought and sold.

Respect for autonomy also places upon us and others the obligation to treat persons as capable of choice unless there is good evidence against viewing them as autonomous. We must not be too ready to assume incompetence. This is too often done with the mentally ill, the mentally incapacitated, children, the elderly, and, in perhaps too many cases, with minority groups, various cultural groups, or even with many women. We must always remember that competence comes in degrees and varieties, and we must work to develop a continuum of competence that makes sense for the various kinds of situations and contexts that might have to be faced in judging one's ability to take autonomous action.

Above all, we must look at enabling circumstances for autonomy that we can change, such as attitudes, language, and cultural barriers, as well as generational barriers and false social and cultural stereotypes and myths. In addition, we need a parallel continuum of coercion and manipulation, for these too can come in varying degrees and often depends on the perspective of the person being coerced. Some people are coerced by mice, but others are not; some mental patients are coerced by threats of further hospitalization, but others are not. Prudential wisdom and ethical, critical alertness are required to work for autonomous action for ourselves and others.

Beneficence is another key ethical principle that should guide health care provision, for it means seeking to promote the good of others and working to not inflict harm or evil—that is, nonmaleficence. The central question for implementing this principle is, How does one know what is the good of another? To assume that one does know this is to possibly fall into the trap of paternalism.

Beneficence and its implementation especially require interpretation and dialogue. The good of a patient can often be discovered in sympa-

thetic discussion with the patient and others. One of the benefits of forming small communities or "provinces" is so that members of these may
develop some understanding of the values and life plans of other members and so that beneficence can be more justly and appropriately
applied. Above all, strong paternalism—that is, acting without consent,
for the presumed good of another—is morally wrong and does, in fact,
violate autonomy and the dignity of the other person. Autonomy and
dignity must always be operative along with beneficence, and beneficence can best be sought in communal contexts and interpretative dialogue.

This brings me to what I consider the best operative ethical principle
for health care and ethical practice in general—namely, the proportionality principle. This principle is essentially that there must be proportion-
ate good to justify permitting the risk of harmful consequences. Further,
this principle can be applied morally only if it does not permit an action
that is against individual dignity and autonomy.[31] The proportionality
principle asks us to be reflective and critically analytical in our ethical
practice. It demands that we ask three crucial questions: (1) What are the
kind and level of the good intended and the kind and level of the harm
risked or permitted? (2) What is the certitude or probability of the good
intended or the harm risked? and (3) What are the actual causal influences in the situation—that is, what factors will really determine the outcomes, and how much force do they have?

Reflecting on these three questions, we can see that in making health
care decisions they would require, first of all, focused, clear treatment
plans, goals, and projected outcomes. Empirical data would be needed,
yet one would also need to recognize that there is, in health care practice
and treatment, many uncertainties. These would need to be clearly recognized and shared with patients and others and dealt with accordingly.
Too often health care providers are afraid to acknowledge uncertainty
and patients mistakenly believe in too unreasonable expectations and
miracles. These misguided attitudes need to be dealt with and overcome
in honest dialogue and assessment of situations.

Further, reflecting on these three questions requires us to really examine the factors that are crucial in an illness as well as those likely to bring
about some definite positive changes. It also demands that we realisti-
cally assess each of our own roles as clinicians, significant others, and
patients in terms of our ability to promote recovery and some restoration
of functionality.

Finally we come back to virtues. Virtues are part of the prudential
wisdom required for applying the principle of proportionality as well as

the principles of autonomy, beneficence, and justice. Virtues should be both personal and professional. I do not believe that one can have one "moral self" for home and another for work. This is "moral schizophrenia," and all of us know that the splitting of the self is unhealthy and unwise.

I have already discussed virtues in the section on interpretation, but I believe there are also some general ones that are necessary for ethical practice in health care and that these are virtues that should be both professional and personal, for practitioners as well as patients. The first of these virtues is honesty—that is, telling the truth as one is best able to discern it in situations in which the person or persons with whom one is interacting have a right to know the truth. Engaging in dishonesty or falsehood is lying or hiding the truth when others have a reasonable expectation of being told the truth. The right to be told the truth is best seen in the context of informed consent, for the correct information is needed for one to have informed consent and to make good decisions. To lie or withhold information is to be disrespectful of both the persons and with whom one is interacting and their autonomy. Honesty is also needed to foster trust between persons whether in personal, therapeutic, or professional relationships.

In the health care environment, to practice honesty as a health care provider is to be open about signs and symptoms, about what impairment one is trying to ease or eliminate, about rationales for treatment strategies, about alternative strategies, about uncertainties and probabilities, about practice guidelines and limitations on care or about treatments and the reasons for these, and of course about financial incentives or disincentives if they are present. For the patient, honesty requires sharing relevant information about habits, values, desires for functionality, and limits of social roles and situations. For the health care providers, it is honest to assume that there is a reasonable expectation of truth and that clients are capable of handling the truth, unless there is very convincing evidence to the contrary. Honesty requires that all parties share any discomfort with possible decisions in terms of their value systems.

Humility, the second virtue, is the ability to acknowledge the limits of one's knowledge and competency. It allows one to overcome professional narcissism—that is, infatuation with one's talents and knowledge. Humility involves the ability to acknowledge uncertainty, to see the validity of other competencies and proposals, and to collaborate with the patient and others in seeking a common and agreed-upon plan of action. It allows one to avoid the situation of the "wise men and the elephant," in which several blind wise men, each of whom was able to experience only a part of an elephant, emphatically asserted their experience of the elephant told them what the elephant was really like. Humility, like honesty, is a virtue needed by everyone in the health care picture, including patients.

Stewardship is a virtue necessary today in health care and in life in general, because there are limits to resources, a common need for these resources, and a need to definitely share resources with others. This virtue requires an ability to recognize one's connectedness and interdependence, to acknowledge that individual well-being is always in a social context and that we need each other's concern and care. It entails the careful, reflective use of one's own and society's resources. It demands tough decisions and courageous action.

Loyalty is commitment to a cause, an idea, a person, or a community. It is a powerful form of love and care. In health care it has always meant the fiduciary responsibility of a health care provider to the well-being of his or her patient. In today's health care environment it also means the patient's loyalty to his or her clinician and to decisions made in concert with others about health care priorities. For all persons it means commitment to a common goal of promoting fair and just access to health care for all and to fair and just use of the distribution of scarce health care resources. Above all, loyalty is reflective and critical and involves our continually asking the question, How can loyalty to others and to the broader community be facilitated?

What, then, is ethics in our new environment of managed care? It is the application of practical wisdom—that is, the right way of acting in difficult and uncertain circumstances for a specific end. It also means ensuring fair access to health care and providing individual patients with reasonable functionality in their circumstances given the resources, values, and talents available. What is ethical practice? It is embracing ambiguity and uncertainty while eschewing paternalistic expertise and attitudes and courageously seeking to deliver quality and reasonable health care to those who need it. It is applying the principle of proportionality in a context of interpretation and community building that requires honesty, humility, and loyalty while seeking justice with courage and evincing an attitude of positive hope and expectation. This is a most difficult task—but, I believe, an ultimately fulfilling one.

17 Untying the Gag: Reason in the World of Health Care Reform

JOHN T. LYSAKER AND MICHAEL SULLIVAN

If instrumental efficacies need to be emphasized, it is not for the sake of instruments but for the sake of that full and more secure distribution of values which is impossible without instrumentalities.
John Dewey, Experience and Nature

In lay discussion as well as scientific, reason has come to be commonly regarded as an intellectual faculty of coordination, the efficiency of which can be increased by methodical use and by the removal of any non-intellectual factors. . . . Reason has never really directed social reality, but now reason has been so thoroughly purged of any specific content that it has finally renounced even the task of passing judgment on man's actions and way of life.
Max Horkheimer, Eclipse of Reason

SINCE HEGEL, we have been reminded of the threats posed by instrumental reason. We blind ourselves to descriptive and normative truths, the argument goes, when we limit the formation of rational practice to the production of means rationalized for the realization of accepted if poorly understood ends. Not only does this procedure foreclose discussion of ends, but, as this century has proven, it often fetishizes means until their management supersedes the realization of the ends they were instituted to bring to fruition. A severe malady in deed and thought, instrumental reason deprives agents, acting individually or collectively, of recourse to rational, democratic discussion about the goods its productive machinery works to secure—for instance, life, liberty, and, in some versions, even happiness.

It is our opinion that in the United States the health care debate is currently hostage to theoretical models ensnared in the webs of instrumental reason. Said more precisely, those currently discussing the future of U.S. health care are blind to the normative dimensions of the controversy as well as the social conditions that form the hinge upon which any plausible solution might swing. Our task here is to outline a path of inquiry that promises a more rational engagement with the multifaceted problems confronting health care practices in the United States.

Gag Rules: The Debate behind the Debate

It is no exaggeration to speak of a health care crisis in the United States. Not only are millions of citizens underinsured or uninsured, not only do many more have limited access to adequate medical treatment and information, but the United States, in comparison to other industrial nations, devotes the highest percentage of its gross domestic product to health care.[1] Moreover—and this testifies to the depth of our crisis—no consensus exists concerning the nature of the problem, let alone what direction reform should take. Not only was this lack of consensus apparent in the salvos that greeted President Clinton's proposed Health Security Act, but it has again been evident in the more recent discussions surrounding the costs and benefits of health maintenance organizations (HMOs).

HMOs began appearing in the 1970s in response to rising medical costs, selling themselves as quality care providers emphasizing preventive medicine and cost control. Two cost-control measures bear notice. First, HMOs precertify only those practices (routine physicals and examinations, prescription of standard medications, x-rays, and so on) that have proven, over time, to be central to quality care. For extraordinary tests and procedures, HMOs require physicians to submit treatment plans for review. HMOs then decide whether they will pay for the proposed treatments or recommend other avenues. The rationale is that decreases in unnecessary treatments and tests should lower costs over time.

Another cost-control measure is incentive-based payment plans for doctors and hospitals, or what has come to be called capitation. After calculating expected costs for a given period, HMOs inspire doctors and hospitals to deliver services at lower costs by agreeing to pay them, often atop a base salary, a percentage of every dollar they save the HMO by spending less than projected. It is therefore in the financial interest of physicians and hospitals to be more efficient, and this should, HMOs argue, pass savings on to patients and those who fund their care, often employers.

It would appear that HMOs have been somewhat successful in controlling medical costs. As reported in the *PR Newswire* for June 19, 1995, "Managed care has helped slow the pace of medical inflation, as measured by the Consumer Price Index. In 1990, the cost of medical care services was rising almost 10 percent a year; last year it went up about 4.5 percent." Likewise, HMOs have managed to slow the rise of premium costs for employers: "In 1988, when employers were paying premiums mostly for traditional insurance plans, their premiums rose at a rate of more than 18 percent. In 1995, when many employers had switched to managed care, premiums went up only 2 percent, and that was after a 1 percent decline the previous year."[2]

It is an open question, of course, whether such cost-saving trends will continue, but for the time being, HMOs have delivered on part of their promise: to control medical costs. But what about their promises concerning quality care? Of late, this has been a matter of intense debate, and the discussion has centered around the following question: Do the cost-control mechanisms employed by HMOs ensure quality care, or do they compromise care in order to contain costs, thereby increasing an organization's profit margin?[3] Perhaps the most scrutinized mechanisms are called gag rules. Let us explore those for a moment.

Strictly speaking, several aspects of managed care have been thrown into the category of gag rules. On the one hand, some HMOs employ gag rules in order to limit physician-patient discussion of treatment options. If an HMO will not cover the treatment, the argument runs, why discuss it? Another type of gag rule prohibits physicians from disclosing the incentives built into their contracts given that particular contractual relationships are not germane to treatment, but solely matters between employer and employees. A third form involves "no-disparagement clauses," clauses designed to prevent physicians from criticizing HMOs' procedures and possibly driving away clients.

Given the range of issues associated with gag rules, it is clear that the term refers less to discrete phenomena than to a general dissatisfaction with the present state of managed care.[4] What has emerged amidst the shouting, however, is a picture of the risks inherent in current managed care practices. In setting limits on what can be discussed between doctors and their patients, HMOs appear to restrict physician autonomy, thus compromising doctors' ability to hunt down remedies for vexing problems. Second, the likelihood of having distant forces evaluate treatment options has eroded patient trust. Clients of HMOs cannot help but wonder whether they have been made aware of all available treatments. Moreover, given that HMO profits hinge upon removing "unnecessary" costs, patients are rightfully afraid that certain decisions are driven by economic interest rather than medical opinion. Third, HMOs appear to establish a conflicts of interest between hospitals or physicians and patients. If hospitals and physicians earn more when they treat less, health care providers have an economic incentive not to be as thorough as possible.

Undoubtedly more could be said about these risks inherent in gag rules, and still other risks associated with managed care could be enumerated. The range of issues one confronts when evaluating managed care is vast. Our goal is not to provide a comprehensive survey of the managed care debate, but rather to find a point of entry into the more general debate surrounding health care reform. What interests us about the recent gag rule controversy is that it makes visible and available for investigation the dominant interests and central conceptions directing— too often unconsciously or at least without notice—our nation's attempts at health care reform. Methodologically, therefore, we invoke the debate over gag rules because it provides a microcosm within which to study the meaning and consequences of dominant health care reform models.

Concern over the impact of gag rules on physicians, patients, and health care in general has led to legislative action. Several states have outlawed restrictions on the discussion of treatment options.[5] Likewise, the Department of Health and Human Services now insists that a doctor caring for a Medicare patient "'may not be limited in counseling or advising the beneficiary' about treatment options that may be appropriate for the patient's condition or disease."[6] States like New York and Oregon are also increasingly demanding that HMOs permit patients to explore physician contracts in order to understand what incentives are driving their health care. All in all, then, it would seem that gag rules will soon be a thing of the past and that the future of managed care will be regulated by state-level and even federal legislation.

The impending removal of gag rules from managed care suggests a victory for those concerned about the quality of health care. It appears that their normative demands have triumphed over fetishized cost-control measures. Although broad consensus exists concerning the undesirability of gag rules, with several HMOs in agreement, we should not lose sight of the fact that wildly divergent visions of the future of U.S. health care undergird the concurrence. Some gag rule opponents argue that gag rules perniciously interfere with physician-patient relationships.[7] Others object that such rules violate consumer rights.[8] Still others, although troubled by gag rules, resist government interference in the marketplace.[9] The rally to bring down gag rules thus hides significant disagreement about health care's deepest ends.

Unfortunately, the gag rule debate ended before these differences in perspectives became conspicuous and a matter for reflection. As a result, the larger project of health care reform missed a golden opportunity to deepen its moral and theoretical underpinnings. Health care reform can go forward only if we know how to choose among our various ends when they prove incompatible. How else will we mediate conflicts among our concerns for physician autonomy, provider profits, consumer choice, cost control, quality care, and technological innovation? In crucial moments, should some goals supersede others? Without a rationale for prioritizing our concerns, such decisions will fall prey to power politics. We should not be misled, therefore, by the surprising consensus that overthrew many gag rules. Promoters of health care reform in the United States are still unsure of what ends they hope to realize. In fact, they are driven by multiple—at times conflicting—concerns. Progress, therefore, depends on public discussion of the fundamental expectations informing current reform proposals. At this point, then, we wish to push past the specifics of the gag rule debate and engage the dominant theoretical models orienting its most vocal participants.

Professions and Markets: Mismanaging Medicine

Although several objections have been voiced and many charges levied in the debate surrounding gag rules, two general theoretical models have been prevalent. On the one hand, several discussants have pitched their claims within a professional model. Professional models emphasize the importance of the physician-patient relationship, arguing that it must form the crux of the debate.[10] Note that this model animates not only those supporting the priority of physician autonomy, but also those who enter the debate as patient advocates. The intuition underlying this position is that the physician-patient relationship forms the backbone of health care, and its demands must take precedence over bureaucratic and market concerns.

On the other hand, many view the matter of reform through the lens of the market, arguing that health care needs to be brought into line with standard business practices. The key to successful reform, they claim, lies in streamlining production techniques, controlling costs, and ensuring consumer satisfaction.[11] As before, this is not a one-sided affair. The market model is invoked by those siding with either consumers or producers, for in both instances health care is regarded as a commodity.[12]

As we argued in the previous section, health care reform must begin with inquiry into these perspectives. We begin with the professional model. In many of the cries for health care reform one finds the notion that control over health care should be returned to those at the center of its practice: physicians. Others, concerned equally with patient and physician autonomy, demand that health care reform begin from reflections on the physician-patient relationship and respect the collaborative autonomy indicative of sound medical treatment. The intuition behind these appeals is a strong one, particularly given the bureaucratic and even autocratic excesses afflicting managed care. As State Senator Gunther of Connecticut has said, "We need to get the provider back in his proper role in the health care system."[13]

As widespread as these intuitions are, little work has been done to develop a reform model that grants physicians significant administrative and clinical autonomy while responding to questions concerning universal access, cost control, and sustainable development. One exception is the work of Eliot Freidson, who advocates for a turn toward a profession-governed health care system.[14] In his view, health care will be managed best by health care professionals operating within the following guidelines. First, a base income floor must be established for physicians in order to control costs. Second, physician-run licensing and review procedures must be established in order to ensure quality care. Third, the profession must cultivate among its membership a spirit of scientific openness to criticism and review as well as a commitment to service over profit.

Freidson has introduced his plan, what he terms "The Professional Labor model," in response to the limits of the free market and bureaucratic approaches. In his mind, market models always allow their concern with profit margins to derail health care, emphasizing material gain over the delivery of the good that defines the nature and purpose of the medical profession—that is, care.[15] And although bureaucratic models of health care management might ensure lower costs, their reliance on standardized methods of diagnosis and treatment cripple physicians' abilities to address their clients' specific needs.[16] As Freidson writes, "[Under bureaucratic models] . . . people are reduced to formally defined categories. They become objects produced by reliable methods at predictable costs. . . . [A bureaucratic model thus] . . . undermines the flexible discretionary judgment that is necessary to adapt services to individual needs."[17]

We find some of Freidson's intuitions quite sound. Profit-driven markets rarely ensure quality or access at the expense of economic gain, and bureaucratic management practices have hindered physicians in their efforts to provide individualized care. On the whole, however, his proposal seems almost surreal. On the one hand, we agree with Freidson's claim that "policy should discourage those who are inclined to devote their efforts primarily to maximizing their income while encouraging those who assign greater value to doing good work for the benefit of others."[18] All professions could benefit from such policy.

But it is preposterous to suggest that a spirit of giving will control malfeasance in the administration of what amounts to monopoly control over a vital human resource. Moreover, it is not as if the medical profession has conducted itself along Franciscanesque lines in recent years. As we have read in *The Hartford Advocate*, "Many physicians will admit that they brought the managed care movement down on themselves with their overuse of testing and new medical technologies. 'Before doctors did whatever they needed to do,' and sometimes that was more than what was really needed, says Dr. Leonard Banco, director of the department of pediatrics at Hartford Hospital and president of the Connecticut chapter of the American Academy of Pediatrics."[19]

Some have suggested that these abuses were due to a rescue mentality, one that advocates doing everything, regardless of cost, to save lives.[20] Others have suggested that third-party payers have shielded physicians and patients from the economic impact of their choices, thus fostering a climate of fiscal irresponsibility.[21] Undoubtedly both points have a certain validity. But one must also acknowledge that physicians have become extremely wealthy as health care costs have escalated, particularly specialists.[22] They have, therefore, a vested interested in maintaining high-cost practices. Moreover, it seems naïve to suggest that they have not been central to the development of our present booming health care industry. We have no reason to believe, therefore, that an egalitarian turn of heart would repossess the medical profession if it were granted monopoly control in health care markets.[23]

Another dramatic flaw in Freidson's proposal is his refusal to address a central aspect of the present health care crisis, access. At its heart, this is a question of economics: who can afford access to adequate medical care, either through employers, privately bought insurance, or fee-for-service arrangements. Freidson's only wave at cost control concerns the establishment of limits on physician salaries. As noted above, this is an important issue, but controlled salaries will not guarantee controlled costs, let alone universal access. First, medical costs reflect the confluence of several factors: advanced machinery, pharmaceutical developments, administrative costs, malpractice insurance, and insurance premiums. Controlling physician salaries is therefore only one aspect of the problem posed by current medical costs.

Second, and irrespective of costs, a physician-run health care system has no decided advantages over any other system when we consider the question of access. The model may secure physician autonomy and individualized care, but these benefits amount to naught if millions of U.S. citizens remain dependent on emergency room and public clinic care, arenas in which individualized, routine (let alone preventive) treatment is out of the question. In short, we see little reason to believe that any professional model will effectively confront the root problems facing health care reform.

The misplaced emphasis lying at the root of professional models becomes most apparent when we reflect on whether it is even meaningful to speak of an autonomous medical profession that might govern itself. Freidson's desire to control physician salaries is curious not only because it underestimates the economic complexities of existing medical costs, but because it supposes that the medical profession is self-directing, when in fact it is more accurate to speak of a multifaceted, rationalized health care industry. In short, health care is not a discrete product that some class of professionals, such as physicians, delivers. Instead, "care" is the product or result of a dynamic complex driven by products, procedures, technologies, persons, and institutions that enters clinical settings only after having traveled the maze that is the U.S. health care industry.

Of course, this maze disappears if we socially isolate the medical profession (or the physician-patient relationship) and regard its contours as the contours of health care per se. And this is precisely what Freidson does, at the cost of obscuring obvious facts. Health care in the United States is constituted by the interaction of various forces: It involves material facts concerning domestic and foreign biomedical technologies and pharmaceutical industries; the various concerns of those agencies; the interests and dollars driving private and government-sponsored research as well as medical school research; the changing face of medical school curricula; the interests, initiatives, and bureaucratic systems of various third-party providers; evolving tax subsidies for employers and employees who purchase insurance; and many other factors.

At the heart of a profession one expects to find a relatively autonomous class of workers who deliver their services to communities without undue dependency on other professions or social forces. Although it may have been the case that in the nineteenth century a "medical profession" conducted its business along self-directed lines, those days are over. Health care no longer is in the hands of *a* profession, but emerges out of complex patterns of social labor. This means that it makes little sense to hold physicians responsible for the depth of the present crisis, and even less sense to suggest with Freidson that doctors conducting themselves responsibly and professionally might lead us out of the thicket choking U.S. health care.

No one group of actors in the present drama is in a position to effectively predict and control the multiple variables at play in the health care industry absent extensive coordination among all relevant groups.[24] Moreover, no one group of actors should direct the drama given that, as we shall show, health care turns on social decisions whose legitimacy and sustainability rest on democratic deliberation. Despite Freidson's misgivings, perhaps our future lies with the market after all.

Market reformers like to remind people that the market has brought us more comfortable and fuel-efficient cars. They are also quick to eulogize price decreases prompted by airline deregulation.[25] Perhaps, it is suggested, a transformation of the medical profession into big business, on a par with or surpassing the auto and airline industries, will yield similar increases in efficiency. For example, large medical conglomerates would not only offer the traditional benefits associated with economies of scale, such as the ability to avoid redundant operations through central consolidation, but they also would have available extensive statistics on treatment outcomes and costs, resulting in effective, streamlined treatment plans. Moreover, market-driven reforms would leave intact the United States' thriving biotechnology industry, thus keeping this country at the vanguard of medical research and innovation, a vanguard that offers its citizens some of the most sophisticated care in the world.

The movement toward more efficient HMOs and other large-scale providers is accompanied, somewhat surprisingly, by claims that individual consumers will be offered high-quality choices. Indeed, markets are lauded not only for increasing efficiency in allocation and production of scarce commodities, but also for providing individuals with greater autonomy. Many suggest that under market conditions individuals are able to choose what percentage of their income will go to which goods. For example, Susan may wish to spend a larger percentage of her income on health insurance and forego increasing her compact disk collection. Fred, on the other hand, may wish to buy less insurance in order to lease a new car every two years. In short, if health care is organized along market lines, Susan and Fred should be able to proceed as they see fit. Market-based reforms not only secure efficiency, therefore, but allow for consumer freedom, thus respecting differences between persons.

"Gag rules" came under attack by market devotees not because they compromise physician autonomy, but rather because they deprive consumers of the information they need to make rational choices, thereby interfering with consumer autonomy. If Susan's doctors are forbidden to discuss treatment options that they consider helpful but the HMO does not support, Susan is denied the opportunity to pursue these treatment options using her own resources. Moreover, if this is done systematically, patients who would otherwise complain and perhaps employ their market influence to enlarge treatment options are prevented from doing so through the cultivation of ignorance. Likewise, if Susan's doctor will not disclose the rules by which his or her own compensation is calculated, then Susan cannot shop plans, electing the one whose form of physician compensation she links with higher quality treatment. Through the ignorance they institute, then, "gag rules" limit consumer choice in a variety of ways. Given these compromises, it seems plausible to argue that the future of health care in the United States should seek freer markets that respect the autonomy of their patrons.

Markets are certainly central features of contemporary capitalist society, but their ubiquity may lull us into mistaking a unique perspective of the world for the world itself. The language of markets employs a special vocabulary to slice up the world. It recognizes goods and services as commodities and individuals and pseudoindividuals (that is, corporations) as consumers and producers. This has proven to be and remains a useful way to look at the world—that is, a useful way when one's goal is to achieve wealth maximization or another set of economic ends. But such a turn of mind has its limits as well, as evidenced by the fact that we are unwilling to commodify everything.[26]

For instance, we refuse to allow babies to be auctioned at market even though we allow race horses to be auctioned. Why? In part because we take the value of human life to exceed any price tag. Also, this society does not allow individuals to sell their free speech rights or their right to vote. Respect for human dignity and the need to insulate democratic institutions from the influence of wealth have led us to resist the commodification of our political agency.

That we resist commodification in certain spheres of life suggests an interesting fact, one often overlooked by market enthusiasts: Treating something within a market model is a matter of choice. The decision to translate goods into commodified terms, thus committing their futures to the plays of the market, is a decision. Given this, we must now ask whether it makes sense, in light of our larger ends, to engage issues of health care within market contexts. Is it rational to pursue health care through market mechanisms, or should some other route be chosen?

Markets tend to be responsive to consumer demand voiced through dollars. The lure of dollars and the air of competitiveness give producers incentives to offer desired goods and services at prices that will undercut the competition. A system with such incentives works to offer consumers a wide range of choices. It is reasonable to think, therefore, that the transformation of the modern health care profession into a form of big business will reward consumers with an increasing array of health care options.

However, it should be noted that markets are responsive only to individuals with dollars, and that means that some impoverished citizens will experience the expanding array of health care options not as an expanding field of choices, but as an expanding field of inaccessible goods. Said bluntly, health care markets not only price out producers, but consumers as well, and thus secure particular freedoms of choice only for those able to buy in the economic sector in question, whether that sector revolves around health care, luxury hotel accommodations, or precious stones.

In response to questions of access, market advocates might observe that although it is sad—even tragic in some instances—that we cannot have all that we want, this is an unavoidable fact of life in a world of scarcity. In other words, scarcity will burden, unavoidably, some people more than others. But note that such truisms cloud the issue, because they treat the exclusions occasioned by the market as fateful dispensations, or the result of natural economic laws playing out the hands we have been dealt.[27] But whether market forces should or will govern the distribution of health care options is a social choice, and thus something for which a society can be held accountable. Moreover, as we have just made evident, to choose the market as the means by which health care options are produced and distributed is in an important sense to sanction—that is, to choose, albeit unwittingly—the exclusions that the market institutes.[28]

Our blindness to the social choices underlying the institution of markets poses a threat to the legitimacy of our society and the integrity of our debates. If commodifying health care is a social choice analogous to our decision not to commodify human infants, its legitimacy rests upon its being the result of democratic deliberation.[29] That the market does not foster such deliberation seems clear. The market formulates its policy options on the basis of demands from dollars, not on the basis of what the people of the United States desire. If all citizens had equal access to that market and therefore could voice an informed opinion through consumption (with buying being analogous to voting), one might argue that a legitimation mechanism underwrites market results. But given that markets are exclusive domains and not truly democratic, no such legitimation process can be said to underwrite existing health care practices.[30]

Although the objection just voiced is sound, it obscures a pivotal point. The issue under discussion is not simply whether markets give the people what they want, but whether people want their health care to be driven by market mechanisms. And clearly this question cannot be raised, let alone decided, by the market. Although the market is well equipped to register consumer preferences for various goods and services—that is, for commodities—it is ill equipped to measure dissatisfaction with the process of commodification itself. When the question concerns whether to commodify health care, therefore, allowing the people to vote with their feet or with their dollars not only excludes several people from the conversation, but forecloses the question concerning whether to commodify health care at the outset.

But perhaps we are misguided in our demand for such a conversation. One might object that since we do not require democratic consensus on the appropriate structure of the automobile industry and remain happy enough to leave selection of our primary form of transportation to market forces, there is no reason for health care to be different. In the first instance, it is not true that we leave big industries like the automobile industry to the fate of the market. Recall, for example, President Carter's historical bailout of Chrysler or President Bush's decision to address the savings and loan crisis. Second, the question concerning the automobile industry is more generally a question of transportation, and one could argue that we should pursue democratic inquiry into the most rational way of securing transportation, particularly given our limited fossil fuel resources and the various externalities associated with automobile usage.

Third, even if most industries are appropriately left to "regulation" by market forces, it does not follow that all goods are of this character. Indeed, to understand the provision of health care as merely one commodity among others is to fail to recognize the special ways in which health care is a condition of the possibility of effective consumer participation in markets.

One's ability to participate in markets, as either a consumer or a producer, depends in part on the maintenance of one's health. Although sheer luck occasionally will provide an individual with the health requisite for gainful employment, an obvious precondition for those who have not inherited sustainable purchasing power is access to basic health care from prenatal stages on.

More generally, although it may be true that markets empower consumers, it is also true that that a consumer culture can provide consumers with its dazzling array of options only if the conditions necessary for market society are maintained, such as safe shopping areas, consumer protection agencies, and communication and transportation infrastructures. In our view, a healthy pool of workers and consumers is similarly a fundamental precondition of a market society.

In the last few pages we have been considering whether it is rational to treat health care as a commodity. We have framed the debate in this way given that the decision to treat anything as a commodity reflects a social choice. And although we have acknowledged that it sometimes makes sense, for reasons of efficiency and respect for consumer autonomy, to allow market forces to dictate the production of certain goods, we have also shown that one must ask, Efficiency and autonomy for whom?

Given that one can participate in markets only with sufficient capital in hand, markets inevitably deny some people access to their resources. But does this make it irrational to treat health care as a commodity? This remains the central question, but one that can be answered only if one knows the nature of the end-in-view. After all, one can rationally adopt means to an end only if one knows the nature of that end—in this instance, health care. At this point, then, we must inquire into the nature of the ends of health care.

The Future of Health Care: Opening a Discussion

Determining the nature of the good we term health is obviously an enormous task, one nobody could hope to complete in the span of a chapter. That such a question must be asked here and now seems equally indubitable, however, for it is not as if one could rationally pursue a course of health care reform without determining the nature of health and its relative importance vis-à-vis other goods.[31] To do so would be akin to building highways without first determining where they are to take us or what else is in need of development. In other words, pursuing health care reform without an inquiry into the nature of the end in question, a procedure the United States has employed for years, strikes us as patently irrational.

In order for the debate over health care reform to press on in a productive fashion, it must inquire into the nature of health. And yet it is not as if we could decide the issue here and now. But then, nor should we; for, as we noted earlier, social policy can be legitimate in a democratic society only if it results from democratic deliberation. What is required at this point, then, is a public discussion concerning the nature and importance of health as well as which combination of available means is best suited for its realization. Since we cannot, in a single chapter, supplant or even imaginatively conduct such a conversation, we think it best to take our analysis down another path. We would like to reflect on what a rational public debate concerning health care reform would involve and how such a debate should (or should not) proceed.

In pursuing rational discourse about social goods, many thinkers, following John Rawls's *Theory of Justice,* imaginatively construct inquiries in order to conclude what rational citizens would choose if actual discussions concerning social reform took place.[32] Beginning with the standpoint of a generic, abstract individual, through a procedure we term hypothetical reflection, one might hope to arrive at a minimal account of social goods. Since all rational agents will want to protect themselves and pursue their own forms of the good life, one can construct an account, the argument suggests, of the goods such goals presuppose. These goods usually turn out to involve physical security, protection of self-determination, and guarantee of subsistence goods or the means to acquire them. Perhaps even health care—or the means to acquire it—should be included.

In our view, approaching health care reform through hypothetical reflections is misguided, for such reflections are unable to address questions of sustainability, legitimation, and ultimately, rationality itself. First, health care reform, if it is to produce sustainable reform, must engage existing ideals and concrete desires. Otherwise policy will enter the civic realm as if from on high and alienate those unconvinced of the soundness of the policy in question. Particularly given our nation's current distrust of the legitimacy and effectiveness of federal legislation, we think it unlikely that change mandated by hypothetically grounded policy wonks will take hold of the general will to the extent required for successful large-scale reform. Nationwide reform requires the cooperation of all interested and relevant parties. Without widespread support, its goals are at risk of subversion.

Second, imaginative constructions of what rational agents would say if they were to engage one another in a dialogue about health care lacks legitimacy altogether. Under the law, hypothetical individuals, no matter how rational, have no standing. No policy, therefore, could base itself on the results of Rawlsian speculations in the area of health care reform. This is not to say that one could not develop a general theory of justice from Rawls's original position. Rather, the claim is that health care reform has little use for such reflections given that the goals of reform involve the production of policy.

Of course one could argue forthrightly for the priority of certain social goods such as health care, pointing out that our nation's commitment to the protection of life and liberty rings hollow without a corresponding commitment to providing adequate health care. But such arguments should be made while participating in live, public debate, and not behind the smoke screen of hypothetical reflection.[33] In short, the debate surrounding health care reform needs to be public, and it needs to engage the concrete beliefs and values of U.S. citizens.

A third problem emerges once one recognizes the minimal nature of the goods that rational individuals would supposedly elect. The apparent strength of hypothetical reflection lies in the fact that it allows us to imagine what goods would be amenable to almost everyone, irrespective of their particular vision of the good life. By proceeding hypothetically one can remain, therefore, true to the spirit of a proceduralist liberalism even while generating a list of primary goods. For example, Daniels argues that a just society requires a health care system that guarantees universal access given that a certain level of health care is needed to ensure "normal species functioning," something in which everyone seems to have an interest.[34]

Yet how will we determine what is entailed by normal species functioning? In the absence of real dialogue, we will no doubt pursue minimal levels in order to avoid possible objections from our hypothetical interlocutors. The irony, however, is that U.S. citizens have shown repeatedly that in certain areas they are not satisfied with securing minimal conditions. For example, they are willing to support the building and upkeep of public parks, even though such spaces have little to do with normal species functioning. Likewise, many are interested in publicly funding the arts even though we could easily function without them.

What this shows, we think, is that many citizens are interested not in living up to a standard of normal species functioning, but in exceeding it. In other words, they are interested in contributing to human flourishing, however they understand that term. In our view, then, we should pursue real dialogue in order to determine just how important health care is to the people of the United States, and we should not, particularly at the outset, chain reform to minimal standards derived from counterfactually driven hypothetical debates.

Similarly, who is to say what will transpire when real dialogue takes place? Hypothetical reflection can imagine that people will defend their interests with consummate logic until the dying end, thus necessitating a compromise around minimal standards. In real discussions, however, those holding many positions defend themselves with specious arguments, thus opening themselves to public refutation. Likewise, people often change their minds when confronted with the concrete consequences of their actions. Hypothetical reflection, however, by rushing ahead to the endgame, forgoes these dynamic and sometimes surprising plays of public will formation. Hypothetical reflection thus imprudently bypasses the opportunities for change and growth often generated by and in authentic exchange.

Alongside these practical constraints, theoretical flaws also afflict those who would approach questions of health care reform from the perspective of abstract, supposedly rational individuals. The first flaw is apparent in what has already been said. How is it that hypothetical reflection will determine what counts as normal functioning? As noted, it will seek minimal standards in order to remain neutral vis-à-vis individual conceptions of the good life. But this is impossible. Given the goal of empowering individual conceptions of the good life, such reflection presupposes the general rightness of a proceduralist liberalism, thus excluding from the conversation all who do not take individual self-determination to be a fundamental good.[35] Hypothetical reflection about what rational individuals will term a primary good is therefore far from a neutral affair.[36]

One might suppose that the goal of empowering individual conceptions of the good life is less a positive goal of hypothetical reflection than an acknowledgment of the fact that consensus about such matters in a pluralist society is a pipe dream. One thus adopts a proceduralist framework in order to minimize stepping on too many normative toes.[37] Note, however, that in doing so one has decided that stepping on normative toes amounts to some kind of grievous harm. Put concretely, it is as if being forced to help pay for a health care system that secures universal access is a greater wrong than leaving forty million people without access to adequate health care. But one can make such a claim only if one has a positive good in mind—here political autonomy—whose realization is frusutrated when an individual is so forced.

In other words, proceduralism embodies a vision of the good life that esteems, often above all else, the worth of individual self-determination in the political sphere. It would seem, therefore, that no proceduralist paths exist that would allow us to elude the thorny, normatively loaded discussion that health care reform has provoked. In short, we do not believe that one can avoid making positive claims about the nature of the good life when arguing for whatever set of primary goods one wishes a society to procure and provide.

Inconsistency aside, there is a more sinister element at work in making the decision to seek a minimal set of goods (or a minimal understanding of particular goods such as health or freedom) in order to protect the freedom of individuals to pursue their own conceptions of the good life. As Catherine Mackinnon has claimed, proceduralist liberals often are willing to forgo significant social reform in order to preserve the integrity of an abstract notion of human freedom. The freedom of self-determination often championed by proceduralist liberals is abstract because it champions a kind of human activity that lacks any determinate content; that is, the issue is not freedom to pursue particular, praiseworthy goods, but some vague notion of freedom per se that some are content to define negatively.[38]

This is troubling given that a defense of this kind of freedom often overrides defenses of reforms that address existing material needs such as health care. Recall, for example, the trade-off we described earlier. Does being forced to help pay for a health care system that secures universal access involve a greater wrong than leaving forty million people without access to adequate health care? Should we defend an abstract notion of freedom at the expense of the concrete suffering of millions of people? Perhaps we should, but if we do we should do so self-consciously and only after public deliberation. Hypothetical reflection denies us this opportunity, however, for it assumes without argument that such trade-offs are not only worthwhile, but tantamount to rationality per se, defending as such reflection does, and without argument, the goods endemic to proceduralist liberalism.[39]

What is most puzzling about hypothetical reflection about what social goods have priority over others is its reversal of the order of rationality. As we noted earlier, one can determine the rationality of a choice only with reference to the end-in-view; that is, X can be termed a rational course of action only when one can determine whether it facilitates the realization of its end, Y. A hyopthetical reflection about which social goods would be termed primary by rational agents supposes, however, that one can act rationally without beginning with certain goods as ends-in-view. This strikes us as absurd, and we have already shown that hypothetical reflection does not in fact proceed in this way. The point bears stressing, however, for it must be the case that a public discussion of health care reform will include a discussion of which goods our society is commited to pursuing. But how should such a discussion proceed?

In our opinion, our country stands in need of a new theoretical conception of and institutional infrastructure for deliberative democaracy. It seems clear that no thick theory of the good will solve all our woes, particularly given our historical commitment to pluralism and individuality. And, as we have just shown, hypothetical lines of inquiry hold little promise for those who would reflect on what course policy should take with regard to health care. But significant theoretical and practical problems lie in store for those who would pursue authentic public debate about which goods should orient the labor of public institutions. Given a nation of 250 million people, town meeting ideals seem out of place if not downright silly. Also, across the last twenty years or so public discussion has evaporated and been replaced by the efforts of political ad agencies that treat candidates and issues like the latest thirst quenchers. There is cause to wonder, therefore, whether our nation is capable of sustained public debate.

Nevertheless, such a debate is unavoidable if we are to confront the health care crisis in a democratic fashion. If such a debate does take place, we would insist that participants proceed without exaggerating the powers of the medical profession or falling prey to the normative bankruptcy of the market's instrumentalized rationality. Our nation must again ask itself whether all citizens deserve access to some basic level of health care. And it must pursue this question rationally, which means that the nation must ask what kind of good health care is—and whether it is one of those goods whose procurement is a social responsibility.

18 Ethical Literacy and Cultural Competence

MARIAN GRAY SECUNDY

THE PROLIFERATION of ethics consultants and medical ethicists in health care settings is both encouraging and troubling. The current turmoil, uncertainty, and change in health care delivery call for serious soul-searching and rigorous analysis of professional roles and responsibilities. This is particularly true for those of us who find ourselves in environments where we must provide advice and counsel to physicians, patients, and increasingly to institutions about a wide variety of ethical concerns and dilemmas. The literature is replete with numerous questions and challenges that we should take seriously as we attempt to chart a course for our profession into the twenty-first century.

The Ethical Consultant

Of most concern are issues relative to the preparation of ethics consultants for and our competence and interest in developing a knowledge, skill, and attitudinal base that will allow us to be of maximum assistance to those seeking guidance and help in resolving dilemmas at the patient-doctor or health care provider level. Of equal concern and not at all unrelated to the previous concern is our capacity, suitability, and obligation to become involved in the increasing number of ethical conflicts that are surfacing in our health care institutions and health care systems in this era of cost containment.

What constitutes "ethical literacy" remains an essential and much-debated focus of inquiry. Is a background and expertise in the disciplines of philosophy, theology, or medicine essential and sufficient? Are humanists, social scientists, or health providers from other disciplines capable of developing the core of knowledge necessary to allow them to serve equally well as ethics consultants? Have we broadened the field to such an extent that we are reaching a level of incompetence and taking on more than we can either chew, digest, or integrate? Many of the questions in this regard were discussed by K. Danner Clouser in 1973 and are still before us.[1]

Clouser asserts in his article: "Medical ethics is not sociology, medical ethics is not history of medicine, medical ethics is not anthropology, nor literature, nor family and community medicine."[2] Although he goes on to state that "ethics is a discipline in and of itself, with its own conceptual framework, its own methods, strategies and purposes," he does not, in this article, go on to elaborate or delineate exactly what those are.

Challenges such as that of Giles Scofield in 1993 touch very sensitive nerve endings. Scofield claims that "ethics consultants have yet to prove that they possess the basic elements of a profession."[3] He takes on those who embrace a wide variety of academic disciplines as foundational to competence and ask, "Can anyone master this body of knowledge?"[4] There are those who see ethicists solely as educators and would restrict and define their roles and responsibilities primarily within that context.[5] Fundamentally, the questions still before us speak to issues of scope of knowledge, scope of responsibility, limitations, and characteristics of ethics consultants.

Criteria for Ethical Literacy

I tend to support an expansive, holistic set of criteria for ethics consultants. Admittedly my own training, primarily as a social worker and secondarily in as a medical humanist, with a concentration in bioethics, informs this point of view. However, in my experiences and observations I have encountered practical and justifiable reasons for this position. Essentially a broader knowledge base serves the patient, the physician, and the institution more completely and meaningfully.

For purposes of ethics consultations, ethical literacy is not grounded solely in an expertise in critical philosophical or in theological analysis or inquiry. Such expertise is necessary, but not, in my opinion, sufficient. Applied ethics or normative ethics in the hands of the ethics consultant carries with it an obligation to know and use much more information in order to provide appropriate analysis or counsel. Of course one must revisit the question of just what it is the consultant ought to do. What type and what depth of knowledge is most useful to the task?

In June of 1989 the Society for Bioethics Consultation listed areas of knowledge and skills one was required to have to provide ethics consultations. They were as follows:

1. Knowledge of medicine and the clinical setting
2. Knowledge of biomedical ethics
3. Knowledge of health care law
4. Knowledge of relevance of various cultural and religious traditions for health care decisions
5. Interpersonal and psychological knowledge and skills[6]

Elaborating on a suggested knowledge base, Fletcher also lists a proposed set of standards.[7] Referencing Larson and Friedson, Scofield lists the basic elements of a profession of bioethics consultant. Ethics consultants should:

1. Exclusively possess a specific body of esoteric knowledge.
2. Apply this knowledge in an objective, reliable, and scientific fashion.
3. Have the ability to regulate and supervise themselves.
4. Be motivated to act in the public interest.[8]

There is general agreement that ethics consultants ought be capable of critical inquiry and analysis. They should be able to delineate moral issues, discuss alternative responses, and, some believe, propose appropriate solutions and responses that conform to a rational and logical moral framework. The extent to which such consultants should propose specific courses of action and to whom they are accountable based upon such recommendations is subject to some debate and controversy.[9] Allegiances to physicians, patients, families, or institutions are all existing models.

Weeks and Nelson describe roles for ethics consultants as liaisons, experts, and fiduciary agents. However, they acknowledge problems of balance and priority.[10] Yeo's main paradigms relative to the role of the bioethicist are useful. He differentiates between the role of educator and that of intervenor and seems to opt for that of the educator, whose task it is to "clarify, facilitate, sort through, and to sort out."[11] In the real world of bioethics consultations, however, we find both operating, and therein lies the problem.

Potential Limitations of Roles

My own view is that there are very few instances in which ethics consultants remain or function in a purist fashion as either educators or intervenors. These roles invariably intertwine, and rarely are there attempts to state which role is operative at any given time. Whether an ethics consultant serves as educator, intervenor, or a combination of the two, the issue of range of expertise remains constant. In order to avoid the serious criticism of overstepping boundaries or misusing authority, the ethics consultant ought be very careful to define his or her role. It may be important to indicate that the task is to clarify issues, to facilitate decision making, or to serve in a liaison capacity, where "expertise" is confined to laying out options.

A greater problem has to do with levels of expertise and depth of knowledge when the role of intervenor is operative. When one intervenes, the functions of direct intervention and influence, of providing moral knowledge, and of role advocacy may seem to suggest a knowledge base that is exact and accurate for all time and for all people. Whatever role the consultant takes, there needs to be an understanding of ethics as more rather than less expansive, as objective rather than subjective, as providing moral options rather than solutions, and as being tuned in to the totality of the human condition and human experience.

I do not believe that consultants must have significant expertise in all areas relevant to each patient's condition. I do suggest that consultants should have a minimum level of literacy or, to use a more popular term, cultural competence. It is also important that ethicists functioning as educators or as intervenors acknowledge that their roles are not neutral. The fiction of neutrality interferes with objective assessments.

Competency Challenges

The task of delineating explicit criteria for competence and expertise is awesome. It is not realistic to expect that a special knowledge base in all essential areas is necessary. As Ruth Macklin has suggested, "Any reflective, thoughtful person is potentially as good a decision-maker as any other."[12] I have some difficulty with the concept of ethicists as decision makers, however, and would recommend that we substitute the concept of adviser instead. Despite significant scholarship and knowledge of philosophy and theology or psychosocial aspects of the human condition, I would also doubt, as does Robert Veatch, that anyone has privileged authority in matters of morality.[13] There is real danger in such assumptions.

On the other hand, concerned, sensitive, logical, and rational persons, using the various knowledge bases of many disciplines, ought be able to use those knowledge bases in constructive ways. In so doing they can better assist health care providers who *are* decision makers to become more informed and aware of the implications, significance, and consequences of their decisions for patients, their families, and themselves. Insofar as possible, consultants should present a full and complete a range of moral options based on historical knowledge of all the great philosophical and theological traditions (inclusive of those not within the Eurocentric locus of Western civilization) and the benefits and consequences of those options to the parties affected.

In a pluralistic society with many cultural and religious traditions, there is no one moral truth. Fundamentally, it is the responsibility of the ethics consultant to keep that fact ever before us. Criticisms and claims that attempt to limit the knowledge bases and disciplines that are brought to bear in the work of the ethics consultant can serve, and perhaps have served, to excuse a failure to be inclusive of all traditions and to be aware of and attentive to the influence of cultural, social, and economic conditions on human behavior. A narrow focus on and allegiance to Western philosophy are definitely more manageable intellectually than is a broader perspective that includes the traditions of the Third World and the cultural differences manifested by minority persons and underserved peoples in contrast to America's "mainstream groups."

Dula cautions us not to underestimate the influence of social and cultural history as a definer of perspectives.[14] We err when we hide behind the pretense of "color blindness" or economic neutrality. Race is alive and well as a social construct in America, and economic issues define who we people are in a major way. The history and culture to be understood and examined are not just those of the patient, however, but those of the health care provider as well. We must be able to say with clarity just whose problem we are confronting and why. It is often the culture of the provider that frames the ethical dilemma brought to the consultant. Brody also reminds us to attend to power issues in our analyses.[15]

My own set of criteria for a holistic, expansive approach to ethics consultation fully incorporates the rigorous methodology of philosophical inquiry and analysis relative to the moral life. It does not eliminate or separate the emotional life from the rational. It includes a requirement of knowing as fully as possible who the players are in any given dilemma. In addition to medical and clinical information, one must have a capacity to know or know how to inquire about patients' beliefs, their everyday lives beyond illness and crisis, and their psychological responses. Admittedly it is not always possible to know all of these things, especially if the setting or the nature of the medical crisis does not allow sufficient time to learn all one needs to know. However, one needs to be able to acknowledge just what it is that one does not know and why. One needs to be able to hypothesize just how what one does not know or understand might inform one's inquiry, analysis, and presentation of alternatives and options. Jonsen, Siegler, and Winslade have developed a schema inclusive of patient preferences and contextual features that is an abbreviated way of describing the essential components of the information required.[16]

An ethics consultation is incomplete if it does not describe and fully identify the patient, the patient's family, and the relevant circumstances of the patient's life as well as the characteristics, beliefs, and preferences of the health care providers involved. For example, when the dilemma presented is that the patient wants to revoke his living will because he distrusts his clinician, it is essential that one know about his racial background, his economic circumstances, and his previous and current experiences and relationships with the health care system before deciding on a set of recommendations. It is important to help the health care team involved to know and understand that the patient, a black man sixty years of age, is typical in his distrust of health care systems and providers. Although he will not talk openly with the white clinical ethicist, he will talk openly with the young black resident in training.

When a patient's family expresses open hostility to the health care team, demanding that everything possibly be done in light of clear and understood medical futility, we need to know that they, too, are dubious about the quality of the care being provided and suspicious of the providers. Their demand, seemingly irrational, may serve as their one way of maintaining some control and dignity in this situation. Their rage overrides their irrationality ability to respond rationally. One cannot discuss this case meaningfully in the context of issues of medical futility only.

Tia Powell's discussion of a patient encounter in the *Journal of Clinical Ethics* demonstrates how the perspectives of the powerful ought not diminish the autonomy of the those who are different in their beliefs and essentially unempowered.[17] When a clinician requests a consultant to find out if he has to follow the patient's prior verbal request that no extraordinary measures be taken, it is necessary to delve into how that clinician's beliefs are influencing his capacity for shared decision making. It is important, as well, to help him get in touch with how those feelings are affecting the quality of care he is providing.

One cannot discuss the efficacy of a third liver transplant for a two-year-old impoverished black child in terms of its clinical efficacy and cost effectiveness without attending to the problems of her mother, who is addicted to crack cocaine. One must examine the mother's ability to give informed consent and monitor the child's aftercare. One must understand the context and social chaos of the family—the horrible living conditions of the inner city, the deteriorating project in which they live, their limited resources, and the deprivation they face on a daily basis. Finally, one must appreciate the political realities of the institution in which the transplants have been done.

The latter issue relates to the complex concerns institutions and health care systems raise in terms of the role and responsibility of an ethics consultant. The driving forces of cost containment represent, in my opinion, a fundamental conflict for the consultant. Which master should he or she serve? To whom does he or she owe loyalty? More often than not, today's ethics consultant often finds him- or herself serving two masters. The ethics consultant has the acknowledged responsibility of defining the patient's interests if not advocating for them. But he or she must also deal with the cold reality of an institution's or system's commitment to cost containment.

As managed care becomes the predominant form of health care delivery, the problems brought to the ethics consultant are more and more frequently intertwined with issues of liability and costs. The real needs of the patient frequently may be placed in the background as the consultant is asked to address the fears and doubts of the health care provider in response to institutional regulations. Such regulations may actually be detrimental to the patient's best interests. Often health care providers acknowledge their own concerns and look to ethicists for help in making decisions they do not wish to make by themselves. In these instances observers caution that consultants should be wary of the potential dangers of political interference and cooption.

When one's paycheck and career are dependent on an institution, just how objective can one be? How can one avoid the temptation of becoming the decision maker rather than the adviser? Shiedermayer and La Puma discuss various roles and responsibilities of the ethics consultant relative to risk management, quality assurance, utilization management, and peer review.[18] Additionally, they talk of functions in the areas of negotiation, mediation, and evaluation of quality indicators. Although they caution ethicists against becoming an institution's sole conscience and urge resistance to participation in the regulatory functions, clearly the complexity of attempting to maintain patient-centered objectivity is real.

Despite responsibilities for ensuring that patients' preferences are considered seriously and that fairness and equity are observed, true limitations are presented by a system that in and of itself is unfair and not reflective of justice as an undergirding and operative principle. These limitations raise serious questions about how one can function in any honest way within that system. These issues also relate to who we are as ethicists in terms of our own prejudices, biases, political orientations, and so on. If we believe that current health care reform and managed care policies are preferable to previous types of health care, are we able or willing to speak to inequities we find to be justified or do not believe exist?

We must clarify how our own beliefs will or will not affect what we say and do as advisers. One might argue that affiliation with a system whose focus is primarily cost containment puts the ethics consultant in an untenable situation. On the other hand, perhaps some focus on issues of justice is better than no focus. We must exercise considerable care and examine who we are as ethics consultants if we are employed by managed care systems. When the shift is away from the primacy and sanctity of the physician-patient relationship and toward cost containment concerns, we must be very cautious.

Recommendations

There is a need for a more definitive code of ethics as well as a set of criteria for "ethical literacy." There should be a specification of essential categories of information. Explicit delineation of just how the policies of any given system may impact patient care is, at minimum, an essential part of the task of ethics consultants. We ought to acknowledge and welcome moral disagreement, refuse to believe in unequivocal moral truths when they are in conflict with the beliefs and cultural mores of persons from cultures other than our own, minimize our commitment to autonomy without attention to communal values, question our passion for individualism when family and group authority are central to others our patients respect, and honor the historical and social realities of lives lived differently than ours. But most especially we must be able to recognize those realities for what they are. Ultimately we must take off the blinders of Western civilization and let in the rays of light from other cultures. The quality and effectiveness of our work as ethics consultants depends on our ability to do just that.

Notes

Selected Bibliography

Contributors

Index

NOTES

Introduction

1. In my own institution, clinician scientists on tenure track in the School of Medicine produced, based on data collected in 1995–97, an average of forty peer-reviewed articles prior to receiving tenure.

2. K. Ryan, "Ethics and Pragmatism in Scientific Affairs," *Bioscience* 29 (1979): 35–37.

3. M. Singer, "The Context of American Philosophy," in *American Philosophy,* ed. M. Singer (Cambridge University Press, 1985), 1–20.

4. See Leon Kass, *Toward a More Natural Science: Biology and Human Affairs* (New York: Free Press, 1985); "The New Biology: What Price Relieving Man's Estate," *Science* 174 (1971): 779–88, and "The Wisdom of Repugnance," *New Republic* 243 (1997): 36–72. My comments on the matter of mistaken criticism of pragmatism in bioethics are in Glenn McGee, *The Perfect Baby: A Pragmatic Approach to Genetics* (New York: Rowman and Littlefield, 1997), chaps. 1, 2, 4, and 5.

5. Paul Root Wolpe, "The Triumph of Autonomy in American Bioethics," in *Bioethics and Society,* ed. R. Devries and J. Subedi (New York: Prentice-Hall, 1998), 38–60.

6. Leon R. Kass, *Toward a More Natural Science: Biology and Human Affairs* (New York: Free Press, 1985), 25–26, 98.

7. I have in mind such works as Charles Bosk, *All God's Mistakes: Genetic Counseling in a Pediatric Hospital* (Chicago: University of Chicago Press, 1994); John Lachs, *Intermediate Man* (Chicago: Hackett Press, 1983); and Arthur Caplan, *Am I My Brother's Keeper?* (Bloomington: Indiana University Press, 1998).

8. James Campbell, *The Community Reconstructs: The Meaning of Pragmatic Social Thought* (Chicago: University of Illinois Press, 1992), 46.

Chapter 1: *Moreno,* Bioethics Is a Naturalism

1. Jonathan D. Moreno, "Do Bioethics Commissions Hijack Public Debate?" *Hastings Center Report,* 26, no. 3: 46.

2. In my book *Deciding Together: Bioethics and Moral Consensus* (New York: Oxford University Press, 1995) I elaborate a view of bioethics as a consensus-oriented enterprise.

3. Sandra B. Rosenthal, *Speculative Pragmatism* (Peru, Illinois: Open Court Publishing Co., 1990).

4. Sandra B. Rosenthal, "Classical American Pragmatism: The Other Naturalism," *Metaphilosophy* 27, no. 4: 399.

5. John Dewey, *The Quest for Certainty: A Study of the Relation of Knowledge and Action* (New York: Minton, Balch, 1929).

6. John Dewey, "The Reflex Arc Concept in Psychology," in *Reconstruction of Philosophy*. Carbondale: Southern Illinois University Press.

7. Richard Rorty, *Philosophy and the Mirror of Nature* (Princeton, New Jersey: Princeton University Press, 1979).

8. Yervant H. Krikorian, *Naturalism and the Human Spirit* (New York: Columbia University Press, 1944).

9. John Ryder, ed., *American Philosophic Naturalism* (Amherst, New York: Prometheus Books, 1994).

10. For an expanded account of this way of viewing the tradition and an alternative view that is a near relation to the one I espouse, see Martha C. Nussbaum, *The Therapy of Desire* (Princeton, N.J.: Princeton University Press, 1994).

11. Albert R. Jonsen and Stephen Toulmin, *The Abuse of Casuistry* (Berkeley, Calif.: University of California Press, 1988).

12. Tom Beauchamp and James Childress, *Principles of Biomedical Ethics*, 4th edition (New York: Oxford University Press, 1995).

13. Christopher Boorse, "On the Distinction between Disease and Illness," in *Concepts of Health and Disease*, ed. Arthur L. Caplan, H. Tristram Engelhardt, Jr., and James J. McCartney (Reading, Mass.: Addison-Wesley, 1981).

14. B. M. Knoppers and S. LeBris, "Recent Advances in Medically Assisted Conception: Legal, Ethical and Social Issues," *American Journal of Law and Medicine* 17, no. 4 (1991): 335.

15. Robert M. Veatch, "Definitions of Life and Death: Should There Be Consistency?" in *Defining Human Life: Medical, Legal and Ethical Implications*, ed. M. W. Shaw and A. E. Doudera (Ann Arbor: AUPHA Press, 1983), 99–113.

16. I owe this insight to John Evans, a Princeton University graduate student who is preparing a dissertation on the sociology of bioethics. Personal communication, 1996.

17. Joseph F. Fletcher, *Situation Ethics* (Philadelphia: Westminster Press, 1966).

Chapter 2: *McGee*, Pragmatic Method and Bioethics

Portions of this chapter were presented to the Harvard/MIT philosophy conference in 1994; the author acknowledges help on earlier drafts from John Lachs, Arthur Caplan, and University of Pennsylvania students in American philosophy in 1998.

1. John Dewey, *Logic: The Theory of Inquiry* (Carbondale: Southern Illinois University Press, 1990), 10.

2. Ibid., 11.

3. Ibid., 32.

4. Ibid., 38.

5. Ibid., 49.

6. Ibid., 48.

7. Ibid., 49.

8. See Larry Hickman, *John Dewey's Pragmatic Technology* (Bloomington: Indiana University Press, 1990).

9. Interestingly, Dewey sets out the matrices of inquiry in a similar way in the earlier and more historical introduction to ethics, entitled *Ethics* (New York: Henry Holt and Company, 1932), focusing first on biology, then turning to the cultural aspects of "moral consciousness through history" (x). In his marginalia Dorian Cairns (in his personal copy of *Ethics* held in the library of Ricahrd M. Zaner at Vanderbilt University) notes from his correspondence with Dewey that Dewey took much of this concept of the rise from biology through culture from Tufts.

10. Dewey, *Logic*, 66. Dewey believed that we tend, in contrast, to think of common sense as the "group of conceptions and beliefs that are currently accepted without question by a given group or by mankind in general" (68), but he was resisting this as but one definition of common sense, one he thought is part of a mixed-up way of dividing "common" from "pure" inquiry.

11. James Campbell, *The Community Reconstructs: The Meaning of Pragmatic Social Thought* (Chicago: University of Illinois Press, 1992), 46.

12. Ibid., 45.

13. Dewey, *Logic*, 76.

14. Ibid., 81.

15. Ibid., 82.

16. Ibid., 84.

17. Ibid., 42.

18. Ibid., 84–5.

19. Ibid., 108.

20. Ibid.

21. Ibid., 119.

22. Ibid., 121.

23. Ibid., 122.

24. As Dewey wrote in *Reconstruction of Philosophy*: "[W]hile saints are engaged in introspection, burly sinners run the world" (Carbondale: Southern Illinois University Press, 1920), 12.

25. Dewey, *Logic*, 137.

26. Ibid., 139.

27. Ibid., 180.

28. Ibid., 181.

29. Ibid., 482.

30. Ibid., 483–84.

31. Ibid., 486.

32. Dewey, *Experience and Nature* (Carbondale: Southern Illinois University Press, 1926), 25.

33. Dewey, *Logic*, 481.

34. Ibid.

35. Ibid., 485.

36. Ibid., 486–87.

37. Ibid., 487.

38. Ibid.

39. See Mark Fox, Glenn McGee, and Arthur Caplan, "Practice Settings for Clinical Ethics Consultation," *Cambridge Quarterly in Healthcare Ethics* (Fall 1998).

40. Dewey, *Logic*, 488.

41. Caroline Whitbeck makes this pragmatic point about abortion well in "The Moral Implications of Regarding Women as People: New Perspectives on Pregnancy and Personhood," in *Abortion and the Status of the Fetus*, ed. W. B. Bondeson (Dordrecht, The Netherlands: D. Reidel, 1983).

42. Dewey, *Logic*, 489.

43. Ibid., 492.

44. Ibid., 503.

Chapter 3: *Fins, Bacchetta, and Miller,* Clinical Pragmatism: A Method of Moral Problem Solving. Orignially published in the *Kennedy Institute of Ethics Journal 7*, no. 2 (June 1997): 129–145.

Work on this chapter was supported in part by a grant from the Emily Davie and Joseph S. Kornfeld Foundation.

1. Tom L. Beauchamp, "Principalism and Its Alleged Competitors," *Kennedy Institute of Ethics Journal* 5 (1995): 181–89.

2. A noteworthy recent treatment of process issues in bioethics may be found in Jonathan D. Moreno, *Deciding Together* (New York: Oxford University Press, 1995).

3. John Dewey, *Reconstruction in Philosophy*, enlarged edition (Boston: Beacon Press, 1957); John Dewey, *The Quest for Certainty*, in *The Later Works*, vol. 4: 1929 (Carbondale: Southern Illinois University Press, 1988); John Dewey, *How We Think* (Buffalo, N.Y.: Prometheus Books, 1991); John Dewey, *Logic: The Theory of Inquiry*, in *The Later Works*, vol. 12: 1938 (Carbondale: Southern Illinois University Press, 1991); and John Dewey, *Theory of Valuation*, in *The Later Works*, vol. 13: 1938–39 (Carbondale: Southern Illinois University Press, 1991). A discussion of the Deweyan influence on clinical pragmatism may be seen in Franklin G. Miller, Joseph J. Fins, and Matthew D. Bacchetta, "Clinical Pragmatism: John Dewey and Clinical Ethics," *Journal of Contemporary Health Law and Policy* 13 (1996): 27–51.

4. Joseph J. Fins and Matthew D. Bacchetta, "Framing the Physician-Assisted Suicide and Voluntary Active Euthanasia Debate: The Role of Deontology, Consequentialism, and Clinical Pragmatism," *Journal of the American Geriatrics Society* 43 (1995): 563–68. Elements of clinical pragmatism may be seen in John C. Fletcher, Charles A. Hite, Paul A. Lombardo, and Mary F. Marshall, eds., *Introduction to Clinical Ethics* (Frederick, Md.: University Publishing Group, 1995).

5. Moreno, 124.

6. Joseph Fins, "Truth Telling and Reciprocity in the Doctor-Patient Relationship: A North American Perspective," *Topics in Palliative Care,* vol. 3 (New York: Oxford University Press, forthcoming).

7. Although we present the method of clinical pragamatism as a linear progression, in practice these steps can be taken simultaneously or in a different sequence. This delineation of method should be seen as a broad outline, not as a rigid checklist, because the process of problem solving should be flexible and tailored to the particular features of a case as they emerge in clinical practice.

8. Michael L. Schwalbe, "Towards a Sociology of Moral Problem Solving," *Journal for the Theory of Social Behavior* 20 (1990): 131–55.

9. Some details of this case have been altered to conceal the identity of the patient. The essential facts remain unchanged.

10. Howard Brody, "Transparency: Informed Consent in Primary Care," *Hastings Center Report* 19, no. 5 (1989): 5–9.

11. According to Roger A. MacKinnon and Robert Michels, *The Psychiatric Interview in Clinical Practice* (Philadelphia: W. B. Saunders Company, 1971), p. 30, "countertransference is operating when the therapist is unable to recognize or refuses to acknowledge the real significance of his attitude and behavior." See also Jay Katz, *The Silent World of Doctor and Patient* (New York: Free Press, 1984), pp. 142–50, on countertransference in medical practice.

12. Joseph Fins, "Breaking the Silence: Futility, Fear, and Anger," in "Futility," *Decisions Near the End of Life,* vol. 7 (Newton, Mass.: Education Development Center, 1997), 26–27.

13. Fins and Bacchetta, 1995.

14. For an example of clinical pragmatism's ability to challenge and transform the ethical perspective of a clinician, see Joseph J. Fins, "Approximation and Negotiation: Clinical Pragmatism and Difference," *Cambridge Quarterly of Healthcare Ethics,* forthcoming. In this article a physician alters his views regarding the applicability of a determination of brain death in a case involving a religious objection.

15. Tom Beauchamp and James F. Childress, *Principles of Biomedical Ethics,* 4th edition (New York: Oxford University Press, 1994), 28–37.

16. Joseph J. Fins, "From Indifference to Goodness," *Journal of Religion and Health* 35 (1996): 245–54.

17. Dewey, *How We Think,* 74.

18. Dewey, *Reconstruction in Philosophy,* 96.

Chapter 4: *Hester,* Habits of Healing

1. *Reconstruction in Philosophy* [1920], in *John Dewey: The Middle Works: 1899-1924,* ed. Jo Ann Boydston, vol. 12 (Carbondale: Southern Illinois University Press, 1988) (referred to below as MW12), 176.

2. Cf. Edmund Pellegrino, "The Anatomy of Clinical Judgments: Some Notes on Right Reason and Right Action," in *Clinical Judgment: A Critical Appraisal,* ed. H. T. Engelhardt, Jr., et al. (Dordrecht, Holland: D. Reidel, 1979), 169–194.

3. We possibly could stretch this point beyond the world of human making and doing, but I need not be so bold given the topic at hand.

4. Cf. C. S. Peirce, "The Fixation of Belief" [1877], in *The Essential Peirce*, ed. Nathan Houser and Christian Kloesel, vol. 1 (1867–1893) (Bloomington: Indiana University Press, 1992); William James, *The Principles of Psychology* [1890], vols. 1 and 2 (New York: Dover, 1950); and John Dewey, *Human Nature and Conduct* [1922], in *John Dewey: The Middle Works: 1899–1924*, ed. Jo Ann Boydston, vol. 14 (Carbondale: Southern Illinois University Press, 1988) (referred to below as MW14).

5. MW14, 121, 123.

6. John Dewey, *Liberalism and Social Action* [1939], in *John Dewey: The Later Works: 1825–1953*, ed. Jo Ann Boydston, vol. 11 (Carbondale: Southern Illinois Univ. Press, 1991), 36–37.

7. John Dewey, *Democracy and Education* [1920], in *John Dewey: The Middle Works: 1899–1924*, ed. Jo Ann Boydston, vol. 9 (Carbondale: Southern Illinois University Press, 1988) (referred to below as MW9), 51.

8. MW9, 51–52 (emphasis mine).

9. Donald Morris, *Dewey and the Behavioristic Context of Ethics* (Bethesda, Md.: International Scholars, 1996), 38.

10. MW9, 53.

11. MW9, 54.

12. John Dewey, *Construction and Criticism* [1939], in *John Dewey: The Later Works: 1825–1953*, ed. Jo Ann Boydston, vol. 5 (Carbondale: Southern Illinois University Press, 1991), 134.

13. This comes from a conversation I had with a Columbia/HCA director who recounted the events of a business retreat at which Rick Scott (former CEO of Columbia/HCA) made a statement to the effect that in the three areas of business practices—service, innovation, and operational efficiency—Columbia was primarily to focus its efforts on operational efficiency. The director, by the way, agreed with Mr. Scott on this point.

14. Cf. George Anders, *Health Against Wealth: HMOs and the Breakdown of Medical Trust* (New York: Houghton Mifflin, 1996).

15. This is not to imply that a naive and unreflective approach has been taken to the development of these computer applications. Quite the contrary, great care has been taken and thoughtful debate has been considered to account for concerns of logicians, physicians, philosophers, and patients. However, important and regrettable reductionism by the computer (at this stage of technology) is inevitable.

16. Richard Zaner, *Ethics and the Clinical Encounter* (Englewood Cliffs, N.J.: Prentice-Hall, 1988), 10.

17. Ibid., 55. Zaner's discussion of "asymmetry" is indebted to both P. B. Lenrow and Edmund Pellegrino.

18. Ibid.

19. Cf. David Rothman, *Strangers at the Bedside* (New York: Basic Books, 1992).

20. See Tom Beauchamp and James Childress, *Principles of Biomedical Ethics*, editions 1–4 (New York: Oxford University Press 1979–1996).

21. A survey taken in the late '70s showed clearly that practices have changed since the early '60s. In 1961 only 12 percent of physicians said that their usual policy is to tell patients when they have cancer; this rose to 98 percent in 1977, an 86 percent jump. However, even as the authors of the study noted, "Many questions still remain. Do physicians tell patients they have 'cancer,' or are euphemisms such as 'tumor' or 'growth' still widely used, and if so what does that mean for the communication process?" (Dennis H. Novack, et al., "Changes in Physicians' Attitudes Towards Telling the Cancer Patient" [1979] in *Ethical Issues in Death and Dying*, ed. Tom Beacuchamp and Rober Veath [Upper Saddle River, N.J.: Prentice-Hall, 1996], 74). The question still remains to this day, not Do physicians talk with patients? but What do they say and why?

22. One hears "routine" answers to this, of course: e.g., medical knowledge is frightening for the patient because it is about the patient, not the physician; it speaks to the patient's condition; or medicine is frightening because it is difficult to understand and takes many years to perfect. But these responses beg the question, for they avoid the hard work—viz., they point to the fact that successful, open communication requires much effort, from both parties.

23. This question is more difficult to answer than the last, but clearly, the definition of 'autonomy' is, at best, "consent" and, at worst, nonexistent.

24. Zaner, 53.

25. John Dewey, "The Unity of the Human Being" [1939], in *John Dewey: The Later Works: 1825–1953*, ed. Jo Ann Boydston, vol. 13 (Carbondale: Southern Illinois University Press, 1991) (referred to below as LW13), 336.

26. John J. McDermott, "Feeling as Insight: The Affective Dimension in Social Diagnosis," in *Hippocrates Revisited*, ed. R. Bulger (New York: Medcom, 1973), 177.

27. William James, "On a Certain Blindness in Human Beings" [1899], in *The Writings of William James*, ed. John J. McDermott (Chicago: University of Chicago Press, 1980), 629–630.

28. LW13, 334.

29. For a more in depth discussion of the idea of "community as healing," see D. Micah Hester, "Community As Healing. . . . ," *Journal of Medicine and Philosophy* 23, no. 4 (1998): forthcoming.

30. MW9, 8.

31. Robert Westbrook has argued that Dewey's conception of "community" appears overly idealistic, thus failing on Dewey's own pragmatic grounds. But as Michael Eldridge has, in turn, pointed out, Dewey's "faith" in democratic community is never *overly* ideal but rather both (1) practically (findable in lived experience) and (2) fallibly (open to error and adjustment) ideal. Eldridge argues on the practical side both that this "sharing of activities" does happen in lived experience and that the awareness—and adjustments that occur because of that awareness—is constitutive of the experience of community. In a simple example, marriage (in the narrowest sense) as a community of two individuals often loses its "feeling"—i.e., the "experience"—of community when important

conflicts arise dividing the partners—e.g., when the goals of each are not shared by the other: a desire to live one place rather than another, the pursuit of one profession over another. During these occasions, we may not say that the community dissolves completely (though at times it may), but certainly the experience of community does. He argues also that (2) Dewey never holds up this notion of community as the Absolute end, that, instead, he asks us to experiment with it and to toss out his hypothesis if it leads to error. Further, Eldridge argues that Dewey's "ideal" of community has never been adequately attempted and implemented. Thus, we cannot say whether or not his conception works. Cf. Michael Eldridge, "Dewey's Faith in Democracy as Shared Experience," in *Transactions of the Charles S. Peirce Society* 32, no. 1 (1996): 11–30.

32. Cf. George H. Mead, *Mind, Self, and Society* [1934] (Chicago: University of Chicago Press, 1962), 154. Here Mead uses the example of a baseball team to illustrate his notion of the "generalized other" that acts as a normative account of community, where individual action is regulated by the imaginative take on what the "generalized other"—i.e., the other taken not as a specific person, but as a community—will do.

33. LW5, 127

34. It is important to note at this point that a social "good" itself must have a certain character to it. In particular, I take the Roycean-Deweyan position that social goods must be, what we might call, "inclusive." That is, goals of a community must be of such a character that they do not intrinsically oppose or deny the worth of an alternative community's ends, unless those ends are themselves exclusive, violent, or stifling of the possibilities for deeply enriching experience, both for the communitt's members and, particularly, non-members—e.g., a band of robber-barons or the Nazi party. Josiah Royce sees this as constitutive of true "loyalty," and Dewey takes this to be the nature of a true democracy. (See Josiah Royce: 1995 , *The Philosophy of Loyalty* [1908] [Nashville: Vanderbilt University Press, 1995], particularly lecture 3, "Loyalty to Loyalty," 48–69; and John Dewey, *The Public and Its Problems* [1927], in *John Dewey: The Later Works: 1825–1953*, ed. Jo Ann Boydston, vol. 2 [Carbondale: Southern Illinois University Press, 1988], 235–372, particularly chapter 5, "The Search for the Great Community," 325–350.) As this discussion pertains to the health care community and its end of "health," I see no intrinsically exclusive character to "health" and, so, find no need to defend the mere possibility that the health care community can become an instance of an "ideal" community as I propose.

35. MW9, 96.

36. Ibid., 97.

37. Ibid., 105.

38. Ibid., 368.

Chapter 5: *Parker,* The Bioethics Committee:

1. Transiency, pluralism, and meliorism are discussed as prominent themes of pragmatist ethics in John J. McDermott, "Pragmatic Sensibility: The Morality of Experience," in *New Directions in Ethics*, ed. J. P. DeMarco and R. Fox (New York: Routledge and Kegan Paul, 1986), 113–34.

2. Visiting Nurse Association of West Michigan, "VNA Ethics Committee Mission Statement," March 10, 1994.

3. The functions of the ethics committee highlighted in the VNA "Ethics Committee Mission Statement" are mirrored in other discussions of ethics committee. Cf. Sigrid Fry-Revere, *The Accountability of Bioethics Committees and Consultants* (Frederick, Maryland: University Publishing Group, 1992), 16–17, and Robert P. Craig, Carl L. Middleton, and Laurence J. O'Connell, *Ethics Committees: A Practical Approach* (St. Louis, Missouri: The Catholic Health Association of the United States, 1986), 2–4. Craig et al. also include "theological reflection" as a function of the ethics committee operating as part of a Roman Catholic health care facility.

4. The term *patient* connotes the characteristic passivity of a recipient of health care in this image.

5. Josiah Royce, "Lecture IX: The Community and the Time-Process," in *The Problem of Christianity*, vol. 2 (New York: The Macmillan Company, 1914), 51–52.

6. Josiah Royce, *The Philosophy of Loyalty*, The Vanderbilt Library of American Philosophy (Nashville: Vanderbilt University Press, 1995), 84–85.

7. The concepts of mediation discussed here appear in Royce's late works and are presented in Frank M. Oppenheim, *Royce's Mature Ethics* (Notre Dame, Ind.: University of Notre Dame Press, 1993) 164–69. Oppenheim's main source is "Spirit of the Community," among the "Royce Papers" at the Harvard University Archives.

8. Josiah Royce, "Spirit of Community," quoted in Oppenheim, *Royce's Mature Ethics*, 164.

9. The most prominent statement of this tradition is within the Hippocratic Oath itself. See the analysis offered in Mary B. Mahowald, "Biomedical Ethics: A Precocious Youth," in *New Directions in Ethics*, 141–57.

10. The three potential sources of increased authority are identified in Sigrid Fry-Revere, 16–17.

Chapter 6: *Mahowald*, Collaboration and Casuistry

An earlier version of this chapter appeared in Herman Parret, ed., *Peirce and Value Theory* (Amsterdam: John Benjamins Publishing Company, 1994), 61–71.

1. Mary B. Mahowald, "The Physician," in *The Power of the Professional Person*, ed. Robert. W. Clarke and Robert P. Lawre (New York: University Press of America, 1988), 126–29.

2. Albert R. Jonsen and Stephen Toulmin, *The Abuse of Casuistry* (Berkeley: University of California Press, 1988), 137–51.

3. Mary B. Mahowald, "Peirce's Concept of Community: Another Interpretation," *Transactions of the Charles S. Peirce Society* 9 (1973): 177.

4. Mary B. Mahowald, "Hospital Ethics Committees: Diverse and Problematic," *Newsletter on Medicine and Philosophy* 88 (1989): 88–94.

5. Jonsen and Toulmin.

6. Ibid., 11.

7. Ibid., 12.

8. Ibid., 251.

9. Charles Sanders Peirce, *Collected Papers*, vol. 1, ed. Charles Hartshorne and Paul Weiss (Cambridge, Mass.: Harvard University Press, 1931), para. 71.

10. Peirce, *Collected Papers*, vol. 1, para. 148.

11. Charles Sanders Peirce, *Collected Papers*, vol. 2, ed. Charles Hartshorne and Paul Weiss (Cambridge, Mass.: Harvard University Press, 1932), para. 654.

12. Peirce, *Collected Papers*, vol. 2, para. 652

13. Charles Sanders Peirce, *Collected Papers*, vol. 5, ed. Charles Hartshorne and Paul Weiss (Cambridge, Mass.: Harvard University Press, 1934), para. 494.

14. Peirce, *Collected Papers*, vol. 5, para. 384.

15. Cf. Peirce, *Collected Papers*, vol. 5, para. 402.

16. Peirce, *Collected Papers*, vol. 2, para. 676.

17. Mary B. Mahowald, "C. S. Peirce: His Concepts of God and Religion," *Transactions of the Charles S. Peirce Society* 12 (1976): 373.

18. Peirce, *Collected Papers*, vol. 1, para. 44

19. Sarah Stueber Bishop, "Explanation in Medicine: The Problem-Oriented Approach," *Journal of Medicine and Philosophy* 5 (1980): 30–54.

20. Charles Sanders Peirce, *Writings of Charles S. Peirce: A Chronological Edition*, vol. 2: 1867–1871 (Bloomington, Ind.: Indiana University Press, 1982), 354.

21. Peirce, *Writings*, vol. 2, 239.

22. Albert R. Jonsen, "Transplantation of Fetal Tissue: An Ethicist's Viewpoint," *Clinical Research* 36 (1988): 215–19..

23. Stanley J. Reiser, Arthur J. Duck, and William Curran, eds., "Selections from the Hippocratic Corpus," *Ethics in Medicine* (Cambridge, Mass.: MIT Press, 1977), 7.

24. Mahowald, "The Physician," 126–29.

Chapter 7: *Trotter*, The Medical Covenant: A Roycean Perspective

1. William F. May, *The Physician's Covenant* (Philadelphia: Westminster, 1983).

2. See John Clendenning, *The Life and Thought of Josiah Royce* (Madison: University of Wisconsin Press, 1985), 34–35, 123, 313, 316–18, 343–44, 359–60. These passages deal with Royce's childhood, with his eldest son's mental illness and death, and with Royce's stroke in 1912.

3. Robert M. Veatch, *A Theory of Medical Ethics* (New York: Basic Books, 1981).

4. H. Tristram Engelhardt, Jr., *The Foundations of Bioethics* (New York: Oxford University Press, 1986). Royce also employs transcendental arguments. For instance, he defines moral life (with Dewey) as the intelligent pursuit of ends, then identifies reasonableness and impartiality as transcendental conditions for such a life. Later, he integrates the notions of reasonableness and impartiality into a sophisticated sign-cognitive theory of moral development, culminating in his theory of genuine loyalty (see Griffin Trotter, *The Loyal Physician* [Nashville: Vanderbilt University Press, 1997], 85–103, 109–35). Royce is not a transcenden-

talist, however. He more frequently employs the methods of empirico-historical analysis and interpretive musement to reach his major conclusions.

5. Baruch A. Brody, *Life and Death Decision Making* (New York: Oxford University Press, 1988).

6. Bernard Gert, *Morality: A New Justification of the Moral Rules* (1966; reprint, New York: Oxford University Press, 1988).

7. Alasdair MacIntyre, *After Virtue* (Notre Dame: University of Notre Dame Press, 1981). Most pragmatists—including Royce—are linked to this category by their emphasis on the role of habit in moral life. Dewey and Royce also stress the relation between cultural norms and individual virtues.

8. Trotter, *The Loyal Physician*, 86–91, 268n.18. See also Josiah Royce, *The Problem of Christianity* (1918; reprint, Chicago: University of Chicago Press, 1968), 343–62 (on the theory of interpretation) and Josiah Royce, *The Philosophy of Loyalty* (1908; reprint, Nashville: Vanderbilt University Press, 1995), 170 (on fallibilism).

9. Josiah Royce, *Race Questions and Other American Problems* (New York: Macmillan, 1908), 3–53. John Dewey, *Art as Experience* (1934; reprint, Carbondale: Southern Illinois University Press, 1989), 327–28, 337.

10. In his middle period, Royce wrote: "Tell me to what you are loyal, and why,— and you tell me at once just what constitutes the really moral aspect of your personality. All the rest is chance, or fortune, or prejudice or barren routine. Tell me, again, wherein and whereto you are loyal, and you will at once explain to me how far you have personally solved the problem about the conflict between personal rights and social duties" (Pittsburgh lectures, unpublished lecture notes, 1910?, Royce Collection, Harvard University Archives, Cambridge, Mass.)

11. I use the term "personalism" in a very broad sense that does not conform precisely to the conceptions of American personalists such as George Holmes Howison and Borden Parker Bowne. Royce and William Ernest Hocking are outstanding representatives of the kind of personalism I have in mind. Hocking wrote that "the center of the universe is everywhere that the divine interest finds a person" (*Human Nature and its Remaking*, 2d ed. [New Haven: Yale University Press, 1923], 424).

12. Royce, *The Philosophy of Loyalty*, 79.

13. This second claim, combined with Royce's doctrine of the great or beloved community, differentiates him from most "self-realization" or "self-actualization" theorists insofar as Roycean moral subjects are ready to sacrifice their lives for the sake of the highest cause, and therefore clearly have a moral ideal that overrides any secular imperative for self-fulfillment. Further, morally mature persons, in Royce's view, will harbor such an expansive notion of personal identity that the traditional distinction between self-realization, as a form of individualism, and abnegation, as self-sacrifice on behalf of a moral community, is no longer coherent. On this point, Royce and Dewey part ways.

14. Royce does not invoke Aristotle's notion of *phronesis* (*Nichomachean Ethics* 1140a24–1140b30; 1142a31–1145a10), but his notion of practical wisdom is in

many respects similar. For both thinkers, practical wisdom requires excellence in deliberating about ends or moral ideals.

15. Royce, *The Philosophy of Loyalty*, 90.

16. Ibid., 9.

17. Josiah Royce, *The Letters of Josiah Royce*, ed. John Clendenning (Chicago: University of Chicago Press, 1970), 548–49. Royce goes on to proclaim in the next few lines that a profession is one of the various causes that are suitable foci of loyalty.

18. Royce did not frequently use the word "covenant." The concept, however, is everywhere in his philosophy. Royce would hold that there is a hierarchy of covenants corresponding to the hierarchy of communities. The highest covenant, in this view, is the covenant of an eternal community—the human covenant with God, embodied in the ideal of the beloved, great community. "Genuine" loyalties are those deriving, ultimately, from devotion to this ideal.

19. Those who doubt that the threat of illness is an identity-forming factor should imagine how their self-image would change if they were rendered immortal and illness free.

20. Royce, *The Problem of Christianity*, 134.

21. Trotter, *The Loyal Physician*, 150–61.

22. Josiah Royce, *War and Insurance* (New York: Macmillan, 1914), 32–35. See also the discussion of the clinical dyad in *The Loyal Physician*, 143–46.

23. See Jacquelyn Ann K. Kegley, *Genuine Individuals and Genuine Communities: A Roycean Public Philosophy* (Nashville: Vanderbilt University Press, 1997), 158–205. For a discussion of Royce and ethnic communities, see Griffin Trotter, "Royce, Community and Ethnicity," *Transactions of the Charles S. Peirce Society* 30 (1994): 231–69.

24. The temporal and conceptual priority of "illness," as the patient's experience of physical disharmony or suffering, over "disease," as defined in the medical model, is discussed in *The Loyal Physician*, as well as in the works of Zaner and Cassell. See Richard M. Zaner, *Ethics and the Clinical Encounter* (Englewood Cliffs, N.J.: Prentice-Hall, 1988), and Eric J. Cassell, *The Nature of Suffering* (New York: Oxford University Press, 1991).

25. Francis W. Peabody, "The Care of the Patient," in Oglesby Paul, *The Caring Physician: The Life of Francis W. Peabody* (Boston: Francis A. Countway Library of Medicine, 1991), 173–4.

26. I discuss problems with profit-oriented economic models of the patient-physician relationship in "Against Customer Service," *The Journal of Emergency Medicine* 16 (1998): 227–33.

27. Trotter, *The Loyal Physician*, 28–33.

28. Josiah Royce, "On Certain Limitations of the Thoughtful Public in America," in *The Basic Writings of Josiah Royce*, ed. John J. McDermott (Chicago: University of Chicago Press, 1969), 1111–34. In the same address, Royce commented that "the human mind, in its present form of consciousness, is simply incapable of formulating all its practical devices under any one simple rule. We have to learn both to work and to wait."

29. Josiah Royce, *Outlines of Psychology* (New York: Macmillan, 1903), 367–68.

30. The principle of beneficence, as interpreted by Royce, would imply what Emanual and Emanual have termed a "deliberative model" of decision making. See Ezekiel J. Emanuel and Linda L. Emanuel, "Four Models of the Physician-Patient Relationship," *JAMA* 267, no. 16 (1992): 2221–26.

31. P. Werner, "Productivity and Quality Management" in *Productivity and Performance Management in Health Care Institutions* (Chicago: American Hospital Publishing, 1989), 83.

32. Contrast the Roycean focus on restoring persons to fruitful community life with the profit orientation of the authors of a text on customer satisfaction, who write:

Organizations that consistently provide excellent service are winners for several reasons. For example:
• They earn customer loyalty, and customer loyalty translates into repeat customers.
• They are less vulnerable to price wars. There is even evidence that they have historically been able to command higher prices without losing market share.
• They don't have to spend as much on marketing because customers spread the good word about them.
• They are profitable.

(Wendy Leebov and Gail Scott, *Service Quality Improvement: The Customer Satisfaction Strategy for Health Care* [Chicago: American Hospital Publishing, 1994], 5–6.)

33. The abstract ideals that define communities are, like all abstract notions, understood (and loved) in terms of concrete examples. We conceive "bird" by thinking about robins and eagles. Likewise, our abstract notion of "care" is constructed from our experiences of caring.

34. Royce, *The Philosophy of Loyalty*, 11, 25–27, 143–46.

35. Royce, *The Problem of Christianity*, 119.

Chapter 8: *Gavin*, On "Tame" and "Untamed" Death: Jamesian Reflections

1. Geoffrey Gorer, "The Pornography of Death," in *Death: Current Perspectives*, ed. Edwin S. Sheneidman (Palo Alto: Mayfield Publishing Company, 1976), 74.

2. Ibid., 76.

3. For the following, see Elisabeth Kübler-Ross *On Death and Dying* (New York: Macmillan, 1970), 34–121.

4. Ibid., 77.

5. Ibid., 99.

6. Ibid., 122.

7. Ibid., 123.

8. Ibid., 123.

9. Ibid., 9.

10. Elisabeth Kübler-Ross, *Questions and Answers on Death and Dying* (New York: Collier Books, Macmillan, 1974), 37.

11. Ibid., 36

12. Ibid., 34.

13. William James, "The Sentiment of Rationality," in *The Writings of William James*, ed. and intro. by John J. McDermott (New York: Modern Library, Random House, 1967), 321.

14. For the following, see Philippe Ariès, *Western Attitudes Toward Death: From the Middle Ages to the Present* (Baltimore: Johns Hopkins University Press, 1974).

15. Ibid., 88–89.

16. Philippe Ariès, "Death Inside Out," in *Death Inside Out* ed. Peter Steinfels and Robert M. Veatch (New York: Harper and Row, 1975), 24.

17. Daniel Callahan, *The Troubled Dream of Life: Living with Mortality* (New York: Simon and Schuster, 1993), 28.

18. Ibid., 52–53.

19. Ibid., 55.

20. Ibid., 223–24, 230.

21. William James, *The Principles of Psychology* (New York: Dover Publications, 1950), 2 vols.; vol. 1, 251.

22. Callahan, *The Troubled Dream of Life*, 13.

23. Ibid., 35.

24. See "A Definition of Irreversible Coma," Report of the Ad Hoc Committee of the Harvard Medical School to Examine the Definition of Brain Death, in *Ethical Issues in Death and Dying*, ed. Tom Beauchamp and Seymour Perlin (Englewood Cliffs, N.J.: Prentice-Hall, 1978), 11–18.

25. See David Lamb, *Death, Brain Death, and Ethics* (Albany: State University of New York Press, 1985), 20.

26. See, for example, Robert M. Veatch, "Defining Death Anew: Technical and Ethical Problems," in Beauchamp and Perlin, *Ethical Issues in Death and Dying*, 18–38; *Death Beyond Whole-Brain Criteria*, ed. Richard Zaner (Dordrecht, The Netherlands: Kluwer Academic Publishers, 1988).

27. See William J. Gavin, *Cuttin' the Body Loose: Historical, Biological, and Personal Approaches to Death and Dying* (Philadelphia: Temple University press, 1995), chap. 3.

28. See Veatch, "Defining Death Anew: Technical and Ethical Problems," in *Ethical Issues in Death and Dying*, 21.

29. Robert M. Veatch, "Defining Death Anew: Policy Options," in *Ethical Issues in Death and Dying*, 81–83.

30. See Robert Olick, "Brain Death, Religious Freedom and Public Policy, New Jersey's Landmark Legislative Initiative," in *Ethical Issues in Death and Dying*, 2d ed., ed. Tom Beauchamp and Robert M. Veatch (Upper Saddle River, N.J.: Prentice-Hall, 1996), 52–60. Some steps of a similar nature have also been taken by New York State.

31. Hans Jonas, "Against the Stream: Comments on the Definition and

Redefinition of Death," in *Ethical Issues in Death and Dying*, 51–52.

32. Ibid., 53.

33. Ibid., 53.

34. Patricia D. White, "Should the Law Define Death?—A Genuine Question," in *Death: Beyond Whole-Brain Criteria*, pp. 104–106.

35. See Don Ihde, *Technics and Praxis* (Dordrecht, The Netherlands: D. Reidel Publishing Company, 1979), 21

36. See Alfred North Whitehead, *Science and the Modern World* (New York: Free Press, 1967), 51.

37. Dena Davis, "Rich Cases: The Ethics of Thick Description," *Hastings Center Report* 21 (July–August 1991): 15.

38. For the following, see Larry Churchill, "The Human Experience of Dying: The Moral Primacy of Stories Over Stages," *Soundings* 62 (Spring 1979): 24–37.

39. Ibid., 27.

40. Ibid., 30.

41. Ibid., 30.

42. Ibid., 31.

43. Ibid., 33.

44. See Paul Ramsey, "The Indignity of 'Death With Dignity,'" in *Death Inside Out*, 81–96.

45. Ibid., 82.

46. Ibid., 82.

47. Ibid., 83.

48. Ibid., 84.

49. Ibid., 89–90.

50. Ibid., 90.

51. Ibid., 95–96.

52. James, *The Principles of Psychology*, vol. 1, 226.

53. William James, *Essays in Radical Empiricism*, in *Essays in Radical Empiricism and A Pluralistic Universe* (Glouster: Peter Smith, 1967), 170, n.

54. On this matter see Steven Goldberg, "The Changing Face of Death: Computers, Consciousness, and Nancy Cruzan," *Stanford Law Review*, 43 (February 1991): 659–84.

55. See Jean-Paul Sartre, *Being and Nothingness, An Essay on Phenomenological Ontology*, trans. and with an intro. by Hazel E. Barnes (New York: Washington Square Press, 1966), pp. 650–81.

56. William James, *The Will to Believe and Other Essays in Popular Philosophy* (New York: Longmans, Green and Co., 1927), 31. Original source: Fitz-James Stephen, *Liberty, Equality, Fraternity*, 2d ed. (London, 1874), 353.

Chapter 9: *Hester*, Significance at the End of Life

1. Nancy Dubler and David Nimmons, *Ethics on Call* (New York: Harmony, 1992), 146

2. Sherwin B. Nuland, *How We Die* (New York: Alfred A. Knopf, 1993), xv, xvii.

3. See William Gavin, *Cuttin' the Body Lose* (Philadelphia: Temple University Press 1995).

4. Nuland and Nimmons, 3–5.

5. James H. Buchanan, *Patient Encounters* (New York: Henry Holt, 1989), 45–50.

6. Richard Seltzer, *Down from Troy*. Boston: Little, Brown, 1992), 284.

7. For a more in-depth discussion of the points in this section, including discussions of PVS, brain death, and the mentally incapacitated, see D. Micah Hester, "Progressive Dying . . . ," *The Journal of Medical Humanities* 19, no. 4 (1998): forthcoming.

8. James does qualify this idea of "significance" with the phrase "for communicable and publicly recognizable purposes." I believe this qualification is made to contrast specifically with remarks he makes elsewhere in such works as *Varieties of Religious Experience*, where he admits to the possibility of a kind of mystical "private" significance in an individual's life. Cf. William James, *Varieties of Religious Experience* (New York: Longman & Greens, 1902), 379–429, Lectures XVI & XVII, "Mysticism." In particular, James's qualifier seems specifically to contrast with his use of the term 'mystical states of consciousness' in *Varieties*, where James begins his definition of this term with the idea that the mystical is "ineffable," "transient," and "passive"—three terms not readily applicable to socially recognizable meaning in life. Since my discussion is concerned with dying as part of lived, social experience, the qualifier is simply redundant.

9. William James, "What Makes a Life Significant?" in *The Writings of William James* [1899], ed. John J. McDermott (Chicago: University of Chicago Press, 1977), 657.

10. Ibid., 656.

11. Ibid. (emphasis mine).

12. Ibid., 657.

13. Ibid.

14. We would be wise to cultivate the ability, particularly as we become elderly and means reduce in number and potency, to find meaning more and more in those activities that youth affords us the luxury of ignoring. As we age and move closer to dying (though I do not wish to restrict this only to the elderly), we should, rather than shaping meaning through the development of long-term goals and activities, attempt to develop significance out of the more immediate pleasures and basic activities of life. As we find our abilities changing, our goals must also. The less stamina and strength we demonstrate, wisdom tells us, the more immediate our ends should become. The sounds of the day, the taste of the food, the movements of the body, all can be sources of meaning. If sight begins to degenerate, simply hearing the song of a bird can be an activity both idealized and appreciated. When a hot day diminishes energy, the pleasure of ice cream can reinvigorate. As muscles begin to weaken, the swinging of the legs and arms in everyday walking can prove defiant against the aging process. In this way we can retain meaning throughout life by pursuing ends appropriate to our means.

15. James, "What Makes a Life Significant?" 653.

16. William James, "On a Certain Blindness in Human Beings" [1899], in *The Writings of William James*, 640.

17. Ibid., 645.

18. Arthur Kleinman, *The Illness Narratives* (New York: Basic Books, 1988), 142.

19. Ibid., 144.

20. Gavin, 123.

21. Oliver Sacks illustrates this sentiment well in speaking of his post-encephalitic patients at the closing of the preface to his book *Awakenings*: "[T]hose who have died are in some sense not dead—their unclosed charts, their letters, still face me as I write. They still live, for me, in some very personal way. They were not only patients but teachers and friends, and the years I spent with them were the most significant of my life. I want something of their lives, their presence, to be preserved and live for others, as examples of human predicament and survival" (Oliver Sacks, *Awakenings*. New York: Harper Perennial, 1990), xxxviii–xxxix).

Also, this is often portrayed by those dying patients who explicitly take on the role of being an example for others so that their death is not "in vain" but instead becomes meaningful to themselves and others. (Cf. Kleinman, 1988, ch. 8, as well as Plato's *Apology*, *Crito*, and *Phaedo*.)

22. I want to make clear that I am not addressing the important and complex issues of chronically ill or injured patients, such as those with long-term renal problems, extensive burns, or other debilitating problems that are difficult (if not impossible) to live with in a way meaningful to the afflicted individual but are not, in themselves, fatal. It is possible to extend my argument to some such cases, but I cannot accomplish that here.

Though also important, I must also leave out a discussion of euthanasia of infants or young children. For a variety of perspectives on the topic see *Euthanasia and the Newborn*, ed. H. Tristram Engelhardt, Jr.(Dordrecht, The Netherlands: D. Reidel, 1987).

23. Some may wish to interject that hospice care is a reasonable alternative to intentional acts of dying (cf. Sandol Stoddard, "Terminal, but Not Hopeless," in *Intervention and Reflection: Basic Issues in Medical Ethics*, ed. Ronald Munson, 5th ed. (Belmont, Calif.: Wadsworth, 1996); and though I do not disagree that hospice offers many patients a viable alternative in their last months of lives, I am arguing that beyond these patients are some people for whom even this alternative is not what is most meaningful, dignified, "best"—e.g., suffering cancer patients with bones so brittle they can break performing simple, everyday movements or patients who respond poorly or are allergic to drug therapy.

24. For further possible objections, see the articles by R. Macklin and by E. Pelligrino in *Ethical Issues in Death and Dying*, ed. Tom Beacuchamp and Rober Veath (Upper Saddle River, N.J.: Prentice-Hall, 1996). For my more in depth response to other possible objections—including issues of technological advances, physician-assisted suicide, and the very question of 'meaning' itself—see Hester, "Progressive Dying. . . ."

25. Gerald D. Coleman, "Assisted Suicide: An Ethical Perspective," in

Euthanasia: The Moral Issues, ed. Robert Baird and Stuart Rosembaum (Buffalo: Prometheus Books, 1987.

26. Daniel Callahan, "When Self-Determination Runs Amok," *Hastings Center Report* 22, no. 2 (1992): 52–55.

27. Ibid., 52.

28. Other possible interpretations of Callahan's statement are easily dismissed, I believe, as either obviously uninteresting or not morally complex enough to address at this time. For example, it is quite ridiculous to believe that physicians or "lay people" have been given a "right" to kill, if we mean by this that they can go around killing without impediment or consequence simply because we have also accepted as a society the "right to die." A "right to die" clearly does not warrant unconsented-to acts of killing. Further, if we simply mean that society has sanctioned the right of a doctor to kill a patient, this is still all predicated on the patient's desire to die, which is clearly a relationship of rights to obligations, not rights to rights.

29. John Dewey, *Human Nature and Conduct* in *The Middle Works,* vol. 14, ed. JoAnn Boydston (Carbondale, Ill.: Southern Illinois University Press, 1988), 16.

30. William James, "The Moral Philosopher and the Moral Life" [1897], in *The Writings of William James,* 617.

31. Margaret Pabst Battin, *The Least Worst Death* (New York: Oxford University Press, 1994).

Chapter 10: *Wilshire,* William James, Black Elk, and the Healing Act

1. Larry Dossey, *Healing Words: The Power of Prayer and the Practice of Medicine* (San Francisco, 1995); Andrew Weil, *Spontaneous Healing: How to Enlist and Enhance the Body's Own Gifts for Maintaining and Healing Itself* (New York, 1995); Bernie Siegel, *Love, Medicine, and Miracles: Lessons Learned about Self-Healing from a Surgeon's Experience with Exceptional Patients* (New York, 1990); O. Carl Simonton, Stephanie Matthew-Simonton, and James Creighton, *Getting Well Again: A Step by Step Self-Help Guide to Overcoming Cancer for Patients and their Families* (Los Angeles, 1978).

2. For example, "History," in *Ralph Waldo Emerson: Selected Essays,* ed. Larzar Ziff (New York, 1982), 158–59.

3. In *Essays in Radical Empiricism,* "The Place of Affectional Facts in a World of Pure Experience," for example, in my *William James: The Essential Writings* (Albany: SUNY Press, 1984), 205.

4. See the penultimate paragraph in "The Place for Affectional Facts. . . ."

5. See "The First Cure," in *Black Elk Speaks: Being the Life Story of a Holy Man of the Oglala Sioux—As Told through John G. Neihardt (Flaming Rainbow)* (1932; reprint, Lincoln: University of Nebraska Press, 1988), 194–203. The complete transcript of Neihardt's interviews with Black Elk has been published in Raymond J. DeMallie, ed., *The Sixth Grandfather: Black Elk's Teaching Given to John G. Neihardt* (Lincoln: University of Nebraska Press, 1984). Neihardt's original edited version was intended to communicate with a wide audience of persons of European extraction, and it largely succeeds in that, I believe. To include much

more would have confounded and confused. In this chapter I follow the original, leaving out, for example, Black Elk's shamanic technique of extracting the source of sickness—"the blue man"—and so on. So obsessed is the Western mentality with discovering "the true nature of the external world"—and so limited is its conception of body-self and mentality and health—that extractions are construed as mere fakery; that is, the shaman may bring a small stone, say, in his mouth, which he then shows after sucking on the patient's body. So thin and abstract is our conception of symbols! A commentary, largely helpful, can be found in Julian Rice, *Black Elk's Story: Distinguishing Its Lokata Purpose* (1991; reprinted Albuquerque: University of New Mexico Press, 1994).

    6. In *The Old Ways* (San Francisco: City Light Boods, 1977).

    7. "Does Consciousness Exist?" in *Essays in Radical Empiricism*, in, for example, my *William James: The Essential Writings* (Albany: SUNY Press, 1984), 176.

    8. Exodus 34:30, King James Version.

    9. Here James should be augmented by what Emerson and Charles Peirce wrote about universals. Early in "The American Scholar" Emerson lamented the loss of the "original unit"—the whole of humanity, the universal Man—"the fountain of power" that "has been so . . . spilled into drops" that it "cannot be gathered." So *individuals* can no longer possess themselves. In viable indigenous societies this is not the case. See also Charles Peirce, particularly "The Law of Mind" (for example, in Justus Buchler, ed., *Philosophical Writings of Peirce* [New York: Dover, 1955]). Ideas are not discrete entities inside individual mind-containers, but are feelings that generalize themselves over time and space and between things and persons and are real and potent. So North Wind is not merely a compendious name for individual gusts of wind coming from the north—gusts that can be measured by a meterologist's instruments. There may be no such gusts inside the tepee at the moment Black Elk draws the North Wind through the boy's body and out his abdomen, but finally and properly understood, it is true that he does so. There is much more to reality than times, places, persons, and animals in their brute particularity. Indeed, "brute particularity" is an abstraction posing as the concrete.

Chapter 11: *Singer,* Mental Illness: Rights, Competence, and Communication

    I am grateful to Raymond Baltch of the New York Mental Hygiene Legal Service for bibliographical assistance in the preparation of this chapter. I am also grateful to Mary Mahowald for reading and commenting on it.

    1. *Rivers v. Katz,* 67 N.Y. 2d 485, 492, 495; N.E. 2d 337, 341, 504; N.Y.S. 2d 74, 78 (1986).

    2. Ellen Wright Clayton, "Rights of the Mentally Ill to Refuse Medication," *American Journal of Law and Medicine* 13, no. 1 (1987): 45–46. Consistent with this, the California Welfare and Institutions Code, sec. 5331, states, "No person may be presumed incompetent because he or she has been evaluated or treated for mental disorder or chronic alcoholism, regardless of whether voluntarily or involuntarily received."

3. In California being "gravely disabled," in the limited sense of being unable, by reason of a mental disorder, to provide for one's own food, clothing, or shelter, is also justification. Welfare and Institutions Code, secs. 5150, 5250, 5260, 5270.15.

4. Clayton, 45–46.

5. Jessica Willen Berg, Paul S. Appelbaum, and Thomas Grisso, "Constructing Competence: Formulating Standards of Legal Competence to Make Medical Decisions," *Rutgers Law Review* 48, no. 2 (Winter 1996): 346.

6. Baruch A. Brody, *Life and Death Decision Making* (New York: Oxford University Press, 1988), 101.

7. Brody, 1988: 101–102.

8. Cf. Beth J. Singer, *Operative Rights* (New York: State University of New York Press, 1993). The term is from Drucilla Cornell, "Two Lectures on the Normative Dimensions of Community in the Law," second lecture, *In Defense of Dialogic Reciprocity*, vol. 54 (1987): 335–43. However, I define it somewhat differently from the way Cornell does.

9. Elyn R. Saks "Competency to Refuse Psychotropic Medication: Three Alternatives to the Law's Cognitive Standard," *University of Miami Law Review* 47, no. 3 (January 1993): 761.

10. Ibid., 760.

11. Ibid., 691.

12. Berg, Appelbaum, and Grisso, 346.

13. Ibid., 346–47.

14. Ibid., 348.

15. Elyn R. Saks, "Competency to Refuse Treatment," *North Carolina Law Review* 69 (1991): 945 and passim.

16. Berg, Appelbaum, and Grisso, 349–50, n. 17.

17. Ibid., 349.

18. Ibid., 351. The reference is to Paul S. Appelbaum and Thomas Grisso, "Assessing Patients' Capacities to Consent to Treatment," *New England Journal of Medicine* 319 (1988), and Paul S. Appelbaum and Thomas Grisso, "The MacArthur Treatment Competence Study I: Mental Illness and Competence to Consent to Treatment," *Law and Human Behavior* 19 (1995).

19. In a provocative article in *The Journal of Clinical Ethics* 5, no. 3 (Fall 1994), Edmund G. Howe reports research based on chaos theory, in which the patterned irregularity and complexity of brain function was measured by electroencephalogram. Using a unit of measure called dimensionality, a mathematical expression of the number of independent variables functioning in a person's brain at a given time, researchers found disrupted patterns of dimensionality in patients who had been diagnosed as schizophrenic. The study in question is reported in T. Elbert et al., "Physical Aspects of the EEG in Schizophrenia," *Biological Psychiatry* 32 (1992). The theory on which it is based is described in T. Elbert et al., "Chaos and Physiology: Deterministic Chaos in Excitable Cell Assemblies," *Physiological Review* 74 (1994). But it is questionable whether such measures will ever be available for the detailed abilities involved in the compe-

tence to make reasonable decisions concerning the acceptance of medication.

20. California Department of Mental Health, *Handbook of Rights for Mental Health Patients*, rev. March 1991.

21. "If a person has been involuntarily committed to a mental institution, then adequate treatment . . . must be provided, for nothing else justifies involuntary commitment." Mary Ann Carroll, Henry G. Schneider, and George R. Wesly, "The Right to Treatment and Involuntary Commitment," in *Ethics in the Practice of Psychology* (Englewood Cliffs, N.J., Prentice-Hall, 1985), 92. This chapter is a slightly altered version of Mary Ann Carroll, "The Right to Treatment and Involuntary Commitment," *The Journal of Medicine and Philosophy* 5, no. 4 (1980).

22. Cf. George Herbert Mead, *Mind, Self, and Society: From the Standpoint of a Social Behaviorist*, ed. Charles W. Morris (Chicago: University of Chicago Press), 1934.

23. "[T]he idea of autonomy has emerged as a central notion in the idea of applied moral philosophy, particularly in the biomedical context. All discussions of the nature of informed consent and its rationale refer to patient (or subject) autonomy. Conflicts between autonomy and paternalism occur in cases involving civil commitment . . . and patient care. . . . Whether or not this is the same concept that appears in the more theoretical discussions remains to be seen, but . . . [i]t would be unwise to assume that different authors are all referring to the same thing when they use the term 'autonomy' . . . in moral and political philosophy." Gerald Dworkin, *The Theory and Practice of Autonomy* (Cambridge: Cambridge University Press, 1988), 4–5.

24. In ordinary language, *judgment* is used to refer to intellectual or moral evaluation or to legal dicta. Following Justus Buchler, I use it as a general term for any sort of appraisal and, more generally, any given idea, interpretation, or understanding. To judge anything is to view it or understand it in a particular way. This means to have a viewpoint or perspective with regard to it, to have or adopt an attitude or position toward it. Cf. Justus Buchler, *Toward a General Theory of Human Judgment* (New York: Columbia University Press, 1951), and Justus Buchler, *Nature and Judgment* (New York: Columbia University Press, 1955). (In Mead's language, *attitude* is a synonym for *perspective*, so taking the attitude of another is adopting that person's perspective.) But, as is commonly done, I also speak of the expression of a judgment as a judgment. Primarily, as the terms *dialogue* and *discussion* make clear, it is verbal communication that is meant. But the fact that we use the word *expression* for this calls attention to the emotive dimension of speech, and although I do not discuss this, we should not forget, especially in the present context, that we pick up cues as to someone's meaning and intent from the nonverbal dimensions of that person's communication and that nonverbal communication is as important as the use of language.

25. Buchler, *Toward a General Theory of Human Judgment* and *Nature and Judgment*.

26. By *community* I mean what I have termed a "normative community": any group or collection of persons who govern their behavior by shared social norms, or are expected to do so. Cf. Singer, *Operative Rights*.

27. The importance of the obligation of staff to respect patients as presump-
tively autonomous and authoritative and to be ready to alter their judgments of
them is underscored by a study reported in *Science* 179 (1973): 250–58. As summarized in the *Hastings Center Report* 3, no. 2 (1973), "Once eight pseudopatients
had gained admission to mental institutions (by saying they heard voices) they
found themselves indelibly labelled with a diagnosis of schizophrenia—in spite
of their subsequent normal behavior. Ironically, it was only the other inmates
who suspected that the pseudopatients were normal. The hospital personnel
were not able to acknowledge normal behavior within the hospital milieu" (15).
Plainly, this inability resulted from a failure to exercise the capacity for dialogic
reciprocity.

28. *Lessard v. Schmidt* 349F. Supp. (1972), p. 1093; Carroll, Schneider, and
Wesly, 93.

29. Carroll, Schneider, and Wesly, 93.

30. D. Richards, *The Moral Criticism of Law* (Belmont, Calif.: Dickenson
Publishing Co., 1977), 219.

31. Carroll, 95.

Chapter 12: *Saatkamp*, Genetics and Pragmatism

1. See Philip Kitcher, *The Lives to Come: The Genetic Revolution and Human
Possibilities* (New York: Simon and Schuster, 1996), and Glenn McGee, *The Perfect
Baby* (New York: Rowman and Littlefield Publishers, Inc., 1997).

2. Two essays that describe characteristics of pragmatism are John J.
McDermott, "Pragmatic Sensibility: The Morality of Experience," in *New
Directions in Ethics: The Challenge of Applied Ethics*, ed. Joseph P. DeMarco and
Richard M. Fox (New York and London: Routledge and Kegan Paul, 1986); and
Henry Samuel Levinson, "Santayana and Making Claims on the Spiritual Truth
about Matters of Fact," *Overheard in Seville: Bulletin of the Santayana Society*, 12
(Fall 1994): 3.

3. Charles S. Peirce, "How to Make Our Ideas Clear, 1878," *Writings of Charles
S. Peirce: A Chronological Edition*, vol. 3 (Bloomington: Indiana University Press,
1986), 266.

4. Michael Hodges, a professor of philosophy at Vanderbilt University, made
a similar point in response to a paper by David Dilworth, a professor of philosophy at SUNY Stony Brook, during the Santayana Society meeting held in conjunction with the Eastern Division Meeting of the American Philosophical
Association, December 27, 1996.

5. Trisomy is a condition in which one chromosome is present in three
copies, whereas all the other chromosomes are diploid. Trisomy 18 (Edwards's
syndrome) is a condition in which a child has three copies of chromosome 18.
Infants are small at birth, grow very slowly, and are mentally retarded. Heart
malformations are almost always present, and the average survival time is two
to four months. Trisomy 18 has a frequency of one in eleven thousand live
births. Trisomy 13 is also lethal, with half of all affected individuals dying in the
first month. Trisomy 21 is Down's syndrome.

6. George Santayana, *Reason in Common Sense* (New York: Scribner's, 1905), 284.

7. Although the principal focus of this chapter is on human genetics, major changes in agricultural production are highly likely due to the new technologies of genetics, and these new production alternatives will raise similar questions, though not as close to home, as those related to the reproduction and raising of human children.

8. There are significant legal and moral issues involved in parent-child relations. Many hospitals are now adopting child assent procedures to ensure that children, not only parents, have a voice in medical treatment, and one anticipates that similar procedures may be adopted in areas of genetic counseling when the future of a child, particularly age fourteen or over, is involved.

Chapter 13: *McGee*, Genetic Enhancement of Families

I acknowledge Peter Ubel, Arthur Caplan, Bette-Jane Crigger, Dan Brock, Eric Juengst, James Gustafson, Monica Arruda, and Erik Parens for comments on early drafts. I am grateful for the support I have received from Vanderbilt Center for Social and Political Thought, the University of Iowa, SUNY Downstate Medical Center, Miami University, and The Hastings Center's Project on the Prospect of Technologies Aimed at the Enhancement of Human Capacities.

1. Peter Kramer, *Listening to Prozac* (New York: HarperCollins, 1994).

2. Lawrence H. Diller, "The Run on Ritalin: Attention Deficit Disorder and Stimulant Treatment in the 1990s," *Hastings Center Report* 26, no. 2 (1996): p. 12.

3. Kathy Davis, *Reshaping the Female Body: The Dilemma of Cosmetic Surgery* (New York: Routledge, 1995).

4. Norman Daniels, *Just Health Care* (New York: Cambridge Univeristy Press, 1986), 28.

5. Glenn McGee, *The Perfect Baby: A Pragmatic Approach to Genetics* (Lanham: Rowman and Littlefield, 1997).

6. Daniel Kevles, *In the Name of Eugenics* (Berkeley: University of California Press, 1984).

7. C. K. Chan, "Eugenics on the Rise: A Report from Singapore," in *Ethics, Reproduction, and Genetic Control*, ed. Ruth Chadwick (London: Croon Helm, 1987), 210–23.

8. Paul Ramsey also makes mention of deadly sins of a different kind in his *Fabricated Man* (New Haven: Yale University Press, 1970).

9. Obviously this advice and counsel takes many forms in many different groups, varying with language, folkways, and styles of communication. One parent's advice may come in the form of constant reassurances and encouragement, whereas another may scold and demean the child when he or she misbehaves.

10. Susan Bordo, *Unbearable Weight: Feminism, Western Culture, and the Body* (Berkeley: University of California Press, 1993).

11. McGee, *The Perfect Baby*.

12. Brian Stableford, *Future Man* (New York: Crown Publishers, 1984), 13–15.

13. We have only to look at the tragic results of the introduction of ultrasound to India to see what thoughtless application of reproductive technologies can mean. Indian women are forced to abort their female fetuses despite the effect on the population and the women. Therefore, the very technology that was created to bring more of reproduction under the control of women came to be an instrument for the oppression of women. It is not the maldistribution of technology that is at issue, but the actual rearticulation of the purposes of that technology.

14. Glenn McGee, "Consumers, Land, and Food: In Search of Food Ethics," in *The Agricultural and Food Sector in the New Global Era*, ed. A. Bonanno (New Dehli: Concept, 1993); Jack Doyle, *Altered Harvest: Agriculture, Genetics and the Fate of the World's Food Supply* (New York: Viking, 1985); David Goodman, *From Farming to Biotechnology: A Theory of Agro-Industrial Development* (New York: Basil Blackwell, 1987); and House Subcommittee on Natural Resources, Agricultural Research, and Environment of the Committee on Science, Space, and Technology, "Field Testing Genetically Engineered Organisms: Hearing before the Subcommittee on Natural Resources, Agricultural Research, and Environment of the Committee on Science, Space, and Technology," 100th Cong., 2d sess., 1988.

15. Hans Jonas, *Bioengineering* (New York: Oxford University Press, 1983).

16. William James, *Talks to Teachers* (New York: Henry Holt, 1907), 11–37.

17. Jeremy Rifkin, The Biotech Century (New York: Putnam, 1998).

18. "The Construction of the Good," in *The Philosophy of John Dewey*, ed. J. McDermott (Chicago: University of Chicago Press, 1981), 577.

19. Richard Lewontin, *Biology as Ideology: The Doctrine of DNA* (New York: HarperCollins, 1993).

20. Ibid., 583.

Chapter 14: *Benjamin,* Pragmatism and the Determination of Death

1. William James, *Pragmatism* (Indianapolis, Hackett, 1981), 31.

2. John Dewey, "The Need for a Recovery of Philosophy," in *John Dewey: The Middle Works, 1899–1924,* ed. Jo Ann Boydston, vol. 10 (Carbondale: Southern Illinois University Press, 1980), 4.

3. Ad Hoc Committee of the Harvard Medical School to Examine the Definition of Death, "A Definition of Irreversible Coma," *Journal of the American Medical Association* 205 (1968): 337–40.

4. President's Commission for the Study of Ethical Problems in Medicine and Biomedical and Behavioral Research, *Defining Death* (Washington: U.S. Government Printing Office, 1981), 73.

5. Multi-Society Task Force on PVS (American Academy of Neurology, Child Neurology Society, American Neurological Association, American Association of Neurological Surgeons, American Academy of Pediatrics, "Medical Aspects of the Persistent Vegetative State," *New England Journal of Medicine* 330 (1994): 1499–1508, 1572–79.

6. See, for example, Karen Gervais, *Redefining Death* (New Haven: Yale University Press, 1986); Gina Kolata, "Ethicists Debating a New Definition of Death," *New York Times,* 21 April 1992.

7. President's Commission, *Defining Death,* 33.

8. Ibid., 40.

9. For an illuminating analysis of complexities that I cannot explore here, see Jeff McMahan, "The Metaphysics of Brain Death," *Bioethics* 9 (1995): 91–126.

10. Council on Ethical and Judicial Affairs, American Medical Association, "The Use of Anencephalic Neonates as Organ Donors," *Journal of the American Medical Association* 273 (1995): 1614. The council, though supporting use of anencephalics as sources of organs, does not consider them dead.

11. President's Commission, *Defining Death,* 41–42.

12. Multi—Society Task Force on PVS, "Medical Aspects of the Persistent Vegetative State," 1578.

13. James, *Pragmatism,* 33.

14. Don Marquis, "Why Abortion Is Immoral," *Journal of Philosophy* 86 (1989): 189. Though I agree with Marquis's general point about what makes killing wrong, I disagree with his extending it to fetuses. If a fetus cannot plausibly be said to have a personal interest in its future, the loss of such a future cannot be a loss to the fetus (though, of course, it may be a loss to others with an interest in the fetus's future).

Chapter 15: *Lachs,* Dying Old as a Social Problem

1. U.S. Bureau of the Census, *Population Projections of the United States, by Age, Sex, Race, and Hispanic Origin: 1993–2050,* by Jennifer Cheeseman Day, Current Population Reports P25–1104 (Washington: U.S. Government Printing Office, 1993).

2. I have in mind such attacks as Leon R. Kass mounts in "Is There a Right to Die?" *Hastings Center Report* 23, no. 1 (1993): 34–43.

3. John Stuart Mill, *On Liberty,* in *Essential Works of John Stuart Mill,* ed. Max Lerner (New York: Bantam Books, 1965).

4. See John Hardwig," Is There a Duty to Die?" *Hastings Center Report* 27, no. 2 (1997): 34–42.

5. For an extended treatment of the consequences of mediation, see my *Intermediate Man* (Indianapolis: Hackett, 1981).

Chapter 16: *Kegley,* Community, Autonomy, and Managed Care

1. Martin Darragh and Pat Milme McCarrick, "Managed Health Care: New Ethical Issues for All," Scope Note 31, *Kennedy Institute of Ethics Journal* 6, no. 2 (1996): 188–89.

2. George Ritzer and David Walczak, "Rationalization and the Deprofessionalization of Physicians," *Social Forces* 12, no. 1 (September 1988): 1–22.

3. Ibid.

4. *Wall Street Journal,* December 4, 1996, A1.

5. Ibid.

6. Robert Kettner, "Managing Care or Costs?" *The Washington Post Weekly Edition*, December 2–8, 1996, 5.

7. See Norman Daniels, "The Articulation of Values and Principles Involved in Health Care Reform," *Journal of Medicine and Philosophy* 19 (October 1994): 425–433.

8. See Natalie S. Glance and A. Haberman, "The Dynamics of Social Dilemmas," *Scientific American* 270 (1994): 76–82.

9. Jeremy Bentham, *An Introduction to the Principles of Morals and Legislation*, ed. J. H. Burns and H. L. A. Hart (London: University of London, Athlone Press, 1970), chap. 1, sec. 4. He writes: "The interests of the community then is what?— The sum of the interests of the several members who compose it" (12).

10. Beth Singer, *Operative Rights* (Albany: State University of New York, 1993), xv.

11. Marian Gray Secundy, "Lack of a Moral Consensus on Health Care: Focus on Minority Elderly," in *It Just Ain't Fair*, ed. Annette Dula and Sara Goering (Westport, Conn.: Praeger, 1994), 62–63.

12. Jacquelyn Ann K. Kegley, "Using Genetic Information: A Radical Problematic for an Individualistic Framework," *Medicine and Law* 15, no. 4 (December 1996).

13. Jacquelyn Ann K. Kegley, *Genuine Individuals and Genuine Communities: A Roycean Public Philosophy* (Nashville: Vanderbilt University Press, 1996).

14. Nancy Ann Jeffrey, "HMO's Say 'Hola' to Potential Customers." *Wall Street Journal*, November 30, 1995, B1.

15. Ellen Severoni, "CHD's Managed Care Feedback Loop Delivery System Charge," presentation at the Third World Congress of Bioethics, San Francisco, California, November 20, 1996.

16. Elizabeth M. Whitley and Gerald F. Heeley, "Mission Possible: Collboration on Managed Care Ethics," presentation at the Third World Congress of Bioethics, San Francisco, California, November 23, 1996.

17. This notion is developed in my book *Genuine Individuals and Genuine Communities*.

18. Although it proceeds from a different background, I found much agreement with the view presented by Andrew Lustig in his "The Common Good in a Secular Society: The Relevance of a Roman Catholic Notion to the Health Care Allocation Debate," *Journal of Medicine and Philosophy* 18, no. 6 (1993): 569–87. Often those coming from a public health perspective also share views somewhat similar to mine. See Dan E. Beauchamp, "Public Health As Social Justice," *Inquiry* 13 (March 1976): 3–14.

19. For a somewhat similar stand on rationing, see U.S. Bishops, "Resolution on Health Care Reform," *Origins* 23: 93–102, and Catholic Health Organization, *With Justice for All? Health Care Rationing* (St. Louis: CCHA, 1991).

20. See D. Eddy, "Principles for making difficult decisions in difficult times." Journal of the American Medical Association, 271 (1994): 1792–98; D. Eddy, "Health System Reform: Will Controlling Costs Require Rationing Services?"

Journal of the American Medical Association 271 (1994): 324–26; and D. Eddy, "Rationing Resources While Improving Quality: How to Get More for Less," *Journal of the American Medical Association* 272 (1994): 817–24.

21. Leonard Fleck, "Just Caring: Rational Democratic Deliberation, Health Care Rationing and Managed Care," presentation at the Third World Congress of Bioethics, San Francisco, November 23, 1996.

22. Leonard Fleck, "Just Caring: Health Reform and Health Care Rationing," *Journal of Medicine and Philosophy* 19 (1994): 435–43.

23. Uwe Reinhardt, "Rationing in Managed Care," *Wall Street Journal*, April 22, 1993, A1.

24. L. Brown, "The National Politics of Oregon's Rationing Plan," *Health Affairs* 10 (Summer 1991): 28–51 (emphasis in the original).

25. D. Eddy, "Principles for Making Difficult Decisions in Difficult Times," *Journal of the American Medical Association* 271 (1994): 1796.

26. Robert Veatch, "The Medical Model: Its Nature and Problems," *Hastings Center Studies* 1 (1973): 39–76; reprinted in Rem Edwards, ed., *Psychiatry and Ethics* (Buffalo: Prometheus Books, . 1982), 88–108.

27. Discussed in Veatch, 90–91.

28. This mode of analysis of illness is based on that provided by Kay Toombs, "The Temporality of Illness: Four Levels of Experience," *Theoretical Medicine* 11 (1990): 227–41.

29. See Rita Kielstein and Hans-Martin Sass, "Using Stories to Assess Value and Establish Medical Directives," *Kennedy Institute of Ethics Journal*, September 3, 1993, 303–25.

30. Singer, xv.

31. For an extensive discussion of a similar principle of proportionality, see Thomas M. Garrett, Harold W. Baillie, and Rosellen M. Garrett, *Health Care Ethics*, 2d ed. (Englewood Cliffs, N.J.: Prentice-Hall, 1993), 58–61.

Chapter 17: *Lysaker and Sullivan*, Untying the Gag: Reason in the World of Health Care Reform

1. For example, it was estimated that in 1995 some 40 million people were uninsured, and therefore dependent on emergency room and free clinic care. Concerning U.S. expenditure, note that in 1991 14 percent of our gross domestic product was spent on health care in comparison to France and Germany's 9 percent and Japan's and Britain's 8 percent. The difference is particularly startling when one recalls that each of these nations guarantees health care services for its citizens.

2. *PR Newswire*, June 19, 1995.

3. We agree with Lisa Belkin's claim that quality concerns have supplanted questions of economic feasibility in the debate over managed care. See her article "The Ellwoods; But What about Quality?" in the "Sunday Magazine" of *The New York Times*, December 8, 1996, section 6, p. 68.

4. A brief examination of newspapers and business journals throughout 1996 will make it evident that across the country multiple aspects of managed care

came under attack, and from several quarters, most prominently patient advocacy groups, the American Medical Association (AMA), professional organizations, and legislators. We take this to mean that widespread discontent with managed care practices has surfaced over the last two years.

5. As of September 1996, these states included California, Colorado, Delaware, Georgia, Indiana, Maine, Maryland, Massachusetts, New Hampshire, New York, Pennsylvania, Rhode Island, Tennessee, Vermont, Virginia, and Washington.

6. Quoted from a CNN web post on December 7, 1996, transcript no. 96120612V26.

7. This is the position of the AMA, as reported in *The Charleston Gazette*, June 28, 1996, p. A-1.

8. This is the position that drove New York's 1996 consumer protection bill (SB 7553). Among other things, the bill required that HMOs make available, upon request, the compensation arrangements they have made with their employees. Ira Ellman and Mark Hall have also argued that consumers should be informed of the "costly variations [among third-party providers] in the standards employed to determine access to costly medical procedures" ("Redefining the Terms of Health Insurance to Accommodate Varying Consumer Risk Preferences," *American Journal of Law and Medicine* 20 [1994]: 192).

9. This objection, reported in "U.S. States Overturning HMO Gay Clauses," *Marketletter*, September 23, 1996, has been voiced by various HMO lobbyists.

10. In an editorial from the *Chicago Sun Times*, July 1, 1996, p. 21, we find: "'Gag-clauses are just one example of the muzzling of HMO doctors that interferes with the doctor-patient relationship,' said Dr. Sidney Wolfe, president of Public Citizen Health Research Group. He's right. Anything that interferes with that relationship undermines health care."

11. Proponents of market-based reform strategies include Regina E. Herzlinger, who advocates attention to customer satisfaction, and Robert E. Moffit, who advocates freeing the health care market from artificial constraints in order to arrive at "true prices." See Regina E. Herzlinger, *Market Driven Health Care: Who Wins and Who Loses in the Transformation of America's Largest Service Industry* (Reading, Pa.: Addison-Wesley Longman, 1997), and Robert Emmet Moffit, "Personal Freedom and Responsibility: The Ethical Foundations of a Market-Based Health Care Reform," *Journal of Medicine and Philosophy* 19, no. 5 (October 1994), 387–405.

12. Eliot Freidson has argued that a third model, a bureaucratic one, informs current discussion. He no doubt argues thus given the rise of managed care. See Eliot Freidson, "The Centrality of Professionalism to Health Care," *Jurimetrics Journal* 30 (Summer 1990): 431–45. We find this characterization of managed care misleading, and in two ways. First, managed care, like insurance, is a market-driven enterprise that regards health care as a commodity to be bought and sold. Granted that HMOs, like insurance companies, complicate the fee-for-service model of exchange, which at one time may have characterized health care markets, but they do not deviate from a basic market understanding of the goods

they produce. Under conditions of managed care, health care remains a commodity whose exchange provides goods and services while generating capital for those who contribute to that exchange on the side of production. Second, bureaucratic models are really parts of professional and market models, for neither can operate at any scale without bureaucratic administrative strategies. We see little sense, therefore, in regarding bureaucratic measures as constituting an independent wing in the arena of health care reform. Instead, bureaucracy will infect any attempt to produce health care in a nation of over 250 million people.

13. Quoted in *The Hartford Advocate*, March 7, 1996, pp. 12ff.

14. Freidson, 431–45.

15. Freidson also argues that health care issues are, for the most part, too complex to ever allow for rational consumer choice, and thus market models presuppose what will never exist: an informed consumer base able to cast informed votes with their feet.

16. As noted before, we find it misleading to speak of a bureaucratic model given that all existing models involve varying degrees of bureaucracy. Given this, we will take Freidson's discontent with these so-called bureaucratic models to involve discontent with managed care.

17. Freidson, 441. Recall that bureaucratic control over physician-patient relationships was and remains a focal concern in the debate surrounding "gag rules."

18. Freidson, 442.

19. *The Hartford Advocate*, March 7, 1996, pp. 12ff.

20. E. Haavi Moreim argues this in his "Of Rescue and Responsibility: Learning to Live with Limits," *Journal of Medicine and Philosophy* 19, no. 5 (October 1994), 455–70.

21. Robert Emmet Moffit argues this in his "Personal Freedom and Responsibility: The Ethical Foundations of A Market-Based Health Care Reform," *Journal of Medicine and Philosophy* 19, no. 5 (October 1994), 471–81.

22. In 1975 the average physician salary was $56,400. In 1984 it had risen to $92,000, and in 1993 it reached $189,000. Although the "real" impact of these increases is open to dispute given adjustments for inflation, the medical profession as a whole undoubtedly experienced steady growth across an almost twenty-year period, a period that simultaneously saw escalating medical costs. Our statistics come from reports published by the American Medical Association. See Martin L. Gonzalez, "Physician Income Trends, 1975–1985," *Socioeconomic Characteristics of Medical Practice* (1986): 17–21. See also James W. Moser, "Trends and Patterns in Physician Income," *Socioeconomic Characteristics of Medical Practice* (1996), 27–33.

23. Following Arnold Relman, one should note that even under fee-for-service conditions a conflict of interest mediates the physician-client relationship, for the physician will always gain economically when more care is given. See Arnold S. Relman, "The Future of Medical Practice," in *In Search of the Modern Hippocrates*, ed. Roger J. Bulger (Iowa City: University of Iowa Press, 1987), 203.

24. The social complexity of health care reform is also insufficiently appreciated

by Troyen Brennan, who, in order to further reform, has "recommended an analytical experiment akin to Rawls's original position, in which physicians must think about how patients should ideally be cared for, while remaining ignorant about the socioeconomic status of the patients for whom the physician would care. Blind to their own and their patients' identities, physicians would design a just system of health care that comports with central values of medical ethics. This approach leads to an ethics of health policy that would resonate with medical ethics, but not necessarily retain the current institutional structure of medical care." See Troyen A. Brennan, "An Ethical Perspective on Health Care Insurance Reform," *American Journal of Law and Medicine* 19, no. 37 (1995), 50. Unfortunately, these physicians would be blind not only to the socioeconomic status of their patients, but to the socioeconomic forces that make the U.S. health care industry what it is. In our view the key is not to imagine reform free of economic forces, but to construct reform policies that openly engage them.

25. Both points have been made by Charles Stein in *The Boston Globe*. See the *Globe's* "Sunday Magazine," June 1, 1997.

26. For an insightful discussion of commodification generally, see Margaret Jane Radin, "Market-Inalienability," *Harvard Law Review* 100 (June 1987), 1915–36.

27. For an interesting attack on the very notion of "natural" economic laws, see David M. Frankford, "Privatizing Health Care: Economic Magic to Cure Legal Medicine," *Southern California Law Review*, November 1992.

28. This is not to say that a state-based single care provider should collectivize existing health care markets. Neither is it to say that health care should be pursued independent of market mechanisms. Rather, our claim at this point is only that the existence of health care markets represents a social choice with definite costs and benefits that are rarely entertained in mainstream discussions concerning health care reform.

29. To term such choices social is simply to acknowledge that they do not allow for individuals to do as they please. If we prefer Edsels to MGs, the sheer fact that others can buy MGs most likely will not interfere with our pursuit of the Edsel life. However, if we prefer that society avoid transportation that burns fossil fuel, the sheer fact that others buy fossil fuel–burning vehicles dashes our hopes for a world free from noxious emissions. It would, of course, be no remedy to suggest that we are free to buy the environmentally benign form of transportation of our choice because, absent a larger social commitment to avoid air pollution from fossil fuels, we could not achieve the end we sought.

30. Moreover, it is not the case that all citizens who have access to various markets have equal access given that more money usually translates into more access. Likewise, informed participation is rarely possible when specialized profession-based industries are involved, and as Freidson has argued, this is certainly the case with medicine.

31. Given that health care reform in the United States currently avoids this question, one of our goals here is to press the normative dimensions of "health" and health care to the fore of the debate.

32. *Just Health Care,* by Norman Daniels (Cambridge: Cambridge University Press, 1985), is the most famous example of a Rawlsian approach to health care reform.

33. We take it that Daniels's primary concern is providing all citizens with access to basic health care. We share his commitment, but wish that he would pursue it without appeals to Rawls's hypothetical line of inquiry.

34. Daniels adds that a society must secure health care if it is to ensure equal opportunity given that many diseases are not the result of blind fate, but affect individuals because they live in a society of their peers. See *Just Health Care,* 3, 42, 45.

35. We can imagine such a position arising in multiple situations, the most obvious involving cultures that do not esteem the value of the individual over the community. Note, though, that one might also—at least in certain circumstances—question the value of political self-determination if one believes that political participation in the United States remains a dramatic rather than a substantive affair. Yes, we vote, one could argue, but for a range of candidates who all promise, in one form or another, "business" as usual. In other words, if one believes that the government is for the most part a cosponsor of corporate interest, one will believe that a "right" to political self-determination is a deceptive way to describe a right to play along with the interests of industry. One might, then, in some circumstances, wish to bypass this right when confronted by those needs (and the needy) that are too often ignored in the bustle of business as usual.

36. This kind of blindness to the inescapably normative dimensions of policy is apparent in pro-choice advocates who think their position leaves room for pro-life advocates. If the issue were simply a matter of individual choice, the pro-choice position would be able to accommodate its rival's hopes and dreams. But given that most pro-lifers suppose that the infant is a person with constitutional rights, allowing abortions will always entail murder in their view, irrespective of the moral outlook of the parties involved.

37. H. Tristram Engelhardt, Jr., has argued along these lines. See his "Health Care Reform: A Study in Moral Malfeasance," *Journal of Medicine and Philosophy* 19, no. 5 (October 1994): 501–16.

38. Although one might argue that proceduralists are defending political freedom per se, this begs the question, shifting the indeterminacy onto the concept "politics." Given that we do not in fact protect political freedoms of all stripes, the question becomes, Freedom for what kind(s) of politics? Until we can answer that question, it is not clear what values we are defending when we rally around "political" freedom.

39. We want to stress that we have not argued, let alone demonstrated, that in the arena of health care reform one should not defend, above all else, the right of individuals to decide for themselves whether they wish to contribute to a system that ensures universal access. We wish to show only (a) that such positions entail concrete, social costs, (b) that a public debate concerning health care reform must address the reasonableness of such costs, and (c) that hypothetical reflection along Rawlsian lines fails to engage these questions.

Chapter 18: *Secundy,* Ethical Literacy and Cultural Competence
    1. K. Danner Clouser, "Some Things Medical Ethics Is Not," *Journal of the American Medical Association* 223, no. 7 (1973): 787–89; Giles R. Scofield, "Ethics Consultation: The Least Dangerous Profession?" *Cambridge Quarterly of Healthcare Ethics* 2 (1993): 417–42.
    2. Clouser, 787.
    3. Scofield, 417.
    4. Ibid., 418.
    5. Judith Wilson Ross, "Commentary: Why Clinical Ethics Consultants Might Not Want to Be Educators," *Cambridge Quarterly of Healthcare Ethics* 2 (1993): 445–48; quote on p. 445.
    6. John Fletcher, "Commentary: Constructiveness Where It Counts," *Cambridge Quarterly of Healthcare Ethics* 2 (1993): 426–33; quote on p. 430.
    7. Fletcher, 431–32.
    8. Scofield. See also M. S. Larson, *The Rise of Professionalism* (Berkeley: University of California Press, 1977); E. Friedson, *Professional Dominance* (New York: Atherton, 1970).
    9. William B. Weeks, and William A. Nelson, "The Ethical Role of the Consultant," *Cambridge Quarterly of Healthcare Ethics* 2 (1993): 477.
    10. Weeks and Nelson, 479.
    11. Michael Yeo, "Prolegomena to Any Future Code of Ethics for Bioethicists," *Cambridge Quarterly of Healthcare Ethics* 2 (1993): 412.
    12. Ruth, Macklin, *Mortal Choices* (New York: Pantheon, 1987), 18. This reference is highlighted by Yeo in his discussion of the role of bioethicists in the *Cambridge Quarterly of Healthcare Ethics* in 1993. See p. 408.
    13. Robert Veatch. "Models for Ethical Medicine in a Revolutionary Age." *Hastings Center Report* 2, no. 3 (1972): 5–7. Also see Yeo, 414.
    14. Annette Dula, "LJ's Religious Craziness," *Journal of Clinical Ethic* 6, no. 1 (Spring 1995): 77-80
    15. Howard Brody, *The Healer's Power* (New Haven: Yale University Press, 1992).
    16. Al Jonsen,, Mark Siegler, and William Winslade, *Clinical Ethics: A Practical Approach to Ethical Decisions in Clinical Medicin,* 3d edition (New York, Mcgraw-Hill, 1992), 11, 17.
    17. Tia Powell. "Religion, Race, and Reason: The Case of LJ," *The Journal of Clinical Ethics* 6, no. 1 (Spring 1995): 73-77.
    18. David Schiedermayer, and John LaPuma, "The Ethics Consultant and Ethics Committees, and Their Acronyms: IRBs, HECs, RM, QA, UM, PROs IPCs, and HREAPs," *Cambridge Quarterly of Healthcare Ethics* 2 (1993): 469–77.

SELECTED BIBLIOGRAPHY

Appelbaum, Paul S., and Thomas Grisso. "Assessing Patients' Capacities to Consent to Treatment." *New England Journal of Medicine* 319, no. 2 (1988): 1635–38.

———. "The MacArthur Treatment Competence Study I: Mental Illness and Competence to Consent to Treatment." *Law and Human Behavior* 19 (1995): 105–126.

Ashley, Benedict M., and Kevin D. O'Rourke. *Healthcare Ethics*, 4th edition. Washington, D.C.: Georgetown University Press, 1997.

Beauchamp, Tom L. "Principalism and Its Alleged Competitors." *Kennedy Institute of Ethics Journal* 5 (1995): 181–89.

Beauchamp, Tom, and James Childress. *Principles of Biomedical Ethics*. 4th edition. New York: Oxford University Press, 1995.

Berg, Jessica Willen, Paul S. Appelbaum, and Thomas Grisso. "Constructing Competence: Formulating Standards of Legal Competence to Make Medical Decisions." *Rutgers Law Review* 48, no. 2 (Winter 1996): 345–396.

Bishop, Sarah Stueber. "Explanation in Medicine: The Problem-oriented Approach." *Journal of Medicine and Philosophy* 5 (1980): 30–54.

Boorse, Christopher. "On the Distinction between Disease and Illness." In *Concepts of Health and Disease*, edited by Arthur L. Caplan, H. Tristram Engelhardt, Jr., and James J. McCartney. Reading, Mass.: Addison-Wesley, 1981.

Brody, Baruch A. *Life and Death Decision Making*. New York: Oxford University Press, 1988.

Brody, Howard. "Transparency: Informed Consent in Primary Care." *Hastings Center Report* 19, no. 5 (1989): 5–9.

Buchanan, James H. *Patient Encounters*. New York: Henry Holt, 1989.

Buchler, Justus. *Toward a General Theory of Human Judgment*. New York: Columbia University Press, 1951.

———. *Nature and Judgment*. New York: Columbia University Press, 1955.

State of California. *Handbook of Rights for Mental Health Patients*. Revised March 1991.

Carroll, Mary Ann. "The Right to Treatment and Involuntary Commitment." *The Journal of Medicine and Philosophy* 5, no. 4, (1980): 278–291.

Carroll, Mary Ann, Henry G. Schneider, and George R. Wesly. "The Right to

Treatment and Involuntary Commitment." In *Ethics in the Practice of Psychology*. Englewood Cliffs, N.J.: Prentice-Hall.

Cassell, Eric J. *The Nature of Suffering*. New York: Oxford University Press, 1991.

Clayton, Ellen Wright. "Rights of the Mentally Ill to Refuse Medication." *American Journal of Law and Medicine* 13, no. 1 (1987): 45–46.

Craig, Robert P., Carl L. Middleton, and Laurence J. O'Connell. *Ethics Committees: A Practical Approach*. St. Louis: Catholic Health Association of the United States, 1986.

DeMarco, Joseph P., and Richard M. Fox, eds. *New Directions in Ethics: The Challenge of Applied Ethics*. New York: Routledge and Kegan Paul, 1986.

Dewey, John. *Democracy and Education* [1916]. New York: Free Press, 1940.

——. *Reconstruction in Philosophy* [1920]. Vol. 12 of *John Dewey: The Middle Works, 1899–1924*, edited by Jo Ann Boydston. Carbondale: Southern Illinois University Press, 1988.

——. *The Public and Its Problems* [1927]. Vol. 2 of *John Dewey: The Later Works, 1825–1953*, edited by Jo Ann Boydston. Carbondale: Southern Illinois University Press, 1988.

——. *Logic: The Theory of Inquiry* [1938]. Vol. 12 of *John Dewey: The Later Works, 1925–1953*, edited by Jo Ann Boydston. Carbondale: Southern Illinois University Press, 1991.

——. *Theory of Valuation* [1939]. Vol. 13 of *John Dewey: The Later Works, 1925–1953*, edited by Jo Ann Boydston. Carbondale: Southern Illinois University Press, 1991.

——. "The Unity of the Human Being [1939]." In *John Dewey: The Later Works, 1825–1953*, vol. 13, edited by Jo Ann Boydston. Carbondale: Southern Illinois University Press, 1991.

Dworkin, Gerald. *The Theory and Practice of Autonomy*. Cambridge: Cambridge University Press, 1988.

Emanuel, Ezekiel J., and Linda L. Emanuel. "Four Models of the Physician-Patient Relationship." *JAMA* 267, no. 16 (1992): 2221–26.

Engelhardt, H. Tristram, Jr. *The Foundations of Bioethics*. New York: Oxford University Press, 1986.

Fins, Joseph J. "From Indifference to Goodness." *Journal of Religion and Health* 35 (1996): 245–54.

Fins, Joseph J., and Matthew D. Bacchetta. "Framing the Physician-Assisted Suicide and Voluntary Active Euthanasia Debate: The Role of Deontology, Consequentialism, and Clinical Pragmatism." *Journal of the American Geriatrics Society* 43 (1995): 563–68.

Fletcher, John C., Charles A. Hite, Paul A. Lombardo, and Mary F. Marshall, eds. *Introduction to Clinical Ethics*. Frederick, Md.: University Publishing, 1995.

Fletcher, Joseph F. *Situation Ethics*. Philadelphia: Westminster, 1966.

Fox, Mark, Glenn McGee, and Arthur Caplan. "Practice Settings for Clinical Ethics Consultation." *Cambridge Quarterly in Healthcare Ethics* 7 (Spring 1998): 308–314.

Fry-Revere, Sigrid, *The Accountability of Bioethics Committees and Consultants.* Frederick, Md.: University Publishing, 1992.

Gert, Bernard. *Morality: A New Justification of the Moral Rules.* 1966. Reprint, New York: Oxford University Press, 1988.

Hickman, Larry. *John Dewey's Pragmatic Technology.* Bloomington: Indiana University Press, 1990.

James, William, "On a Certain Blindness in Human Beings." In *The Writings of William James,* edited by John J. McDermott. Chicago: University of Chicago Press, 1980.

Jonsen, Albert R. "Transplantation of Fetal Tissue: An Ethicist's Viewpoint." *Clinical Research* 3 (1988): 215–19.

Jonsen, Albert R., and Stephen Toulmin. *The Abuse of Casuistry.* Berkeley: University of California Press, 1988.

Katz, Jay. *The Silent World of Doctor and Patient.* New York: Free Press, 1984.

Knoppers, B. M., and S. LeBris. "Recent Advances in Medically Assisted Conception: Legal, Ethical and Social Issues." *American Journal of Law and Medicine* 17, no. 4 (1991): 329–361.

Krikorian, Yervant H., *Naturalism and the Human Spirit.* New York: Columbia University Press, 1944.

Leebov, Wendy, and Gail Scott. *Service Quality Improvement: The Customer Satisfaction Strategy for Health Care.* Chicago: American Hospital, 1994.

Light, Donald, and Glenn McGee. "On the Social Embeddedness of Bioethics." In *Bioethics and Society,* edited by R. DeVries. Engelwood Cliffs, N.J.: Prentice-Hall, 1998.

McDermott, John J. "Feeling as Insight: The Affective Dimension in Social Diagnosis." In *Hippocrates Revisited,* edited by R. Bolger. New York: Medcom, 1973.

McGee, Glenn, "Reforming Research Ethics: A Bill of Rights," *Chronicle of Higher Education,* June 1996.

———. "Genetic Testing, Ethics, and the Public Health Interest." *Academic Physician and Scientist* (July/August 1997): 2–3.

———. *The Perfect Baby: A Pragmatic Approach to Genetics.* New York: Rowman & Littlefield, 1997.

———. "Breaking Bioethics: An Introduction." *Cambridge Quarterly in Healthcare Ethics* 7, no. 4 (Spring 1998): 414–417.

———. "Ethics and Genetics in the Next 100 Years." In *Global Perspectives on Genetics,* edited by D. Macer. New York: UNESCO Press, 1998.

McGee, Glenn, ed.. *The Human Cloning Debate.* San Francisco: Berkeley Hills Press, 1998.

MacIntyre, Alisdair. *After Virtue.* Notre Dame, Ind.: University of Notre Dame Press, 1981.

MacKinnon, Roger A., and Robert Michels. *The Psychiatric Interview in Clinical Practice.* Philadelphia: W. B. Saunders, 1971.

Mahowald, Mary B. "C. S. Peirce: His Concepts of God and Religion." *Transactions of the Charles S. Peirce Society* 12 (1976): 367–398.

————. "The Physician." In *The Power of the Professional Person*, edited by Robert. W. Clarke and Robert P. Lawre. New York: University Press of America, 1988.

————. "Hospital Ethics Committees: Diverse and Problematic." *Newsletter on Medicine and Philosophy* 88 (1989): 88–94.

May, William F. *The Physician's Covenant*. Philadelphia: Westminster, 1983.

Mead, George Herbert. *Mind, Self, and Society*. 1934. Reprint, Chicago: University of Chicago Press, 1962.

Miller, Franklin G., Joseph J. Fins, and Matthew D. Bacchetta. "Clinical Pragmatism: John Dewey and Clinical Ethics." *Journal of Contemporary Health Law and Policy* 13 (1996): 27–51.

Moreno, Jonathan D. "Do Bioethics Commissions Hijack Public Debate?" *Hastings Center Report* 26, no. 3 (May 1996): 47.

————. *Deciding Together: Bioethics and Moral Consensus*. New York: Oxford University Press, 1995.

Nussbaum, Martha C. *The Therapy of Desire*. Princeton, N.J.: Princeton University Press, 1994.

Oppenheim, Frank M. *Royce's Mature Ethics*. Notre Dame, Indiana: University of Notre Dame Press, 1993.

Parret, Herman, ed. *Peirce and Value Theory*. Amsterdam: John Benjamins, 1994.

Peirce, Charles Sanders. *Collected Papers*. Edited by Charles Hartshorne and Paul Weiss. Vols. 1, 2, and 5. Cambridge, Mass.: Harvard University Press, 1931, 1932, 1934.

————. *Writings of Charles S. Peirce, A Chronological Edition*. Vol. 2, 1867–1871. Bloomington: Indiana University Press, 1982.

Pellegrino, Edmund. "The Anatomy of Clinical Judgments: Some Notes on Right Reason and Right Action." In *Clinical Judgment: A Critical Appraisal*, edited by H. Tristram Engelhardt, Jr., et al. Dordrecht, Holland: D. Reidel, 1979.

Reiser, Stanley J., Arthur J. Duck, and William Curran, eds. "Selections from the Hippocratic Corpus." In *Ethics in Medicine*. Cambridge: Mass.: MIT Press, 1977.

Richards, David A. J. *The Moral Criticism of Law*. Belmont, Calif.: Dickenson, 1977.

Rorty, Richard. *Philosophy and the Mirror of Nature*. Princeton, N.J.: Princeton University Press, 1979.

Rosenthal, Sandra B. *Speculative Pragmatism*. Peru, Ill.: Open Court, 1990.

————. "Classical American Pragmatism: The Other Naturalism," *Metaphilosophy* 27, no. 4 (March 1996): 19–28.

Royce, Josiah. *Outlines of Psychology*. New York: Macmillan, 1903.

————. *The Philosophy of Loyalty* [1908]. Nashville: Vanderbilt University Press, 1995.

————. *War and Insurance*. New York: Macmillan, 1914.

————. *The Problem of Christianity*. 1918. Reprint, Chicago: University of Chicago Press, 1968.

————. "On Certain Limitations of the Thoughtful Public in America." In *The*

Basic Writings of Josiah Royce, edited by John J. McDermott. Chicago: University of Chicago Press, 1969.

———. *The Letters of Josiah Royce*. Edited by John Clendenning. Chicago: University of Chicago Press, 1970.

Ryder, John, ed. *American Philosophic Naturalism in the Twentieth Century*. Amherst, N.H.: Prometheus Books, 1994.

Sacks, Oliver. *An Anthropologist on Mars*. New York: Alfred A. Knopf, 1995.

Saks, Elyn R. "Competency to Refuse Psychotropic Medication: Three Alternatives to the Law's Cognitive Standard." *University of Miami Law Review* 47, no. 3 (January, 1993): 689–761.

———. "Competency to Refuse Treatment." *North Carolina Law Review* 69, no. 4 (1991): 945–999.

Schwalbe, Michael L. "Towards a Sociology of Moral Problem Solving. *Journal for the Theory of Social Behavior* 20 (1990): 131–55.

Singer, Beth J. *Operative Rights*. New York: State University of New York Press, 1993.

Smith, Edward, ed. *The Human Genome Project: A Look Back After Five Years*. New York: Cambridge University Press, 1998.

Trotter, Griffin. *The Loyal Physician*. Nashville: Vanderbilt University Press, 1997.

Veatch, Robert M. *A Theory of Medical Ethics*. New York: Basic Books, 1981.

———. "Definitions of Life and Death: Should There Be Consistency?" In *Defining Human Life: Medical, Legal and Ethical Implications*, ed. M. W. Shaw and A. E. Doudera. Ann Arbor, Mich.: AUPHA, 1983.

Werner, J. P. "Productivity and Quality Management." In *Productivity and Performance Management in Health Care Institutions*. American Hospital, 1989.

Whitbeck, Caroline. "The Moral Implications of Regarding Women as People: New Perspectives on Pregnancy and Personhood." In *Abortion and the Status of the Fetus*, ed. W. B. Bondeson. Dordrecht, Holland: D. Reidel, 1983.

Zaner, Richard M. *Ethics and the Clinical Encounter*. Englewood Cliffs, N.J.: Prentice-Hall, 1988.

CONTRIBUTORS

MATTHEW D. BACCHETTA, M.B.A., M.A., is a member of the Cornell University Medical College Class of 1998.

MARTIN BENJAMIN teaches in the Philosophy Department and the Center for Ethics and the Humanities in the Life Sciences at Michigan State University. He is author of *Splitting the Difference: Compromise and Integrity in Ethics and Politics* (University Press of Kansas, 1990) and coauthor (with Joy Curtis) of *Ethics in Nursing* (Oxford, 1991). He is currently writing a book on contemporary pragmatism.

JOSEPH J. FINS, M.D., F.A.C.P., is director of medical ethics at the New York Hospital, assistant professor of medicine and medicine in psychiatry at Cornell University Medical College, associate for medicine at the Hastings Center, and Soros Faculty Scholar at the Project on Death in America.

WILLIAM J. GAVIN is professor of philosophy at the University of Southern Maine, where he has taught for the past thirty years. His areas of interest include American philosophy, especially William James, and biomedical ethics, especially the field of death and dying. Gavin is the author, coauthor, or editor of five books and has published over seventy-five articles and reviews on diverse topics. His two most recently published books are *William James and the Reinstatement of the Vague* (1992), and *Cuttin' the Body Loose: Historical, Biological and Personal Approaches to Death and Dying* (1995), both published by Temple University Press.

D. MICAH HESTER concentrates efforts in the areas of classic American philosophy and bioethics, as well as on issues in computer technologies. He has read papers before the Society of Health and Human Values, the Society for the Advancement of American Philosophy, and the American Academy of Religions. Forthcoming articles will appear in *The Journal of Medical Humanities* and *The Journal of Medicine and Philosophy*. Hester is also preparing several anthologies, including a reissue of John Dewey's *Essays in Experimental Logic*, a collection of critical essays on Dewey's logical theory, a textbook on computer ethics, and a critical reader on the philosophy of William Ernest Hocking.

JACQUELYN ANN K. KEGLEY is the Trustees' Outstanding Professor of Philosophy and Senior Associate at the Kegley Institute of Ethics at California State University, Bakersfield. Her many previous publications include *Introduction to Logic* (with Charles W. Kegley) (Charles E. Merrill, 1978; University Press of America, 1982), *Paul Tillich on Creativity* (editor) (University Press of America, 1989), and *Genuine Individuals and Genuine Communities: A Roycean Public Philosophy* (Vanderbilt University Press, 1997).

JOHN LACHS is Centennial Professor of Philosophy at Vanderbilt University. His works include *Intermediate Man* (Hackett, 1981), *The Relevance of Philosophy to Life* (Vanderbilt University Press, 1995), and *In Love with Life: Reflections on the Joy of Living and Why We Hate to Die* (Vanderbilt University Press, 1998).

JOHN T. LYSAKER is assistant professor of philosophy at the University of Oregon. His research moves across continental and American traditions and concerns issues of rationality, truth, and aesthetics. He has written articles on the public and private aspects of self-creation, art, and politics, and on the future of critical theory in liberal democracy.

MARY B. MAHOWALD is professor at the University of Chicago in the Department of Obstetrics and Gynecology, Committee on Genetics, MacLean Center for Clinical Medical Ethic, and the College. Her books include *An Idealistic Pragmatism* (Nijhoff, 1972), *Women and Children in Health Care* (Oxford, 1993), *Philosophy of Woman* (Hackett, 1994), *Disability, Difference, and Discrimination* (with A. Silvers and D. Wasserman) (Rowman & Littlefield, 1998), and *Genes, Women, and Equality* (Oxford, forthcoming). She has been principal investigator on grants from the National Institutes of Health on *The Human Genome Project and Women* and from the U.S. Department of Energy on *Implications of the "Geneticization" of Health Care for Primary Caregivers*.

GLENN MCGEE is associate director for education and assistant professor in the Center for Bioethics of the University of Pennsylvania and teaches American philosophy in the Penn Philosophy Department. He is the author of *The Perfect Baby: A Pragmatic Approach to Genetics* (Rowman & Littlefield, 1997), editor of *The Human Cloning Debate* (Berkeley Hills, 1998), and has authored fifty-two articles and reviews in bioethics and philosophy. He is on the editorial board of *Theoretical Medicine*, is editor of *Penn Bioethics* and of "Breaking Bioethics" for the *Cambridge Quarterly in Healthcare Ethics* and MS-NBC. McGee is senior research fellow at both Georgetown's Kennedy Institute and the Dartmouth Ethics Institute. In 1998 he was a member of the CDC Working Group on Genetic Testing and Public Health, the American Bar Association Bioethics Board, the American Association of Health Plans task force on ethical issues in managed care, the National Advisory Board on Ethics in Reproduction, and the Hastings Center group on enhancement technologies. He directs www.bioethics.net.

FRANKLIN G. MILLER is associate professor of Medical Education at the University of Virginia School of Medicine and senior research fellow of the Kennedy Institute of Ethics. He serves on the Institutional Review Board (IRB) of the intramural research program of the National Institute of Mental Health and the Ethics Committee of the NIH Clinical Center. In addition, he serves on the Ethics Committee of the Hospice and Home Care Program of the Jewish Social Services Agency of Metropolitan Washington, D.C. Miller is consultant ethicist to the New York Hospital, working as codirector of a project to improve the care of dying patients. His major research interests are death and dying, ethical issues in clinical research, professional integrity, and the application of philosophical pragmatism to clinical ethics.

JONATHAN D. MORENO is the Emily Davie and Joseph S. Kornfeld Professor of Biomedical Ethics and Director of the Center for Biomedical Ethics at the University of Virginia. Among Moreno's books are *Deciding Together: Bioethics and Moral Consensus* (Oxford University Press, 1995), *Ethics in Clinical Practice* (Little, Brown and Co., 1994), and *Arguing Euthanasia* (Touchstone/Simon & Schuster, 1995). Currently he is a consultant to the National Bioethics Advisory Commission. Moreno is currently preparing a second edition of *Ethics in Clinical Practice* that will be published by Aspen. He is also writing a book on bioethics and national security. Moreno has published over 100 papers and book chapters, and is a member of the editorial boards of *Bioethics*, *The Journal of Clinical Ethics*, and the *Health Care Ethics Committee Forum*.

KELLY A. PARKER teaches in the Philosophy and Liberal Studies Programs at Grand Valley State University in Allendale, Michigan. His research and teaching focus on environmental philosophy, American pragmatism, and applied ethics. He is the author of numerous journal articles, as well as *The Continuity of Peirce's Thought* (Vanderbilt University Press, 1998).

HERMAN J. SAATKAMP, JR., is dean of the School of Liberal Arts, Indiana University and Purdue University at Indianapolis. He serves as the general editor of the Vanderbilt Library of American Philosophy and also as the general editor of *The Works of George Santayana*, a critical edition supported by the National Endowment for the Humanities and published by MIT Press.

MARIAN GRAY SECUNDY is a professor of ethics and the director of the Program in Clinical Ethics, Howard University College of Medicine, Department of Community Health and Family Practice. Dr. Secundy's research interests are in the areas of ethical dimensions of patient care, socialization of the medical student, literature and medicine, and minority aging. She has recently completed both an anthology and an annotated bibliography of materials by African American writers, which address issues of health, illness, aging, and loss and grief.

BETH J. SINGER is professor of philosophy emerita at Brooklyn College of the City University of New York. Her publications include *Operative Rights* (SUNY Press, 1993), in which she develops an original theory of rights as social institutions. In some of her other writings she has applied the basic principles of this theory to a variety of topics, including conflict resolution and the treatment of ethnic minorities.

MICHAEL SULLIVAN is a Ph.D. candidate in philosophy at Vanderbilt University and has a Juris Doctor degree from Yale University Law School. In his work, he has studied the pragmatic basis for pursuing questions of ethics in legal and public policy formulation. He has written articles on reforming legal rationality and on reconsidering the import of critical theory to modern political practice.

C. GRIFFIN TROTTER, M.D., Ph.D., is an assistant professor of ethics in the Department of Internal Medicine and the Center for Health Care Ethics at Saint Louis University. In addition to his academic responsibilities, Dr. Trotter is a practicing emergency medicine physician. Dr. Trotter has published numerous articles and book chapters in the fields of philosophy, emergency medicine, and medical ethics. He is the author of *The Loyal Physician: Roycean Ethics and the Practice of Medicine* (Vanderbilt University Press, 1997).

BRUCE WILSHIRE has long been interested in the overlap between philosophies of life and philosophies of healing. His writings include three books and a dozen or so articles on William James. A professor of philosophy at Rutgers University, he shares James's many interests and sees how multifaceted and interconnected any sincere human endeavor is. He has written ten books including *William James and Phenomenology* (AMS Press, 1977); *Role Playing and Identity* (Indiana University Press, 1982); *The Moral Collapse of the University* (New York University Press, 1989); *Wild Hunger: Nature's Excitements and Their Addictive Distortions* (Rowman & Littlefield, 1998); and the forthcoming *The Pull of Primal Life: New Essays on American Philosophers*.

INDEX